The A–Z Reference Book of the New GMS Contract

Comprising:

1. **Standard General Medical Services Contract**

2. **Statutory Instrument 2004 No. 291: The National Health Service (General Medical Services Contracts) Regulations 2004**

3. **GMS Statement of Financial Entitlements**

4. **Delivering Investment in General Practice (Guidance)**

(For England)

£30.72

For Butterworth Heinemann:

Commissioning Editor: Heidi Harrison
Development Editor: Catherine Jackson
Project Manager: Andy Hannan
Design and production: Helius and Julian Howell

The A–Z Reference Book
of the New GMS Contract

Andrew Dearden MBBCh MRCGP

Principal GP, Cardiff;
Chairman GPC, Wales;
Member, UK Negotiating Team, GPC, UK

2004

ELSEVIER
BUTTERWORTH
HEINEMANN

First published 2004

ISBN 0 7506 8839 4

British Library Cataloguing in Publication Data
A catalogue record for this book is available from the British Library

Library of Congress Cataloging in Publication Data
A catalog record for this book is available from the Library of Congress

Notice
Medical knowledge and best practice in this field are constantly changing. As new research and experience broaden our knowledge, changes in practice, treatment and drug therapy may become necessary or appropriate. Readers are advised to check the most current information provided (i) on procedures featured or (ii) by the manufacturer of each product to be administered, to verify the recommended dose or formula, the method and duration of administration, and contraindications. It is the responsibility of the practitioner, relying on their own experience and knowledge of the patient, to make diagnoses, to determine dosages and the best treatment for each individual patient, and to take all appropriate safety precautions. To the fullest extent of the law, neither the publisher nor the editors assume any liability for any injury and/or damage.

The Publisher

The publisher's policy is to use paper manufactured from sustainable forests

Printed in Spain

Dedication

To all those who are now working to make the new GMS contract work for doctors and patients and who hopefully may find this book useful.

Including Sue and Colin, Theresa and Chris.

Acknowledgements

To all those who worked many unsociable hours to complete the new contract and all the documents and paperwork that make the contract work, thank you. This includes those who work within the GPC, the BMA and the various Departments of Health. This book is a reflection of your hard work.

Contents

Contents

Contents

Contents

Contents

Contents

Contents

Contents

Contents

Contents

Contents

Abbreviations

A&E accident and emergency
ADPF adjusted disease prevalence factor
ADS attribution data set
APMS alternative providers of medical services
AWP Allocations Working Paper
BMA British Medical Association
CFSMS Counter Fraud and Security Management Services
CHAI Commission for Healthcare Audit and Inspection
CHD coronary heart disease
CMR current market rate
COPD chronic obstructive pulmonary disease
CPI contractor population index
CRB Criminal Records Bureau
CRP Contractor Registered Population
CVI childhood vaccinations and immunisations
DES directed enhanced services
DH Department of Health
DRS delayed retirement scheme
ECRC enhanced criminal record certificate
EEA European Economic Area
FCS Flexible Career Scheme
FHSAA Family Health Service Appeals Authority
FIS Family Income Supplement
FYOIP Five-Year-Olds Immunisation Payment
GIG Gross Investment Guarantee
GMS general medical services
GMSCL GMS cash-limited
GMSNCL GMS non-cash-limited
GP general practitioner
GPAQ General Practice Assessment Questionnaire
GPC General Practitioner Committee
GS Global Sum

GSE	Global Sum Equivalent
GSMP	global sum monthly payment
IANI	Intended Average Net Income
IAS	Improved Access Scheme
IAU	Interim Aspiration Utility
ICBS	Indicative Contractor Budget Spreadsheet
IM&T	information management and technology
IPQ	Improving Patient Questionnaire
IT	information technology
IWL	Improving Working Lives
LA	Local Authority
LMC	Local Medical Committee
LSP	Local Service Provider
MPIG	Minimum Practice Income Guarantee
NASP	National Application Service Providers
NCAA	National Clinical Assessment Authority
NES	National Enhanced Service
NHS	National Health Service
NHSC	NHS Confederation
NPfIT	National Programme for IT
OOHDF	Out-of-Hours Development Fund
PA	Personally Administered
PCAS	Primary Care Access Survey
PCO	Primary Care Organisation
PCT	Primary Care Trust
PCTMS	Primary Care Trust medical services
PMS	personal medical services
PPA	Prescription Pricing Authority
PWSI	practitioner with a special interest
QMAS	Quality Management and Analysis System
QOF	quality and outcomes framework
QPREP	quality preparation
QuIP	quality information preparation
QuIP	quality information preparation
RS	Returners' Scheme

Abbreviations

ScHARR	School of Health and Related Research
SFE	Statement of Financial Entitlement
SHA	Strategic Health Authority
SLA	Service Level Agreement
SLS	Selected List Scheme
TSC	Technical Steering Committee
TYOIP	Two-Year-Olds Immunisation Payment
UB	Unified Budget

How to use this book

What I have tried to do, as much as possible is to follow the traditional A to Z format. There are several sections, however, where this is very difficult due to the fact that they have been written in a logical sequence and often refer to preceding paragraphs. Where this occurs I have left the section as a whole to make it easier to read and follow the line of thought, but will then make references to other related sections elsewhere in the book.

Each section will contain the relevant sections from the above documents (if there are any) in the following order:

> The Regulations, then
> The Statement of Financial Entitlement, then
> The Standard Contract, and finally
> Delivering Investment in General Practice (Guidance).

This was correct at the time of printing. Modifications of the documents especially in the SFE and Regulations occurs regularly. We strongly suggest that this book is used in tandem with any and all updates of the documents published.

Access

See also: Quality and outcome · Enhanced services

Statement of Financial Entitlement

6. IMPROVED ACCESS SCHEME

6.1 Direction 3(1)(a) of the Directed Enhanced Services (DES) Directions requires each Primary Care Trust (PCT) to establish (if it has not already done so), operate and, as appropriate, revise an Improved Access Scheme (IAS) for its area, the underlying purpose of which is to improve patient access to primary medical services, and which may comprise or include –

(a) arrangements for ensuring that patients requiring routine appointments will, on request, be able to see face-to-face, by the end of –
　(i) the first normal working day after the day on which the request was made, a health care professional, and
　(ii) the second normal working day after the day on which the request was made, a general practitioner; and
(b) arrangements to address specific local health needs or requirements in respect of access to primary medical services locally.

6.2 As part of its Improved Access Scheme, a PCT must, each financial year, offer to enter into arrangements with each contractor in its area (unless it already has such arrangements with the contractor in respect of that financial year), thereby affording the contractor a reasonable opportunity to participate in the Scheme during that financial year. However, before entering into any such arrangements, the PCT must satisfy itself of the matters set out in direction 3(2)(a) and (b) of the DES Directions.

6.3 The plan setting out any arrangements that the PCT enters into, or has entered into, with a particular contractor ("an IAS plan") must cover the matters set out in direction 4(2) (a) to (d) of the DES Directions.

Improved Access Scheme Implementation Payments

6.4 If, as part of a General Medical Services (GMS) contract, a contractor and a PCT have agreed an IAS plan, the PCT must in respect of the financial year 2004/05 pay to the contractor under its GMS contract an Improved Access Scheme Implementation Payment of £2580.50 multiplied by the contractor's Contractor Population Index (CPI). This amount is to fall due –

(a) if the plan is agreed on or was agreed before 1 April 2004, on 30 April 2004; and
(b) if the plan is agreed after 1 April 2004, on the first date after the plan is agreed on which one of the contractor's Payable Global Sum Monthly Payments (GSMPs) falls due.

Improved Access Scheme Reward Payments

6.5 If, as part of a GMS contract a contractor and a PCT have agreed an IAS plan, the PCT must in respect of the financial year 2004/05 pay to the contractor under its GMS contract an Improved Access Scheme Reward Payment if, in the reasonable opinion of the PCT, during that financial year the contractor has fulfilled its obligations under that plan.

6.6 If the plan –
(a) is agreed on or was agreed before 1 April 2004 and has effect for the whole of the financial year 2004/05, the amount payable is £2580.50, multiplied by the contractor's CPI at the start of the last quarter;
(b) has effect for only part of the financial year 2004/05, the amount payable is £2580.50, multiplied by –
   (i) the contractor's CPI either for the last quarter or, if the plan ceases to have effect before 1 January 2005, for when the plan ceased to have effect, and
   (ii) the fraction produced by dividing the number of days for which the plan had effect during the financial year 2004/05 by 365.

6.7 The payment is to be treated for accounting and superannuation purposes as gross income of the contractor in the financial year 2004/05 but is to fall due on 30 April 2005.

6.8 Improved Access Scheme Reward Payments, or any part thereof, are only payable if the contractor satisfies the following conditions –
(a) the contractor must make available to the PCT any information which the PCT does not have but needs, and the contractor either has or could reasonably be expected to obtain, in order to form its opinion on whether the contractor has fulfilled its obligations under the IAS plan;
(b) the contractor must make any returns required of it (whether computerised or otherwise) to the Exeter Registration System, and do so promptly and fully; and
(c) all information supplied pursuant to or in accordance with this paragraph must be accurate.

6.9 If the contractor breaches any of these conditions, the PCT may, in appropriate circumstances, withhold payment of any or any part of an Improved Access Scheme Reward Payment that is otherwise payable.

● Achievement points and payments

See also: Quality and outcomes · Aspiration payments · Disease prevalence

----

Statement of Financial Entitlement

Voluntary

5.1 Participation in the Quality and Outcomes Framework (QOF) is voluntary, and if a contractor decides not to participate in the QOF, this Section will not apply to it.

5.2 Aspiration Payments are payments based on the total number of points that a contractor has agreed with a Primary Care Trust (PCT) that it is aspiring towards under the QOF during the financial year 2004/05. This total is its Aspiration Points Total. The points available are set out in the QOF indicators in the QOF, which have numbers of points attached to particular performance indicators (negative points totals in relation to indicators are always to be disregarded).

5.3 If a contractor is to have an Aspiration Points Total, this is to be agreed between it and the PCT for when its contract takes effect. However, if the contract is to take effect on or after 2 February 2005, no Aspiration Points Total is to be agreed for the financial year 2004/05. Contractors which do not have an Aspiration Points Total will nevertheless be entitled to Achievement Payments under the QOF if they participate in the QOF.

5.4 Achievement Payments are payments based on the points total that the contractor achieves under the QOF during the financial year 2004/05 (which is its Achievement Points Total). The payments are to be made in respect of all Achievement Points actually achieved, whether or not the contractor was seeking to achieve those points when its Aspiration Points Total was agreed.

CALCULATION OF POINTS TOTALS

5.5 The QOF is divided into four principal domains, which are: the clinical domain; the organisational domain; the patient experience domain; and the additional services domain.

Calculation of points in the clinical domain

5.6 The clinical domain contains ten clinical areas, for each of which there are a number of indicators set out in tables in Section 2 of the QOF.

These indicators contain standards against which the performance of the contractor will be assessed.

5.7 Some of the indicators simply require particular tasks to be accomplished (i.e. the production of disease registers), and the standards contained in the indicators do not have, opposite them in the tables, percentage figures for Achievement Thresholds. The points available in relation to these indicators are only obtainable (and then in full) if the task is accomplished. Guidance on what is required to accomplish these tasks is given in Section 2 of the QOF.

5.8 Other indicators have designated Achievement Thresholds. The contractor's performance against the standards set out in these indicators is assessed by a percentage – generally of the patients suffering from a particular disease in respect of whom a specific task is to be performed or a specific outcome recorded. Two percentages are set in relation to each indicator –
(a) a minimum percentage of patients, which represents the start of the scale (i.e. with a value of zero points); and
(b) a maximum percentage of patients, which is the lowest percentage of eligible patients in respect of whom the task must be performed or outcome recorded in order to qualify for all the points available in respect of that indicator.

5.9 If a contractor has achieved a percentage score in relation to a particular indicator that is the minimum set for that indicator, or is below that minimum, it achieves no points in relation to that indicator. If a contractor has achieved a percentage score in relation to a particular indicator that is between the minimum and the maximum set for that indicator, it achieves a proportion of the points available in relation to that indicator. The proportion is calculated as follows.

5.10 First, a calculation will have to be made of the percentage the contractor actually scores (D). This is calculated from the following fraction: divide –
(a) the number of patients registered with the contractor in respect of whom the task has been performed or outcome achieved (A); by
(b) the number produced by subtracting from the total number of patients registered with the contractor with the relevant medical condition (B) the number of patients to be excluded from the calculation on the basis of the provisions in the QOF on exception reporting (C).
The provisions on exception reporting are set out in Section 2.2 of the QOF. This fraction is then multiplied by 100 for the percentage score. The calculation can be expressed as:

$$\frac{A}{(B-C)} \times 100 = D$$

5.11   Once the percentage the contractor actually scores has been calculated
(D), subtract from this the minimum percentage score set for that
indicator (E), then divide the result by the difference between the
maximum (F) and minimum (E) percentage scores set for that indicator,
and multiply the result of that calculation by the total number of points
available in relation to that indicator (G). This can be expressed as:

$$\frac{(D-E)}{(F-E)} \times G$$

5.12   The result is the number of points to which the contractor is entitled in
relation to that indicator.

Calculation of points in the organisational domain

5.13   This domain is itself split into five further sub-domains: records and
information about patients; information for patients; education and
training; practice management; and medicines management. Section 3 of
the QOF contains a number of indicators for each of these sub-domains,
which in turn contain standards against which the performance of the
contractor will be assessed.

5.14   The standards set relate either to a task to be performed or an outcome
to be achieved. The points available in relation to these indicators are
only obtainable (and then in full) if the task is in fact accomplished or
the outcome achieved. Guidance on what is required to accomplish the
task or achieve the outcome is given in Section 3 of the QOF.

Calculation of points in the patient experience domain

5.15   This domain, in Section 4 of the QOF, contains essentially two indicators,
both of which relate to patient experience: the first is about the length of
patient consultations; the second, split into three levels, is about patient
surveys.

5.16   The points available in relation to the first indicator will only be
obtainable (and then in full) if the relevant outcomes recorded in that
indicator are achieved.

5.17   The points available in relation to the second indicator will only be
obtainable if –
(a) the task set out in the lowest performance level is accomplished, i.e.
the contractor has undertaken an approved patient survey; and
(b) in the course of that survey, at least 25 questionnaires per 1000
patients registered with the contractor have been returned by
patients.

For each additional level of performance that is reached, the additional points available in relation to that level are obtainable, so a contractor reaching the highest level of performance achieves the points available for all three levels of performance.

5.18 Guidance on what is required to gain the points set out in this domain is given in Section 4 of the QOF.

Calculation of points in the additional services domain

5.19 The additional services domain relates to the following Additional Services: cervical screening services; child health surveillance; maternity services; and contraceptive services. For each of these services, there are a number of indicators, set out in tables in Section 5 of the QOF, which contain standards against which the performance of the contractor will be assessed.

5.20 The child health surveillance and maternity medical services indicators require particular services to be offered – and the points available in relation to these indicators will only be obtainable (and then in full) if the service is offered to the relevant target population. The contraceptive services indicators and all but one of the cervical screening services indicators require particular tasks to be performed in relation to a target population, and the points available in relation to these indicators will only be obtainable (and then in full) if the task is accomplished. One of the cervical screening services indicators has a designated achievement threshold, and the method for calculating points in relation to this indicator is the same as the method for calculating points in relation to this type of indicator in the clinical domain. Guidance on what is required to gain the points set out in this domain is given in Section 5 of the QOF and Annex F.

Calculation of points in relation to the Holistic Care Payment

5.21 Contractors will be entitled to a proportion of 100 points as the basis of a Holistic Care Payment. This is a payment designed to recognise breadth of achievement across the clinical domain.

5.22 In order to calculate the points in respect of this Payment, the contractor's points totals in each of the clinical areas in the clinical domain are to be ranked on the basis of the proportion it scores of the points available in that clinical area, the highest proportion being ranked first. The proportion that is third-to-last is the proportion of 100 points to which it is entitled as the basis of its Holistic Care Payment.

Calculation of points in relation to the Quality Practice Payment

5.23   Contractors will also be entitled to a proportion of 30 points as the basis of a Quality Practice Payment, designed to recognise breadth of achievement across the organisational, patient experience and additional services domains.

5.24   In order to calculate the points in respect of this Payment, the contractor's points totals in each of the sub-domains in the organisational, patient experience and additional services domains are to be ranked on the basis of the proportion it scores of the points available in that sub-domain, the highest proportion being ranked first. For these purposes, the sub-domains –
   (a) in the organisational domain are under the headings –
      (i)   records and information about patients,
      (ii) information for patients,
      (iii) education and training,
      (iv) practice management, and
      (v)   medicines management;
   (b) in the patient experience domain are the length of consultations indicator and the patient survey indicator. For the patient survey indicator, the ranked proportion is to be the proportion of the maximum number of points available in relation to this indicator (i.e. if the highest performance level is achieved); and
   (c) in the additional services domain are the four different additional services in that domain.

5.25   The proportion that is ranked third-to-last is the proportion of 30 points to which it is entitled as the basis of its Quality Practice Payment. Additional services which the contractor does not provide must nevertheless be included in the ranking.

Calculation of points in relation to QOF Access Payment

5.26   The relevant access targets are those referred to in paragraph 6.1(a). Achievement in relation to these targets in the four months from December 2004 to March 2005 inclusive will enable contractors to score up to 8 data points (4 in relation to access to GPs and 4 in relation to access to health care professionals) under the Primary Care Access Survey during that four month period. Practices scoring –
   (a) 6, 7 or 8 data points in respect of achieving these access targets during that period;
   (b) at least 3 data points in relation to access to GPs during that period; and

(c) at least 3 points in relation to access to health care professionals during that period,

will be entitled to 50 points as the basis of a QOF Access Payment.

CALCULATION OF PAYMENTS

Calculation of Monthly Aspiration Payments

5.27   Aspiration Payments are based on a contractor's Aspiration Points Total. As indicated in paragraph 5.3, if a contractor is to have an Aspiration Points Total for the financial year 2004/05, this is to be agreed between it and the PCT for when its contract takes effect.

5.28   If the PCT and the contractor have agreed an Aspiration Points Total for the contractor, that total is to be divided by three. The resulting figure is to be multiplied by £75, and then by the contractor's CPI. The resulting amount, which is the annual amount of the contractor's Aspiration Payment, is then to be divided by twelve for the contractor's Monthly Aspiration Payment.

5.29   The PCT must thereafter pay the contractor under its GMS contract its Monthly Aspiration Payment monthly. The Monthly Aspiration Payment is to fall due on the last day of each month. However, if the contractor's contract took effect on a day other than the first day of a month, its Monthly Aspiration Payment in respect of that first part month is to be adjusted by the fraction produced by dividing –
(a) the number of days during the month in which the contractor was participating in the QOF; by
(b) the total number of days in that month.

5.30   The amount of a contractor's Monthly Aspiration Payments is thereafter to remain unchanged throughout the financial year 2004/05, even when its CPI changes or if the contractor ceases to provide an Additional Service and as a consequence is less likely to achieve the Aspiration Points Total that has been agreed.

Conditions attached to Monthly Aspiration Payments

5.31   Monthly Aspiration Payments, or any part thereof, are only payable if the contractor satisfies the following conditions –
(a) the contractor's Aspiration Points Total on which the Payments are based must be realistic, agreed with the PCT and broken down for the PCT by the contractor into a standard format, provided nationally;
(b) the contractor must make available to the PCT any information which the PCT does not have but needs, and the contractor either

has or could reasonably be expected to obtain, in order to calculate the contractor's Monthly Aspiration Payments;

(b) the contractor must make any returns required of it (whether computerised or otherwise) to the Exeter Registration System, and do so promptly and fully;

(d) once it is possible for accredited computer systems to generate monthly returns relating to achievement of the standards contained in the indicators in the QOF –

    (i) contractors utilising accredited computer systems must make available to the PCT anonymised, aggregated monthly returns relating to their achievement of the standards contained in the indicators in the QOF, and in the standard form provided for by such systems, and

    (ii) contractors not utilising accredited computer systems must make available to the PCT similar monthly returns, in such form as the PCT reasonably requests (for example, PCTs may reasonably request that contractors fill in manually a printout of the standard spreadsheet which is produced by accredited systems in respect of monthly achievement of the standards contained in the indicators in the QOF);

(e) from December 2004, the contractor must make available to the PCT, under the Primary Care Access Survey, returns relating to its data points scores in relation to the access targets referred to in paragraph 6.1(a); and

(f) all information supplied pursuant to or in accordance with this paragraph must be accurate.

5.32 If the contractor breaches any of these conditions, the PCT may, in appropriate circumstances, withhold payment of any or any part of a Monthly Aspiration Payment that is otherwise payable.

Payment of Achievement Payments

5.33 Achievement Payments are to be based on the Achievement Points Total to which a contractor is entitled at the end of the financial year 2004/05, as calculated in accordance with this Section.

5.34 The date in respect of which the assessment of achievement points is to be made is 31 March 2005, subject to the following exceptions –

(a) as indicated in paragraph 5.26 above, the arrangements for making the assessment in respect of the QOF Access Payment are different. Achievement of the access targets will be assessed over a four month period from December 2004 to March 2005 inclusive;

(b) if a contractor is under an obligation, under its GMS contract, to provide an additional service for part of the financial year but ceases

providing that service before the end of the financial year –
(i) permanently, or
(ii) temporarily, but does not then resume providing the service before the end of the financial year,

the assessment of the Achievement Points to which it is entitled in respect of that service is to made in respect of the last date in the financial year on which it was under an obligation, under its GMS contract, to provide that service; and

(c) if a GMS contract terminates before the end of the financial year, the assessment of the Achievement Points to which it is entitled is to be made in respect of the last date in the financial year on which it was under an obligation, under its GMS contract, to provide essential services.

5.35 In order to make a claim for an Achievement Payment, a contractor must make a return in respect of the information required of it by the PCT in order for the PCT to calculate its Achievement Payment.

5.36 On the basis of that return, but subject to any revision of the Achievement Points total that the PCT may reasonably see fit to make –
(a) to correct the accuracy of any points total; or
(b) having regard to any guidance issued by the Department of Health,

the PCT is to calculate the contractor's Achievement Payment as follows.

5.37 The parts of the Achievement Payment that relate to the clinical domain and the additional services domain are calculated in a different way from the parts relating to the other domains. As regards –
(a) the clinical domain, first a calculation needs to be made of an Adjusted Practice Disease Factor for each disease area, and this is then multiplied by £75 and by the contractor's Achievement Points total in respect of the disease area to produce a cash amount for that disease area. Then the cash totals in respect of all the individual disease areas in the domain are to be added together to give the cash total in respect of the domain. A fuller explanation of the calculation of Adjusted Practice Disease Factors is given in Annex G; and
(b) the additional services domain, the Achievement Points total in respect of each additional service is to be assessed in accordance with the guidance in Annex F, and a calculation is to be made of the cash total in respect of that domain in the manner set out in that guidance.

5.38 As regards all the other Achievement Points gained by the contractor, the total number of them is to be multiplied by £75.

5.39 The cash totals produced under paragraphs 5.37 and 5.38 are then added together and multiplied by the contractor's CPI –

(a) at the start of the final quarter of the financial year 2004/05;

(b) if its contract takes effect after the start of the final quarter of the financial year 2004/05, on the date the contract takes effect; or

(c) if its contract has terminated, its CPI immediately before the contract terminated (i.e. its most recently established list size).

5.40 If the contractor's GMS contract had effect –

(a) throughout the financial year 2004/05, the resulting amount is the provisional total for the contractor's Achievement Payment for the financial year 2004/05; or

(b) for only part of the financial year 2004/05, the resulting amount is to be adjusted by the fraction produced by dividing the number of days during the financial year 2004/05 for which the contractor's GMS contract had effect by 365, and the result of that calculation is the provisional total for the contractor's Achievement Payment for the financial year 2004/05.

5.41 From these provisional totals, the PCT needs to subtract the total value of all the Monthly Aspiration Payments made to the contractor under its GMS contract in the financial year 2004/05. The resulting amount (unless it is a negative amount or zero, in which case no Achievement Payment is payable) is the contractor's Achievement Payment for the financial year 2004/05.

5.42 This Achievement Payment is to be treated for accounting and superannuation purposes as gross income of the contractor in the financial year 2004/05 but is to fall due –

(a) if the PCT is considering revising the contractor's Achievement Points Total in accordance with paragraph 5.36, on 30 June 2005; and

(b) in all other cases, on 30 April 2005.

Conditions attached to Achievement Payments

5.43 Achievement Payments, or any part thereof, are only payable if the contractor satisfies the following conditions –

(a) the contractor must make the return required of it under paragraph 5.35;

(b) the contractor must ensure that all the information that it makes available to the PCT in respect of the calculation of its Achievement Payment is based on accurate and reliable information, and that any calculations it makes are carried out correctly;

(c) the contractor must ensure that it is able to provide any information that the PCT may reasonably request of it to demonstrate that it is entitled to each Achievement Point to which it says it is entitled, and the contractor must make that information available to the PCT on request;

(d) the contractor must make any returns required of it (whether computerised or otherwise) to the Exeter Registration System, and do so promptly and fully;

(e) the contractor must co-operate fully with any reasonable inspection or review (including the PCT's QOF annual review) that the PCT or another relevant statutory authority wishes to undertake in respect of the Achievement Points to which it says it is entitled; and

(f) all information supplied pursuant to or in accordance with this paragraph must be accurate.

5.44 If the contractor breaches any of these conditions, the PCT may, in appropriate circumstances, withhold payment of all or part of an Achievement Payment that is otherwise payable.

Guidance

GENERAL

3.44 This section of the chapter sets out how achievement points are calculated in each of the domains. Contractors will be legally entitled under the Statement of Financial Entitlement (SFE) to receive payments in accordance with the rules summarised in this section. The method for calculating points varies by domain and each is considered in turn.

(i) Clinical points

3.45 The contractor achieves all the points available for a disease register if it can produce a disease register. This must be accurate to the contractor's best knowledge. If the contractor does not have a register then it is not possible to calculate achievement points against any of the other clinical indicators in that disease area or to calculate prevalence.

3.46 The remaining clinical indicators have achievement thresholds. The number of points achieved is dependent on achievement between these thresholds. This is illustrated in the worked example in Figure 6.

3.47 Contractors should ensure that they use the correct Read codes in their patient records, because Quality Management and Analysis System (QMAS) works by recognising and counting records with the relevant Read codes. Failure to use the correct Read codes may result in under-payments because those patients would not be counted. Contractors must also make sure they do not omit Read code information where patients have not been treated in line with the QOF indicators as this would constitute fraud. Contractors will be able to see if data are

---

> ### Figure 6 Calculating clinical points
>
> 80% of the practice's patients with hypertension have had their blood pressure recorded in the past 9 months (indicator BP 5). The minimum threshold for this indicator is 25%, the maximum is 90%. The total number of points available for this indicator is 20.
>
> The calculation is:
>
> $$\frac{(80-25)}{(90-25)} \times 20 = \frac{55}{65} \times 20 = 0.85 \times 20 = 17$$
>
> The contractor has achieved 17 points for its performance against indicator BP 5.

---

incorrect or missing by looking at the monthly reports on the QMAS system and should act to ensure the data are corrected.

(ii) Organisational points

3.48   As with the clinical disease register points, the organisational indicators are either achieved in full, in which case the contractor receives all the points, or not. A proportion of points will not be given for partial achievement. For example, for indicator Education 9, all the contractor's staff must have had an appraisal. The contractor cannot achieve half the points if only half the staff have had an appraisal.

(iii) Patient experience points

3.49   The same all-or-nothing rule applies to calculating points arising from the patient experience indicators. To achieve the patient survey indicators, the SFE requires the contractor to:
(i)   ensure that at least 25 questionnaires per 1000 patients are returned by patients. Given current list sizes, this threshold is in line with the 50 per doctor set out in the *New GMS Contract 2003 Supplementary Documents*
(ii)   use an accredited patient survey. Two patient surveys have already been accredited for use against the patient survey indicators of the QOF. They are:
(a)   Improving Patient Questionnaire (IPQ), developed by Exeter University and available at http://latis.ex.ac.uk/cfep/ipq.htm
(b)   General Practice Assessment Questionnaire (GPAQ), developed by the National Primary Care Research and Development Centre in Manchester and available at http://www.gpaq.info

Use of other surveys will not count towards quality achievement. However, further validated patient surveys are expected to be formally accredited for use in the QOF over the next few months. Details of these will be sent to all GPs and PCTs, and posted on the DH, GPC, NHS Confederation and NatPaCT websites.

(iv) Additional services points

3.50　The first cervical screening indicator (CS1) has achievement thresholds and is measured in the same way as the clinical indicators. The remaining additional services indicators are either achieved in full, or not, as with the organisational indicators.

3.51　The additional services indicators each have a target population. These are:
(i)　Cervical screening: women aged 25 to 64 years
(ii)　Child health surveillance: children aged under 5 years
(iii) Maternity services: women aged under 55 years
(iv) Contraceptive services: women aged under 55 years.
The pounds per point for each of the indicators in these additional services will be adjusted by the relative size of the contractor's target population, compared to the national average. This is to protect contractors with large target populations and adequately reward them for their greater workload. The calculation is as follows:

$$\frac{\text{(contractor's target population)} \div \text{(contractor's registered population)}}{\text{(national average target population)} \div \text{(national average registered population)}}$$

3.52　Where a contractor opts out of an additional service during the year, its achievement against that indicator will be measured at the date of opt-out. However, the achievement will still be paid with the rest of the achievement payment in the first quarter of the following year.

3.53　Figure 7 provides a worked example of how points for additional services are calculated, using child health surveillance as an example.

(v) Holistic care points

3.54　Holistic care payments reward breadth of quality achievement in the clinical domain. They are calculated by ranking the points scored in all the clinical areas on the basis of the proportion of points scored out of the total available. The third lowest

---

Figure 7 Worked example of additional services points

The contractor's registered list size is 6000 patients. Of these, 450 are children under the age of 5.

The national average registered list size is 5891 patients. The national average registered population of children under 5 is 375.

The adjustment is calculated as follows:

$$\frac{(450 \div 6000)}{(375 \div 5891)} = \frac{0.075}{0.064} = 1.18$$

This is applied to the £75 per point the contractor receives for the child health surveillance additional service indicators:

£75 × 1.18 = £88.37

Therefore the contractor receives £88.37 for each child health surveillance additional service indicator point it achieves.

Figure 8 Worked example of holistic care points

A contractor achieves the following results in the clinical domain:

	Points	Possible points	Proportion
CHD	85	121	70.25%
Stroke/TIA	15	31	48.39%
Hypertension	65	105	61.90%
Diabetes	50	99	50.51%
COPD	16	45	35.56%
Epilepsy	4	16	25.00%
Hypothyroidism	8	8	100.00%
Cancer	6	12	50.00%
Mental health	0	41	00.00%
Asthma	50	72	69.44%

The third lowest ranking disease area is COPD, where the contractor scores 35.56% of the possible points available.

So the contractor receives 35.56% of the 100 holistic care points, or 35.56 points.

proportion is the proportion of the 100 points to which the contractor is entitled. This is illustrated in Figure 8.

(vi) Quality practice payments

3.55   Quality practice payments reward breadth of quality achievement across the organisational, patient experience and additional services domains. They are calculated by ranking the points scored in all five organisational areas, the two patient experience areas, and the four additional service areas, on the basis of the proportion of points scored out of the total available. The third lowest figure determines the proportion of the 30 points to which the contractor is entitled. This is illustrated in Figure 9.

Figure 9   **Worked example of holistic care points**

A contractor achieves the following results in the organisational, patient experience and additional services domains:

	Points	Possible points	Proportion
Records	80	85	94.12%
Patient communications	8	8	100.00%
Education and training	13	29	44.83%
Practice management	15	20	75.00%
Medicines management	35	42	83.33%
Length of consultation	30	30	100.00%
Patient survey	40	70	57.14%
Cervical screening	16	22	72.73%
Child health surveillance	6	6	100.00%
Maternity services	6	6	100.00%
Contraceptive services	2	2	100.00%

The third lowest ranking area is cervical screening, where the contractor scores 72.73% of the possible points available.

So the contractor receives 72.73% of the 30 quality practice points, or 21.82 points.

(vii) Access bonus points

3.56   Contractors that deliver access for patients to a GP within 48 hours and to a primary care professional within 24 hours in line with the NHS Plan and Priorities and Planning Framework 2003/06 target are recognised by the award of 50 bonus points. More information on how to achieve and sustain the 24/48-hour access target is available in a PCT toolkit at http://www.doh.gov.uk/waitingbookingchoice/pcaccess

3.57 From 2005/06, improving access under the QOF will be assessed annually based on performance across the year using practice data already collected by PCTs for the monthly Primary Care Access Survey (PCAS). Measurement will be assessed against a total of 24 data points: 12 for access to GPs and 12 for access to a primary care professional. The assessment will include some tolerance to take account of unavoidable short-term dips in performance, for example through sickness absence or an outbreak of flu.

3.58 Practices scoring 21 to 24 data points will be awarded 50 quality points, provided that there were no more than two failures on either GP or primary care professional access. Practices scoring less than 21 points will receive no award.

3.59 A transitional arrangement is required for 2004/05 because the 24/48-hour access target is for achievement by December 2004. For that year only assessment will be based only on the 4 months from December 2004 to March 2005. Measurement will be on the basis of up to 8 data points: access to a GP within 48 hours each month and access to a primary care professional within 24 hours each month. Practices scoring 6 to 8 data points, with no more than one failure on access to a GP or access to a primary care professional, will be awarded 50 quality points.

CALCULATING ACHIEVEMENT PAYMENTS

3.60 The achievement payment will be calculated automatically by the QMAS IT system, in the following way:
  (i) points achievement is assessed on National Quality Achievement Day (31 March) by the QMAS system. QMAS will automatically use the data on it at 31 March to create an achievement report for each practice and send it directly to the PCT. Practices will be able to see the report, and must confirm by 7 April that it is correct, using a form on QMAS. Delays in confirming that the data are right, or in submitting data from paper-based practices, will lead to delays in PCTs making payments
  (ii) for the clinical domain, the £75 per point in 2004/05 (£120 in 2005/06) is multiplied by the Adjusted Disease Prevalence Factor (ADPF) for each disease area and this is in turn multiplied by the points achieved in each disease area
  (iii) for the additional services domain, the £75 per point is adjusted by the relative size of the contractor's target population
  (iv) for the other domains (except the additional services domain), the £75 pounds per point in 2004/05 (£120 in 2005/06) is multiplied by the points scored, including points for the holistic care and quality practice payments and access bonus

(v)   these payments are added together and adjusted by the contractor's list size relative to the national average (currently 5891). This produces the total QOF payment

(vi) the aspiration payment is deducted from the total QOF payment to produce the achievement payment. Should this be negative the full amount will be deducted from the following year's aspiration payment in monthly instalments. The PCT normally confirms the payment (section G of this chapter sets out exceptional circumstances when this may not happen) and ensures it is paid as a lump sum by the end of April. PCTs must verify all achievement claims before authorising them for payment. The assumption in verification will be that the claim is correct and can be authorised for payment, unless there is evidence to the contrary, e.g. from the annual review

(vii) in line with the joint letter of 30 May 2003 from Dr John Chisholm and Mike Farrar, contractors that do not take part in the QOF, or that achieve less than 100 points, will see a reduction in their final global sum payment. This amounts to £7500 in 2004/05, or £12,000 in 2005/06, adjusted by the contractor's list size relative to the national average of 5891.

3.61   To ensure consistency of calculation, contractors that do not use the QMAS system will need to supply records of achievement against the 146 QOF indicators to PCTs, which will then ensure calculation of the achievement payment and make payments accordingly. Verification of such records, and manual input by the PCT of the data into QMAS, will take considerable time and effort. As a consequence, achievement payments for such contractors will be delayed. For these reasons PCTs and practices are strongly advised to use the QMAS system, and PCTs will want to offer support to paper-based practices so that they become computerised.

3.62   Contractors are entitled to receive an aspiration payment in respect of each day for which they have submitted data to the QMAS, once the system is in place. They need not have agreed an aspiration payment to be eligible for an achievement payment. Contractors whose contracts start or end during the year receive a payment in respect of the days for which the contract runs.

3.63   Figure 10 provides a worked example.

Figure 10	**Worked example of achievement payment**

The contractor's registered list size is 6000 patients.

Relative list size factor = 6000/5891 = 1.02

1. Clinical domain

Adjusted Practice Disease Factor		£ per point	Points	Payment
CHD	1.16	£87.00	90	£7830.00
Stroke	1.02	£76.50	15	£1147.50
Hypertension	1.10	£82.50	50	£4125.00
Diabetes	1.14	£85.50	63	£5386.50
COPD	0.85	£63.75	15	£956.25
Epilepsy	0.89	£66.75	5	£333.75
Hypothyroidism	0.90	£67.50	7	£472.50
Cancer	1.06	£79.50	6	£477.00
Mental Health	0.87	£65.25	20	£1305.00
Asthma	0.91	£68.25	50	£3412.50
Total			**321**	**£25,466.00**

2. Organisational domain

	Points scored	Payment
Records	78	£5850.00
Patient communication	7	£525.00
Education and training	26	£1950.00
Practice management	15	£1125.00
Medicines management	34	£2550.00
Total	**160**	**£12,000.00**

3. Patient experience domain

	Points scored	Payment
Length of consultation	30	£2250.00
Patient surveys	55	£4125.00
Total	**85**	**£6375.00**

4. Additional services domain (assumes average relative target population)

	Points	Payment
Cervical screening	20	£1500.00
Child health surveillance	6	£450.00
Maternity services	6	£450.00
Contraceptive services	2	£150.00
Total	**34**	**£2550.00**

Continued

5. Holistic care payment

The third lowest clinical area score is hypertension. The proportion of points scored is 47.62% (50 points scored out of a possible total of 105). **Therefore, the contractor scores 47.62 holistic care payment points, leading to a payment of £3571.50 (= 47.62 × £75).**

6. Quality practice payment

The third lowest sub-domain score in the other domains is Medicines Management. The proportion of points scored is 80.95% (34 points scored out of a possible total of 42). **Therefore, the contractor scores 24.29 quality practice payment points (80.95% of 30 points), leading to a payment of £1821.75 (= 24.29 × £75).**

7. Access bonus

The contractor met the access target and so qualifies for the access bonus of £3750.

FINAL PAYMENT

Clinical domain	£25,466.00
Organisational domain	£12,000.00
Patient experience domain	£6,375.00
Additional services domain	£2,550.00
Holistic care payment	£3,571.50
Quality practice payment	£1,821.75
Access bonus	£3,750.00
Total	**£55,534.25**

The contractor's total raw payment for the QOF is £55,534.25.

This is then adjusted by relative list size (1.02) to give a total gross QOF achievement payment of £56,561.79.

The contractor's aspiration was 525 points. **It has therefore already received an aspiration payment of £13,367.85. This figure is deducted from the achievement total to arrive at the total payable to the practice:**

£56,561.79 – £13,367.85 = £43,193.94

The contractor is paid £43,193.94 as its net achievement payment for the year.

CALCULATION OF QOF PAYMENTS FOR END OF YEAR

3.64 If a contract starts or ends in-year and the practice is participating in the QOF, then its achievement against the QOF indicators is measured for the period that the contract is running. The practice's achievement total is calculated as normal. This total is then adjusted pro rata according to the length of time the contract ran during the year. This is to avoid paying for quality twice in the event of practice splits. The amount of aspiration payment the practice has already received is deducted from this total, and the resulting figure is the final achievement payment due to the practice. In 2004/05 the payment will not be adjusted by prevalence if the contract ends before 14 February 2005. In subsequent years it will be adjusted by the previous year's prevalence figures. Figure 11 provides a worked example.

Figure 11 **QOF payments for contracts ending in-year**

The contractor's total QOF payment is £42,575.00. This is adjusted according to the number of days the contract has run during the year.

$$£42,575.00 \times \frac{201}{365} = £42,575.00 \times 0.55 = £23,445.41$$

The contractor has already received £10,281.25 in aspiration payments. These are deducted from the adjusted QOF total to give the final achievement payment.

£23,445.41 − £10,281.25 = £13,164.16

The contractor's final achievement payment is £13,164.16.

3.65 The flowchart in Figure 12 summarises the annual visit and achievement payment process.

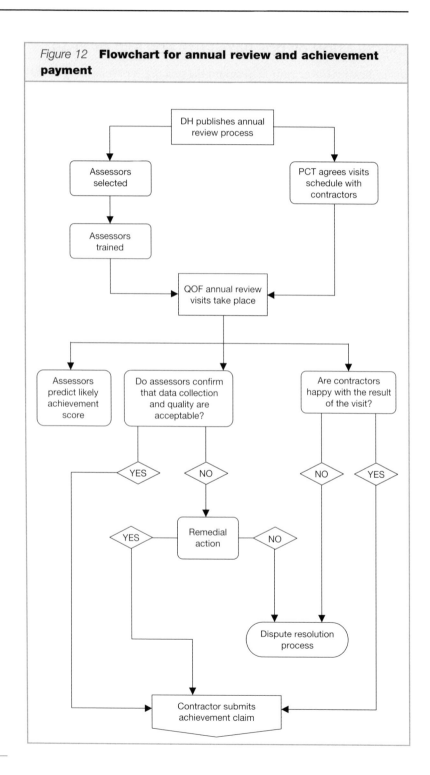

Figure 12 **Flowchart for annual review and achievement payment**

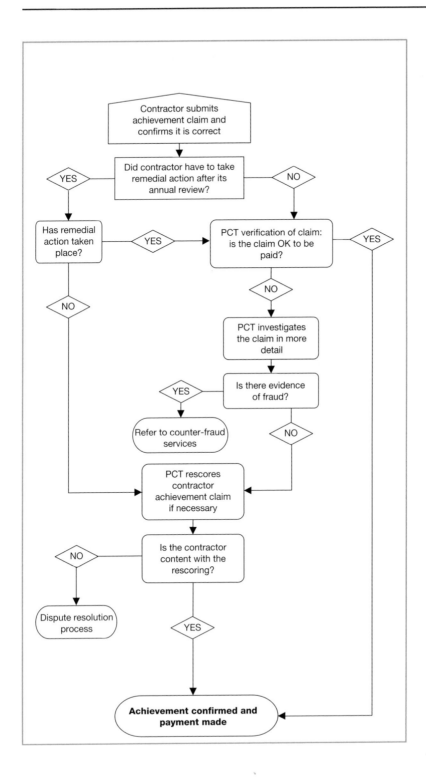

Additional services

Regulations

1.   Additional services generally
The contractor shall provide, in relation to each additional service, such facilities and equipment as are necessary to enable it properly to perform that service.

2.   Cervical screening

(1)   A contractor whose contract includes the provision of cervical screening services shall –
(a) provide all the services described in sub-paragraph (2); and
(b) make such records as are referred to in sub-paragraph (3).

(2)   The services referred to in sub-paragraph (1)(a) are –
(a) the provision of any necessary information and advice to assist women identified by the Primary Care Trust (PCT) as recommended nationally for a cervical screening test in making an informed decision as to participation in the NHS Cervical Screening Programme;
(b) the performance of cervical screening tests on women who have agreed to participate in that Programme;
(c) arranging for women to be informed of the results of the test; and
(d) ensuring that test results are followed up appropriately.

(3)   The records referred to in sub-paragraph (1)(b) are an accurate record of the carrying out of a cervical screening test, the result of the test and any clinical follow-up requirements.

3.   Contraceptive services

(1)   A contractor whose contract includes the provision of contraceptive services shall make available to all its patients who request such services the services described in sub-paragraph (2).

(2)   The services referred to in sub-paragraph (1) are –
(a) the giving of advice about the full range of contraceptive methods;
(b) where appropriate, the medical examination of patients seeking such advice;
(c) the treatment of such patients for contraceptive purposes and the prescribing of contraceptive substances and appliances (excluding the fitting and implanting of intrauterine devices and implants);

(d) the giving of advice about emergency contraception and, where appropriate, the supplying or prescribing of emergency hormonal contraception or, where the contractor has a conscientious objection to emergency contraception, prompt referral to another provider of primary medical services who does not have such conscientious objections;

(e) the provision of advice and referral in cases of unplanned or unwanted pregnancy, including advice about the availability of free pregnancy testing in the practice area and, where appropriate, where the contractor has a conscientious objection to the termination of pregnancy, prompt referral to another provider of primary medical services who does not have such conscientious objections;

(f) the giving of initial advice about sexual health promotion and sexually transmitted infections; and

(g) the referral as necessary for specialist sexual health services, including tests for sexually transmitted infections.

4. Vaccinations and immunisations

(1) A contractor whose contract includes the provision of vaccinations and immunisations shall comply with the requirements in sub-paragraphs (2) and (3).

(2) The contractor shall –

(a) offer to provide to patients all vaccinations and immunisations (excluding childhood vaccinations and immunisations) of a type and in the circumstances for which a fee was provided for under the 2003/04 Statement of Fees and Allowances made under regulation 34 of the National Health Service (General Medical Services) Regulations 1992 other than influenza vaccination;

(b) provide appropriate information and advice to patients about such vaccinations and immunisations;

(c) record in the patient's record kept in accordance with paragraph 73 of Schedule 6 any refusal of the offer referred to in paragraph (a);

(d) where the offer is accepted, administer the vaccinations and immunisations and include in the patient's record kept in accordance with paragraph 73 of Schedule 6 –

   (i) the patient's consent to the vaccination or immunisation or the name of the person who gave consent to the vaccination or immunisation and his relationship to the patient,

   (ii) the batch numbers, expiry date and title of the vaccine,

   (iii) the date of administration,

   (iv) in a case where two vaccines are administered in close succession, the route of administration and the injection site of each vaccine,

(v) any contraindications to the vaccination or immunisation, and

(vi) any adverse reactions to the vaccination or immunisation.

(3)   The contractor shall ensure that all staff involved in administering vaccines are trained in the recognition and initial treatment of anaphylaxis.

5.   Childhood vaccinations and immunisations

(1)   A contractor whose contract includes the provision of childhood vaccinations and immunisations shall comply with the requirements in sub-paragraphs (2) and (3).

(2)   The contractor shall –

(a) offer to provide to children all vaccinations and immunisations of a type and in the circumstances for which a fee was provided for under the 2003/04 Statement of Fees and Allowances made under regulation 34 of the National Health Service (General Medical Services) Regulations 1992;

(b) provide appropriate information and advice to patients and, where appropriate, their parents, about such vaccinations and immunisations;

(c) record in the patient's record kept in accordance with paragraph 73 of Schedule 6 any refusal of the offer referred to in paragraph (a);

(d) where the offer is accepted, administer the vaccinations and immunisations and include in the patient's record kept in accordance with paragraph 73 of Schedule 6 –

(i)   the name of the person who gave consent to the vaccination or immunisation and his relationship to the patient;

(ii) the batch numbers, expiry date and title of the vaccine;

(iii) the date of administration;

(iv) in a case where two vaccines are administered in close succession, the route of administration and the injection site of each vaccine;

(v)   any contraindications to the vaccination or immunisation; and

(vi) any adverse reactions to the vaccination or immunisation.

(3)   The contractor shall ensure that all staff involved in administering vaccines are trained in the recognition and initial treatment of anaphylaxis.

6.   Child health surveillance

(1)   A contractor whose contract includes the provision of child health surveillance services shall, in respect of any child under the age of five for whom it has responsibility under the contract –

(a) provide all the services described in sub-paragraph (2), other than any examination so described which the parent refuses to allow the child to undergo, until the date upon which the child attains the age of 5 years; and

(b) maintain such records as are specified in sub-paragraph (3).

(2) The services referred to in sub-paragraph (1)(a) are –

(a) the monitoring –

(i) by the consideration of any information concerning the child received by or on behalf of the contractor, and

(ii) on any occasion when the child is examined or observed by or on behalf of the contractor (whether pursuant to paragraph (b) or otherwise),

of the health, well-being and physical, mental and social development (all of which characteristics are referred to in this paragraph as "development") of the child while under the age of 5 years with a view to detecting any deviations from normal development;

(b) the examination of the child at a frequency that has been agreed with the PCT in accordance with the nationally agreed evidence based programme set out in the fourth edition of *Health for all Children*.

(3) The records mentioned in sub-paragraph (1)(b) are an accurate record of –

(a) the development of the child while under the age of 5 years, compiled as soon as is reasonably practicable following the first examination of that child and, where appropriate, amended following each subsequent examination; and

(b) the responses (if any) to offers made to the child's parent for the child to undergo any examination referred to in sub-paragraph (2)(b).

7. Maternity medical services

(1) A contractor whose contract includes the provision of maternity medical services shall –

(a) provide to female patients who have been diagnosed as pregnant all necessary maternity medical services throughout the antenatal period;

(b) provide to female patients and their babies all necessary maternity medical services throughout the postnatal period other than neonatal checks;

(c) provide all necessary maternity medical services to female patients whose pregnancy has terminated as a result of miscarriage or abortion or, where the contractor has a conscientious objection to the termination of pregnancy, prompt referral to another provider of primary medical services who does not have such conscientious objections.

(2)   In this paragraph –
"antenatal period" means the period from the start of the pregnancy to the onset of labour;
"maternity medical services" means –
(a) in relation to female patients (other than babies) all primary medical services relating to pregnancy, excluding intra partum care, and
(b) in relation to babies, any primary medical services necessary in their first 14 days of life;
"postnatal period" means the period starting from the conclusion of delivery of the baby or the patient's discharge from secondary care services, whichever is the later, and ending on the fourteenth day after the birth.

8.   Minor surgery

(1)   A contractor whose contract includes the provision of minor surgery shall comply with the requirements in sub-paragraphs (2) and (3).
(2)   The contractor shall make available to patients, where appropriate –
(a) curettage;
(b) cautery; and
(c) cryocautery of warts, verrucae and other skin lesions.

(3)   The contractor shall ensure that its record of any treatment provided under this paragraph includes the consent of the patient to that treatment.

─────

Standard Contract

GENERAL

53.   In relation to each *additional service* it provides, the Contractor shall provide such facilities and equipment as are necessary to enable it properly to perform that service.

54.   Where an *additional service* is to be funded under the *global sum*, the Contractor must provide that *additional service* at such times, within *core hours*, as are appropriate to meet the reasonable needs of its patients. The Contractor must also have in place arrangements for its patients to access such services throughout the *core hours* in case of emergency.

55.   The Contractor shall provide the *additional services*[1] set out in clause 56 to –
55.1   its *registered patients*; and
55.2   persons accepted by it as *temporary residents*;

---

1   Delete from the list at clause 56 any of the *additional services* that the Contractor is not going to be providing under the Contract to the persons specified in clause 55.

56.　The Contractor shall provide to the patients specified in clause 55 –

　　56.1 [*cervical screening services*];
　　56.2 [*contraceptive services*];
　　56.3 [*vaccinations and immunisations*];
　　56.4 [*childhood vaccinations and immunisations*];
　　56.5 [*child health surveillance services*];
　　56.6 [*maternity medical services*];
　　56.7 [*minor surgery*].

57.　The Contractor shall provide the *additional services* set out in [...] to [...][2]

58.　The Contractor shall provide to the patients specified in clause 57 –

　　58.1 [*cervical screening services*];
　　58.2 [*contraceptive services*];
　　58.3 [*vaccinations and immunisations*];
　　58.4 [*childhood vaccinations and immunisations*];
　　58.5 [*child health surveillance services*];
　　58.6 [*maternity medical services*];
　　58.7 [*minor surgery*].

59.　[In addition to the *additional services* specified in clauses 55, 56, 57 and 58 the Contractor shall provide *child health surveillance services* to [*specify here any patients/categories of patients (other than patients who are recorded as being on the Contractor's list of patients) to whom the Contractor was providing child health surveillance services, either under regulation 28 of the National Health Service (General Medical Services) Regulations 1992 or pursuant to a default contract, on or immediately before the date this contract is to be entered into (see article 24 and 25 of the Transitional Order) (see articles 24 and 25 of the Transitional Order)*]. The requirement to provide this *additional service* to the patients specified in this clause shall cease on the date on which any *opt-out* of *child health surveillance services* in respect of the Contractor's own registered patients commences pursuant to Part 10 of the Contract.][3]

60.　[In addition to the *additional services* specified in clauses 55, 56, 57 and 58, the Contractor shall provide *contraceptive services* to [*specify here any*

2　Clauses 57 and 58 only need to be included if the parties agree that the Contractor will provide additional services that are not funded by the global sum. If the parties do so agree, details need to be inserted at clause 57 of the patients to whom such services will be provided, and where particular additional services specified in clause 58 are to be provided to particular patients (e.g. maternity medical services is to be provided to one group of patients and minor surgery is to be provided to a different group of patients), the spaces in square brackets at clause 57 should be completed to make it clear which additional services included at clause 58 are to be provided to which patients: any additional services that the Contractor will not be providing to patients specified in clause 57 need to be deleted from clause 58.

3　This clause only needs to be included if the Contractor must provide such services pursuant to article 24 or 25 of *the Transitional Order*: if neither article applies to the Contractor, this clause can be deleted.

patients/categories of patients (other than patients who are recorded as being on the Contractor's list of patients) to whom the Contractor was providing contraceptive services, either under regulation 29 of the National Health Service (General Medical Services) Regulations 1992 or pursuant to a default contract, on or immediately before the date this contract is to be entered into (see articles 24 and 25 of the Transitional Order)]. The requirement to provide this *additional service* to the patients specified in this clause shall cease on the date on which any *opt-out* of *contraceptive services* in respect of the Contractor's own registered patients commences pursuant to Part 10 of the Contract.]⁴

61.   [In addition to the *additional services* specified in clauses 55, 56, 57 and 58, the Contractor shall provide *maternity medical services* to [*specify here any patients/categories of patients (other than patients who are recorded as being on the Contractor's list of patients) to whom the Contractor was providing contraceptive services either under regulation 31 of the National Health Service (General Medical Services) Regulations 1992 or pursuant to a default contract, on or immediately before the date the Contract is to be entered into (see articles 24 and 25 of the Transitional Order)]*. The requirement to provide this *additional service* to the patients specified in this clause shall cease on the date on which any *opt-out* of *maternity medical services* in respect of the Contractor's own registered patients commences pursuant to Part 10 of the Contract.]⁵

62.   [Nothing in clauses 59 to 61 shall prevent the Contractor from subsequently terminating its responsibility for patients not registered with the Contractor pursuant to clauses 225 to 229.]

63.   [...]⁶

64.   [...]

65.   [...]

66.   [...]

67.   [...]

---

4   This clause only needs to be included if the Contractor must provide such services pursuant to article 24 or 25 of *the Transitional Order*: if neither article applies to the Contractor, this clause can be deleted.

5   This clause only needs to be included if the Contractor must provide such services pursuant to article 24 or 25 of *the Transitional Order*: if neither article applies to the Contractor, this clause can be deleted.

6   Clause 54 makes provision in respect of *additional services* funded by the *global sum* in respect of the times during which *additional services* are to be provided to patients. In relation to *additional services* that are not funded by the *global sum* (specified in clause 58), the parties will need to specify here the times during which such services are to be provided: there is further space in the clauses below to include such further detail as is necessary.

Cervical screening[7]

68. The Contractor shall –
   68.1 provide the services described in clause 69; and
   68.2 make such records as are referred to in clause 70.

69. The services referred to in clause 68 are –
   69.1 the provision of any necessary information and advice to assist women identified by the PCT as recommended nationally for a cervical screening test in making an informed decision as to participation in the NHS Cervical Screening Programme;
   69.2 the performance of cervical screening tests on women who have agreed to participate in that Programme;
   69.3 arranging for women to be informed of the results of the test;
   69.4 ensuring that test results are followed up appropriately.

70. The records referred to in clause 68 are an accurate record of the carrying out of a cervical screening test, the result of the test and any clinical follow-up requirements.

Contraceptive services[8]

71. The Contractor shall make available the following services to all of its patients who request such services –
   71.1 the giving of advice about the full range of contraceptive methods;
   71.2 where appropriate, the medical examination of patients seeking such advice;
   71.3 the treatment of such patients for contraceptive purposes and the prescribing of contraceptive substances and appliances (excluding the fitting and implanting of intrauterine devices and implants);
   71.4 the giving of advice about emergency contraception and, where appropriate, the supplying or prescribing of emergency hormonal contraception or, where the Contractor has a conscientious objection to emergency contraception, prompt referral to another provider of primary medical services who does not have such conscientious objections;
   71.5 the provision of advice and referral in cases of unplanned or unwanted pregnancy, including advice about the availability of free pregnancy testing in the *practice area* and, where appropriate, where the Contractor has a conscientious objection to the termination of

---

7   Clauses 68 to 70 are required by *the Regulations* only where the Contract includes the provision of *cervical screening services*. If the Contractor is not providing *cervical screening services*, these clauses should be deleted.

8   Clause 71 is required by *the Regulations* only where the Contract includes the provision of contraceptive services. If the Contractor is not providing *contraceptive services*, this clause should be deleted.

pregnancy, prompt referral to another provider of primary medical services who does not have such conscientious objections;

71.6 the giving of initial advice about sexual health promotion and sexually transmitted infections; and

71.7 the referral as necessary for specialist sexual health services, including tests for sexually transmitted infections.

Vaccinations and immunisations[9]

72. The Contractor shall –

72.1 offer to provide to patients all vaccinations and immunisations (excluding *childhood vaccinations and immunisations*) of a type and in the circumstances for which a fee was provided for under the 2003/04 Statement of Fees and Allowances made under regulation 34 of the National Health Service (General Medical Services) Regulations 1992 other than influenza vaccination;

72.2 provide appropriate information and advice to patients about such vaccinations and immunisations;

72.3 record in the patient's record kept in accordance with clauses 417 to 425 any refusal of the offer referred to in clause 72.1;

72.4 where the offer is accepted, administer the vaccinations and immunisations, and include in the patient's record kept in accordance with clauses 417 to 425 –

72.4.1 the patient's consent to the vaccination or immunisation or the name of the person who gave consent to the vaccination or immunisation and his relationship to the patient;

72.4.2 the batch numbers, expiry date and title of the vaccine;

72.4.3 the date of administration;

72.4.4 in a case where two vaccines are administered in close succession, the route of administration and the injection site of each vaccine;

72.4.5 any contraindications to the vaccination or immunisation; and

72.4.6 any adverse reactions to the vaccination or immunisation.

73. The Contractor shall ensure that all staff involved in administering vaccines are trained in the recognition and initial treatment of anaphylaxis.

---

9 Clauses 72 and 73 are required by *the Regulations* only where the Contract includes the provision of *vaccinations and immunisations*. If the Contractor is not providing *vaccinations and immunisations*, these clauses should be deleted.

Childhood vaccinations and immunisations[10]

74.　The Contractor shall –

74.1　offer to provide to children all vaccinations and immunisations of a type and in the circumstances for which a fee was provided for under the 2003/04 Statement of Fees and Allowances made under regulation 34 of the National Health Service (General Medical Services) Regulations 1992;

74.2　provide appropriate information and advice to patients and, where appropriate, their parents about such vaccinations and immunisations;

74.3　record in the patient's record kept in accordance with clauses 417 to 425 any refusal of the offer referred to in clause 74.1;

74.4　where the offer is accepted, administer the vaccinations and immunisations, and include in the patient's record kept in accordance with clauses 417 to 425 –

74.4.1　the name of the person who gave consent to the vaccination or immunisation and his relationship to the patient;

74.4.2　the batch numbers, expiry date and title of the vaccine;

74.4.3　the date of administration;

74.4.4　in a case where two vaccines are administered in close succession, the route of administration and the injection site of each vaccine;

74.4.5　any contraindications to the vaccination or immunisation; and

74.4.6　any adverse reactions to the vaccination or immunisation.

75.　The Contractor shall ensure that all staff involved in administering vaccines are trained in the recognition and initial treatment of anaphylaxis.

Child health surveillance[11]

76.　The Contractor shall, in respect of any child under the age of five for whom it has responsibility under the Contract –

76.1　provide the services described in clause 77, other than any examination so described which the parent refuses to allow the

---

10　Clauses 76 to 78 are required by *the Regulations* only where the Contract includes the provision of *childhood vaccinations and immunisations*. If the Contractor is not providing *childhood vaccinations and immunisations*, these clauses should be deleted.

11　Clauses 79 to 80 are required by the *Regulations* only where the Contract includes the provision of *child health surveillance services*. If the Contractor is not providing *child health surveillance services*, these clauses should be deleted.

child to undergo, until the date upon which the child attains the age of 5 years; and

76.2 maintain such records as are specified in clause 78.

77. The services referred to in clause 76.1 are –

77.1 the monitoring –

77.1.1 by the consideration of any information concerning the child received by or on behalf of the Contractor, and

77.1.2 on any occasion when the child is examined or observed by or on behalf of the Contractor (whether pursuant to clause 77.2 or otherwise),

of the health, well-being and physical, mental and social development (all of which characteristics are referred to in clauses 77 to 79 as "development") of the child while under the age of 5 years with a view to detecting any deviations from normal development;

77.2 the examination of the child at a frequency that has been agreed with the PCT in accordance with the nationally agreed evidence based programme set out in the fourth edition of *Health for all Children* (David Hall and David Elliman, January 2003, Oxford University Press, ISBN 0-19-85188-X).

78. The records referred to in clause 76.2 are an accurate record of –

78.1 the development of the child while under the age of 5 years, compiled as soon as is reasonably practicable following the first examination of that child and, where appropriate, amended following each subsequent examination; and

78.2. the responses (if any) to offers made to the child's *parent* for the child to undergo any examination referred to in clause 77.2.

Maternity medical services[12]

79. The Contractor shall –

79.1 provide to female patients who have been diagnosed as pregnant all necessary maternity medical services throughout the antenatal period;

79.2 provide to female patients and their babies all necessary maternity medical services throughout the postnatal period other than neonatal checks;

79.3 provide all necessary maternity medical services to female patients whose pregnancy has terminated as a result of miscarriage or

12 Clauses 79 to 80 are required by *the Regulations* only where the Contract includes the provision of *maternity medical services*. If the Contractor is not providing *maternity medical services*, these clauses should be deleted.

abortion or, where the Contractor has a conscientious objection to the termination of pregnancy, prompt referral to another provider of primary medical services, who does not have such conscientious objections.

80.   In clause 79 –

80.1 "antenatal period" means the period from the start of the pregnancy to the onset of labour,

80.2 "maternity medical services" means –

80.2.1 in relation to female patients (other than babies) all primary medical services relating to pregnancy, excluding intra partum care, and

80.2.2 in relation to babies, any primary medical services necessary in their first 14 days of life, and

80.3 "postnatal period" means the period starting from the conclusion of delivery of the baby or the patient's discharge from secondary care services, whichever is the later, and ending on the fourteenth day after the birth.

Minor surgery[13]

81.   The Contractor shall make available to patients, where appropriate, curettage and cautery and, in relation to warts, verrucae and other skin lesions, cryocautery.

82.   The Contractor shall ensure that its record of any treatment provided pursuant to clause 81 includes the consent of the patient to that treatment.

Guidance

2.49   Under new GMS there are seven additional services. This section summarises the contractual requirements in Schedule 2 of the GMS Regulations, which are set out in Table 5, and the opt-out rules.

Commissioning Additional Services

2.50   PCTs and contractors should note the following points about the provision of additional services:

---

13   Clauses 79 and 81 are required by *the Regulations* only where the Contract includes the provision of *minor surgery*. If the Contractor is not providing *minor surgery*, these clauses should be deleted.

Table 5 **Additional services**		
1. Cervical screening	1.	Providing information and advice to women
	2.	Performing cervical screening tests, arranging for women to be informed of the results, ensuring appropriate follow-up
	3.	Keeping an accurate record of tests and follow-up
	4.	Carrying out screening in accordance with the guidance relating to the NHS Cervical Screening Programme
2. Contraceptive services	1.	Providing advice about the full range of contraceptive methods
	2.	Where appropriate, examining patients seeking contraceptive advice
	3.	Treating patients for contraceptive purposes and prescribing contraceptive substances and appliances, or referral for the fitting of intrauterine devices or implants, which are enhanced services
	4.	Providing advice about emergency contraception and where appropriate supplying or prescribing emergency hormonal contraception. Where the GMS contractor has a conscientious objection to emergency contraception it must promptly refer to a contractor which has no such objection
	5.	Providing advice in cases of unplanned or unwanted pregnancy, including advice about the availability of free pregnancy testing in the practice area. Where the GMS contractor has a conscientious objection to termination it must promptly refer the patient to a contractor which has no such objection
	6.	Giving initial advice about sexual health promotion and sexually transmitted infections
	7.	Referral as necessary for specialist sexual health services, including tests for sexually transmitted infections

Table 5 – continued	
3. Vaccinations and immunisations	1. Providing all necessary vaccinations and immunisations (except flu and childhood vaccinations and immunisations and certain travel vaccines) set out in the 2002/03 Red Book
	2. Providing necessary information and advice to patients, and where appropriate to parents, about such vaccinations and immunisations
	3. Recording in the patient's records consent to, or refusal of, an offer; the batch numbers, expiry date and title of any vaccine given; the date of administration; where two vaccines are administered in close succession, the injection site of each vaccine; any contraindications to immunisation; any adverse reactions to a dose of vaccine
	4. All staff involved in administering vaccines must be trained in the recognition and initial treatment of anaphylaxis in accordance with *Immunisation Against Infectious Disease* (1996) and updates thereof
	5. Ensuring all vaccines are stored in accordance with the manufacturer's instructions and the publication *Immunisation against Infectious Disease* and updates thereof
	6. Ensuring all refrigerators in which vaccines are stored have a minimum/maximum thermometer and that readings are taken on all working days. (This requirement, and point (5) above, apply for all vaccinations provided by the contractor including flu and childhood vaccinations and immunisations)
4. Childhood vaccinations and immunisations	1. Providing all necessary childhood vaccinations and immunisations in accordance with the 2002/03 Red Book
	2. Requirements for the vaccinations and immunisations additional service also apply

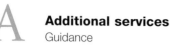
Table 5 – continued	
5. Child health surveillance	1. Monitoring the health, well-being and physical, mental and social development of children under 5 to detect any deviations from normal development
	2. Examining the child at a frequency that has been agreed with the PCT, in accordance with the publication *Health for all Children*
	3. Keeping an accurate record of the sdevelopment of the child while under 5
6. Maternity medical services	1. Providing through the antenatal period all necessary maternity medical services to pregnant women
	2. Providing throughout the postnatal period all necessary maternity medical services to patients and their babies other than neonatal checks
	3. Providing all necessary maternity medical services to women whose pregnancy has terminated as a result of miscarriage or abortion. Where the contractor has a conscientious objection to the termination of pregnancy, it must promptly refer the patient to another provider of primary medical services which does not have ssuch conscientious objections
7. Minor surgery	1. Curettage, cautery and cryocautery of warts, verrucae, and other skin lesions
	2. Must ensure patient consent is recorded

(i) PCTs must ensure that sufficient additional services are in place from 1 April 2004. They may therefore wish to review expected provision with this in mind by the end of January 2004 and draw up plans for filling gaps in services as a result of historic or future opt-outs to take effect from 1 April 2004

(ii) contractors do not have to provide an additional service if they are not currently providing the equivalent service under old GMS

(iii) if contractors are providing the equivalent of that service, they are required to continue to do so under their new GMS contract. However, PCTs may agree with the contractor, before the formal opt-out rules apply, for the contractor to opt out of some or all additional services. Contractors may therefore wish to consider now, if they have not done so already, whether they may wish to opt out of any additional services

(iv) PCTs and contractors should ideally reach provisional agreement on additional services by early January 2004. In agreeing opt-outs by February 2004, before the contract is signed in March 2004, the PCT must also ensure that alternative provision is in place.

Additional services pricing

2.51 Contractors are funded through the global sum for the provision of additional services and the tariff for opting out is set out in Table 6. The percentage reduction is only from the global sum, not the global sum and Minimum Practice Income Guarantee (MPIG) combined.

Tariffs for opting out

Table 6 **Tariffs for opting out of additional services**	
Additional service	% deduction from the global sum
Cervical screening	1.1
Child health surveillance	0.7
Minor surgery	0.6
Maternity medical services	2.1
Contraceptive services	2.4
Childhood immunisations and pre-school booster	1.0
Vaccinations and immunisations	2.0

2.52 There is no fixed price for PCTs to use when they re-commission additional services that contractors have opted out of; however, the opt-out tariff offers a useful benchmark. The exception is where a contractor is re-commissioned by the PCT for providing additional services it had previously opted out of, in which case the opt-out tariff price (i.e. the percentage of the global sum at the time) must automatically apply. This is only the case when the re-provisioned contract is solely for the contractors' registered patients rather than a wider contract to provide, for example, cervical cytology across multiple contractor areas. Where PCTs are re-commissioning additional services they may wish to do so for a fixed time period rather than for an unlimited duration.

● Additional services – general

See also: Additional services · Childhood immunisations – target payments · Global sum

● Additional services – opt-outs

Regulations

1.   **Opt-outs of additional services: general**

(1)   In this Schedule –

"opt-out notice" means a notice given under sub-paragraph (5) to permanently opt out or temporarily opt out of the provision of the additional service;

"permanent opt-out" in relation to the provision of an additional service that is funded through the global sum, means the termination of the obligation under the contract for the contractor to provide that service; and "permanently opt out" shall be construed accordingly;

"permanent opt-out notice" means an opt-out notice to permanently opt out;

"preliminary opt-out notice" means a notice given under sub-paragraph (2) that a contractor wishes to temporarily opt out or permanently opt out of the provision of an additional service;

"temporary opt-out" in relation to the provision of an additional service that is funded through the global sum, means the suspension of the obligation under the contract for the contractor to provide that service for a period of more than 6 months and less than 12 months and includes an extension of a temporary opt-out and "temporarily opt out" and "temporarily opted out" shall be construed accordingly; and

"temporary opt-out notice" means an opt-out notice to temporarily opt out.

(2)   A contractor who wishes to permanently or temporarily opt out shall give to the relevant Primary Care Trust (PCT) in writing a preliminary opt-out notice which shall state the reasons for wishing to opt out.

(3)   As soon as is reasonably practicable and in any event within the period of 7 days beginning with the receipt of the preliminary opt-out notice by

the PCT, the PCT shall enter into discussions with the contractor concerning the support which the PCT may give the contractor, or concerning other changes which the PCT or the contractor may make, which would enable the contractor to continue to provide the additional service and the PCT and the contractor shall use reasonable endeavours to achieve this aim.

(4) The discussions mentioned in sub-paragraph (3) shall be completed within the period of 10 days beginning with the date of the receipt of the preliminary opt-out notice by the PCT or as soon as reasonably practicable thereafter.

(5) Subject to sub-paragraph (9), if following the discussions mentioned in sub-paragraph (3), the contractor still wishes to opt out of the provision of the additional service, it shall send an opt-out notice to the PCT.

(6) An opt-out notice shall specify –

    (a) the additional service concerned;
    (b) whether the contractor wishes to –
        (i) permanently opt out, or
        (ii) temporarily opt out;
    (c) the reasons for wishing to opt out;
    (d) the date from which the contractor would like the opt-out to commence, which must –
        (i) in the case of a temporary opt-out be at least 14 days after the date of service of the opt-out notice, and
        (ii) in the case of a permanent opt-out must be the day either 3 or 6 months after the date of service of the opt-out notice, and
    (e) in the case of a temporary opt-out, the desired duration of the opt-out.

(7) Where a contractor has given two previous temporary opt-out notices within the period of 3 years ending with the date of the service of the latest opt-out notice (whether or not the same additional service is concerned), the latest opt-out notice shall be treated as a permanent opt-out notice (even if the opt-out notice says that it wishes to temporarily opt out).

(8) Paragraph (2) applies following the giving of a temporary opt-out notice and paragraph (3) applies following the giving of a permanent opt-out notice or a temporary opt-out notice which pursuant to sub-paragraph (7) is treated as a permanent opt-out notice.

(9) No temporary opt-out notice may be served by a contractor prior to 1 April 2004.

2. Temporary opt-outs and permanent opt-outs following temporary opt-outs

(1) As soon as is reasonably practicable and in any event within the period of 7 days beginning with the date of receipt of a temporary opt-out notice under paragraph 1(5), the PCT shall –

(a) approve the opt-out notice and specify in accordance with sub-paragraphs (3) and (4) the date on which the temporary opt-out is to commence and the date that it is to come to an end ("the end date"); or

(b) reject the opt-out notice in accordance with sub-paragraph (2), and shall notify the contractor of its decision as soon as possible, including reasons for its decision.

(2) A PCT may reject the opt-out notice on the ground that the contractor –

(a) is providing additional services to patients other than its own registered patients or enhanced services; or

(b) has no reasonable need temporarily to opt out having regard to its ability to deliver the additional service.

(3) The date specified by the PCT for the commencement of the temporary opt-out shall wherever reasonably practicable be the date requested by the contractor in its opt-out notice.

(4) Before determining the end date, the PCT shall make reasonable efforts to reach agreement with the contractor.

(5) Where the PCT approves an opt-out notice, the contractor's obligation to provide the additional service specified in the notice shall be suspended from the date specified by the PCT in it's decision under sub-paragraph (1), and shall remain suspended until the end date unless –

(a) the contractor and the PCT agree in writing an earlier date, in which case the suspension shall come to an end on the earlier date agreed;

(b) the PCT specifies a later date under sub-paragraph (6), in which case the suspension shall end on the later date specified;

(c) sub-paragraph (7) applies and the contractor refers the matter to the NHS dispute resolution procedure or the court, in which case the suspension shall end –

(i) where the outcome of the dispute is to uphold the decision of the PCT, on the day after the date of the decision of the Secretary of State or the court,

(ii) where the outcome of the dispute is to overturn the decision of the PCT, 28 days after the decision of the Secretary of State or the court, or

(iii) where the contractor ceases to pursue the NHS dispute resolution procedure or court proceedings, on the day after the date that the contractor withdraws its claim or the procedure is or proceedings are otherwise terminated by the Secretary of State or the court;

(d) sub-paragraph (9) applies and –

(i) the PCT refuses the contractor's request for a permanent opt-out within the period of 28 days ending with the end date, in which case the suspension shall come to an end 28 days after the end date,

(ii) the PCT refuses the contractor's request for a permanent opt-out after the end date, in which case the suspension shall come to an end 28 days after the date of service of the notice, or

(iii) the PCT notifies the contractor after the end date that the relevant SHA has not approved its proposed decision to refuse the contractor's request to permanently opt out under sub-paragraph (14), in which case the suspension shall come to an end 28 days after the date of service of the notice under this paragraph.

(6) Before the end date, a PCT may, in exceptional circumstances and with the agreement of the contractor, notify the contractor in writing of a later date on which the temporary opt-out is to come to an end, being a date no more than 6 months later than the end date.

(7) Where the PCT considers that –

(a) the contractor will be unable to satisfactorily provide the additional service at the end of the temporary opt-out; and

(b) it would not be appropriate to exercise its discretion under sub-paragraph (6) to specify a later date on which the temporary opt-out is to come to an end or the contractor does not agree to a later date,

the PCT may notify the contractor in writing at least 28 days before the end date that a permanent opt-out shall follow a temporary opt-out.

(8) Where a PCT notifies the contractor under sub-paragraph (7) that a permanent opt-out shall follow a temporary opt-out, the permanent opt-out shall take effect immediately after the end of the temporary opt-out.

(9) A contractor who has temporarily opted out may, at least 3 months prior to the end date, notify the relevant PCT in writing that it wishes to permanently opt out of the additional service in question.

(10) Where the contractor has notified the PCT under sub-paragraph (9) that it wishes to permanently opt out, the temporary opt-out shall be followed by a permanent opt-out beginning on the day after the end date unless the PCT refuses the contractor's request to permanently opt out by giving a notice in writing to the contractor to this effect.

(11) A PCT may only give a notice under sub-paragraph (10) with the approval of the relevant Strategic Health Authority (SHA).

(12)   Where a PCT seeks the approval of a SHA to a proposed decision to refuse a permanent opt-out, it shall notify the contractor of having done so.

(13)   If the relevant SHA has not reached a decision as to whether or not to approve the PCT's proposed decision to refuse a permanent opt-out before the end date, the contractor's obligation to provide the additional service shall remain suspended until the date specified in sub-paragraph (5)(d)(ii) or (iii) (whichever is applicable).

(14)   Where after the end date the relevant SHA notifies the PCT that it does not approve the PCT's proposed decision to refuse a permanent opt-out, the PCT shall notify the contractor in writing of this fact as soon as is reasonably practicable.

(15)   A temporary opt-out or permanent opt-out commences, and a temporary opt-out ends, at 08.00 on the relevant day unless –
   (a) the day is a Saturday, Sunday, Good Friday, Christmas Day, or a Bank Holiday, in which case the opt-out shall take effect on the next working day at 08.00; or
   (b) the PCT and the contractor agree a different day or time.

3.   Permanent opt-outs

(1)   In this paragraph –
   "A day" is the day specified by the contractor in its permanent opt-out notice to a PCT for the commencement of the permanent opt-out;

   "B day" is the day 6 months after the date of service of the permanent opt-out notice; and

   "C day" is the day 9 months after the date of service of the permanent opt-out notice.

(2)   As soon as is reasonably practicable and in any event within the period of 28 days beginning with the date of receipt of a permanent opt-out notice under paragraph 1(5) (or temporary opt-out notice which is treated as a permanent opt-out notice under paragraph 1(7)), the PCT shall –
   (a) approve the opt-out notice; or
   (b) reject the opt-out notice in accordance with sub-paragraph (3),
   and shall notify the contractor of its decision as soon as possible, including reasons for its decision where its decision is to reject the opt-out notice.

(3)   A PCT may reject the opt-out notice on the ground that the contractor is providing an additional service to patients other than its registered patients or enhanced services.

(4) A contractor may not withdraw an opt-out notice once it has been approved by the PCT in accordance with sub-paragraph (2)(a) without the PCT's agreement.

(5) If the PCT approves the opt-out notice under sub-paragraph (2)(a), it shall use its reasonable endeavours to make arrangements for the contractor's registered patients to receive the additional service from an alternative provider from A day.

(6) The contractor's duty to provide the additional service shall terminate on A day unless the PCT serves a notice under sub-paragraph (7) (extending A day to B day or C day).

(7) If the PCT is not successful in finding an alternative provider to take on the provision of the additional service from A day, then it shall notify the contractor in writing of this fact no later than 1 month before A day, and –

(a) in a case where A day is 3 months after service of the opt-out notice, the contractor shall continue to provide the additional service until B day unless at least 1 month before B day it receives a notice in writing from the PCT under sub-paragraph (8) that despite using its reasonable endeavours, it has failed to find an alternative provider to take on the provision of the additional service from B day;

(b) in a case where A day is 6 months after the service of the opt-out notice, the contractor shall continue to provide the additional service until C day unless at least 1 month before C day it receives a notice from the PCT under sub-paragraph (11) that it has made an application to the relevant SHA under sub-paragraph (10) seeking its approval of a decision to refuse a permanent opt-out or to delay the commencement of a permanent opt-out until after C day.

(8) Where in accordance with sub-paragraph (7)(a) the permanent opt-out is to commence on B day and the PCT, despite using its reasonable endeavours has failed to find an alternative provider to take on the provision of the additional service from that day, it shall notify the contractor in writing of this fact at least 1 month before B day, in which case the contractor shall continue to provide the additional service until C day unless at least 1 month before C day it receives a notice from the PCT under sub-paragraph (11) that it has applied to the relevant SHA under sub-paragraph (10) seeking the approval of the relevant SHA to a decision to refuse a permanent opt-out or to postpone the commencement of a permanent opt-out until after C day.

(9) As soon as is reasonably practicable and in any event within 7 days of the PCT serving a notice under sub-paragraph (8), the PCT shall enter into discussions with the contractor concerning the support that the PCT may

give to the contractor or other changes which the PCT or the contractor may make in relation to the provision of the additional service until C day.

(10) The PCT may, if it considers that there are exceptional circumstances, make an application to the relevant SHA for approval of a decision to –
(a) refuse a permanent opt-out; or
(b) postpone the commencement of a permanent opt-out until after C day.

(11) As soon as practicable after making an application under sub-paragraph (10) to the SHA, the PCT shall notify the contractor in writing that it has made such an application.

(12) On receiving an application under sub-paragraph (10) for approval of a decision to refuse a permanent opt-out, the SHA shall –
(a) approve the PCT's application;
(b) reject the PCT's application, but nonetheless recommend a different date for the commencement of the permanent opt-out which shall be later than C day; or
(c) reject the PCT's application.

(13) On receiving an application under sub-paragraph (10) for approval of a decision to postpone the commencement of a permanent opt-out until after C day, the SHA shall –
(a) approve the PCT's application;
(b) reject the PCT's application, but nonetheless recommend –
(i) that the permanent opt-out commence on an earlier date to that proposed by the PCT in its application, or
(ii) that the permanent opt-out be refused; or
(c) reject the PCT's application.

(14) The relevant SHA shall notify the PCT and the contractor in writing of its decision under sub-paragraph (12) or (13) as soon as is practicable, including reasons for its decision.

(15) Where the SHA –
(a) approves a decision to refuse an opt-out under sub-paragraph (12)(a); or
(b) recommends that a permanent opt-out be refused under sub-paragraph (13)(b)(ii),
the PCT shall notify the contractor in writing that it may not opt out of the additional service.

(16) Where a PCT notifies a contractor under sub-paragraph (15), the contractor may not serve a preliminary opt-out notice in respect of that additional service for a period of 12 months beginning with the date of service of the PCT's notice under sub-paragraph (15) unless there has

been a change in the circumstances of the contractor which affects its ability to deliver services under the contract.

(17)   Where the SHA –
(a) recommends a different date for the commencement of the permanent opt-out under sub-paragraph (12)(b);
(b) approves a PCT's application to postpone a permanent opt-out under sub-paragraph (13)(a); or
(c) recommends an earlier date to that proposed by the PCT in its application under sub-paragraph (13)(b)(i),
the PCT shall in accordance with the decision of the SHA notify the contractor in writing of its decision and the notice shall specify the date from which the permanent opt-out shall commence.

(18)   Where the SHA rejects the PCT's application under sub-paragraph (12)(c) or (13)(c), the PCT shall notify the contractor in writing that there shall be a permanent opt-out and the permanent opt-out shall commence on C day or 28 days after the date of service of the PCT's notice, whichever is the later.

(19)   If the relevant SHA has not reached a decision on the PCT's application under sub-paragraph (10) before C day, the contractor's obligation to provide the additional service shall continue until a notice is served on it by the PCT under sub-paragraph (17) or (18).

(20)   Nothing in sub-paragraphs (1) to (19) above shall prevent the contractor and the PCT from agreeing a different date for the termination of the contractor's duty under the contract to provide the additional service and accordingly, varying the contract in accordance with paragraph 104(1) of Schedule 6.

(21)   The permanent opt-out takes effect at 08.00 on the relevant day unless –
(a) the day is a Saturday, Sunday, Good Friday, Christmas Day, or a Bank Holiday, in which case the opt-out shall take effect on the next working day at 08.00; or
(b) the PCT and the contractor agree a different day or time.

Guidance

2.53   Chapter 2 of *Investing in General Practice* explained that opt-outs can either be temporary or permanent. PCTs and contractors should note that the formal procedure exists so as to provide contractual certainty in the event of local disagreement. Its use embodies a failure to maintain good local relationships that are essential in any contracting arrangement. It is always cheaper and less bureaucratic for both parties,

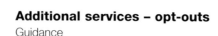

as well as being better for ongoing relationships, if the PCT and contractor can simply reach agreement and, where opt-outs are agreed, come to a mutually acceptable start date.

2.54 The formal procedures for temporary and permanent opt-outs are similar; key differences are that:

(i) temporary opt-outs are designed to enable contractors to cope with temporary workload pressures. As a result they need to be processed and effected quickly; and they normally last for between 6 and 12 months

(ii) permanent opt-outs require more planning by the PCT, and so the PCT may specify a start date of 3 months from receipt of the permanent opt-out notice; and it may extend this by up to two further periods each of 3 months.

Temporary opt-out procedure

2.55 Table 7 summarises the temporary opt-out process.

Table 7 Temporary opt-out procedure for additional services	
Stage	**Process**
1. Informal discussion	1. Contractor talks to PCT – or submits preliminary notice – about wanting to opt out of a specific service on a temporary basis
	2. Within 7 days the PCT discusses possible solutions to avoid need for opting out
	3. Normally within 10 days discussions are complete and the contractor either decides to submit a formal opt-out notice, or agrees to continue to provide the service
	4. Temporary opt-out is for a period of less than a year
2. Temporary opt-out notice	1. The contractor submits a formal opt-out notice
	2. The notice must set out the service concerned; reasons for wanting to opt out; preferred start date – not less than 14 days from the notice date – and preferred duration normally
	Continued

Table 7 – continued	
Stage	**Process**
	6–12 months. A separate notice must be submitted for each service
	3. PCT will want to start planning for re-provision, unless it has good grounds for rejecting the notice
3. PCT decision	1. PCT must make a decision within 7 days
	2. It can accept the notice, in which case the PCT specifies the start and end date. Normally these will be those set out in the notice or otherwise agreed
	3. Or it can decline, for example if the contractor is providing additional services to patients other than its own or any enhanced services, or it does not agree that the contractor's workload is a temporary problem
	4. If the opt-out notice is the third notice from the contractor – for either temporary or permanent opt-out, in relation to any service – within 3 years, the PCT can treat the notice as a request for permanent opt-out
4. Making temporary opt-outs permanent	1. Both sides should review progress towards the contractor re-providing the service
	2. Contractor can seek to make a temporary opt-out permanent. To do so it must notify PCTs 3 months before the end date of a temporary opt-out. The PCT can only refuse by seeking SHA permission
	3. Alternatively, the PCT may notify the contractor that a permanent opt-out is to follow before the temporary opt-out end-date, where it considers the contractor will not be able to provide the service satisfactorily at the end of the temporary opt-out. The contractor can appeal against such decisions to the SHA. In this case the end date of the temporary opt-out will be extended whilst dispute resolution is followed

Permanent opt-out procedure

2.56 Permanent opt-out is subject to the procedure summarised set out in Table 8. The detailed procedure is complicated and it is particularly important that reference is made to the full text of the Contract Regulations.

Table 8 **Permanent opt-out procedure for additional services**	
Stage	Process
1. Informal discussion	1. The contractor talks to PCT – or submits preliminary notice – about wanting to opt out of a specific service on a permanent basis
	2. Within 7 days the PCT discusses possible solutions to avoid need for opt-out
	3. Normally within 10 days discussions are complete and the contractor either submits a formal notice or agrees to continue providing the service
2. Permanent opt-out notice	1. The contractor submits a formal opt-out notice
	2. The notice must set out the service concerned and reasons for wanting to opt out. A separate notice must be submitted for each service
	3. On receipt the PCT is advised to start planning for re-provision – unless the PCT is planning to reject the notice because the contractor is providing enhanced services, or additional services other than to its own patients
3. PCT decision	1. The PCT must make a decision as soon as possible and in any event within 28 days
	2. It can approve the opt-out. In which case the opt-out is that requested by the contractor in its opt-out notice (which will either be the date 3 or 6 months after receipt of the notice, or an otherwise agreed date). Once approved, the contractor cannot withdraw the notice without the PCT's agreement

Continued

Table 8 – continued	
Stage	**Process**
	3. The PCT and contractor should discuss how best to inform patients of the changes. If requested by the PCT, the contractor must inform its registered patients of an opt-out and the arrangements made for them to receive the additional service by placing a notice in the surgery, and/or including details in a revised patient leaflet
	4. Or the PCT can reject the notice, for example if the contractor is providing enhanced services or additional services to patients registered with other contractors. In this situation it need not seek SHA agreement, but the contractor can appeal to the SHA
4. PCT extension notices	The PCT can extend the start date before which permanent opt-out occurs, by up to two further periods each of 3 months where the start date is 3 months after service of the notice or one period of 3 months where the start date is 6 months after service of the opt-out notice. This is to allow further time for re-commissioning. The PCT needs to give notice of these to the contractor at least 1 month before the expected start date of the opt-out
	At the end of the period, if despite using reasonable endeavours the PCT cannot find an alternative provider, the PCT can, if it considers there are exceptional circumstances, seek SHA approval to reject the opt-out, or for a further extension
5. SHA determination	1. The SHA must consider such applications by the PCT to reject or delay opt-out as soon as it can
	2. The SHA may decide that there are exceptional circumstances preventing the opt-out, e.g. in very rural areas where it has not been possible,

Continued

Table 8 – continued	
Stage	Process
	despite the PCT's reasonable endeavours, for it to re-commission from another provider without detriment to NHS patients
	3. The SHA may recommend a different start date for an opt-out, in which case it will start from that date
	4. The SHA may refuse the PCT's application and so the opt-out start date will be 9 months after the date of the opt-out notice, or 28 days after the contractor is notified of the SHA decision, whichever is the later. The PCT must act in accordance with the SHA's decision
	5. Where an SHA approves a decision to refuse a permanent opt-out, or itself recommends that a permanent opt-out be refused, that contractor is not normally entitled to submit another opt-out notice (for either a permanent or temporary opt-out) for a period of 12 months following the SHA decision

2.57   SHAs are advised to start planning for their new role so that arrangements are in place to discharge their functions under both procedures by April 2004.

● Additional services – payment mechanisms

See also: Global sum

Additional services – transitional services

Regulations

29. Additional services

(1) Where the contract is with one of the persons specified in paragraph (2), the contract must, subject to regulation 17, provide for the contractor to provide in core hours to the contractor's registered patients and persons accepted by it as temporary residents, such of the additional services as are equivalent to services which that medical practitioner or practitioners was or were providing to his or their patients on the date that the contract is entered into except to the extent that –

(a) the provision of any of those services by that medical practitioner or practitioners is due to come to an end on or before the date on which services are required to start being provided under the contract; or

(b) prior to the signing of the contract, the Primary Care Trust (PCT) has accepted in writing a written request from the contractor that the contract should not require it to provide all or any of those additional services.

(2) The persons referred to in paragraph (1) are –

(a) an individual medical practitioner who, on 31 March 2004, was providing services under section 29 of the Act (general medical services);

(b) two or more individuals practising in partnership at least one of whom was, on 31 March 2004, a medical practitioner providing services under that section; or

(c) a company in which one or more of the shareholders was, on 31 March 2004, a medical practitioner providing services under that section.

(3) This regulation applies only to contracts under which services are to be provided from 1 April 2004.

Administrative procedures

Statement of Financial Entitlement

Overpayments

21.1 Without prejudice to the specific provisions elsewhere in this Statement of Financial Entitlement (SFE) relating to overpayments of particular payments, if a Primary Care Trust (PCT) makes a payment to a contractor under its GMS contract pursuant to this SFE and –
(a) the contractor was not entitled to receive all or part thereof, whether because it did not meet the entitlement conditions for the payment or because the payment was calculated incorrectly (including where a payment on account overestimates the amount that is to fall due);
(b) the PCT was entitled to withhold all or part of the payment because of a breach of a condition attached to the payment, but is unable to do so because the money has already been paid; or
(c) the PCT is entitled to repayment of all or part of the money paid, the PCT may recover the money paid by deducting an equivalent amount from any other payment payable pursuant to this SFE, and where no such deduction can be made, it is a condition of the payments made pursuant to this SFE that the contractor must pay to the PCT that equivalent amount.

Underpayments and late payments

21.2 Without prejudice to the specific provisions elsewhere in this SFE relating to underpayments of particular payments, if the full amount of a payment that is payable pursuant to this SFE has not been paid before the date on which the payment falls due, then unless –
(a) this is with the consent of the contractor; or
(b) the amount of, or entitlement to, the payment, or any part thereof, is in dispute,
once it falls due, it must be paid promptly (see regulation 22 of the 2004 Regulations).

21.3 If the contractor's entitlement to the payment is not in dispute but the amount of the payment is in dispute, then once the payment falls due, pending the resolution of the dispute, the PCT must –
(a) pay to the contractor, promptly, an amount representing the amount that the PCT accepts that the contractor is at least entitled to; and
(b) thereafter pay any shortfall promptly, once the dispute is finally resolved.

21.4 However, if a contractor has –
   (a) not claimed a payment to which it would be entitled pursuant to this
        SFE if it claimed the payment; or
   (b) claimed a payment to which it is entitled pursuant to this SFE but a
        PCT is unable to calculate the payment until after the payment is due
        to fall due because it does not have the information or computer
        software it needs in order to calculate that payment (all reasonable
        efforts to obtain the information, or make the calculation, having
        been undertaken),
   that payment is (instead) to fall due at the end of the month during
   which the PCT obtains the information or computer software it needs in
   order to calculate the payment.

21.5 Furthermore, for the first quarter to which this SFE relates, if a PCT is
   unable to calculate any payment payable pursuant to this SFE that falls
   due before the end of that quarter because it does not have the
   information or computer software it needs in order to calculate that
   payment (all reasonable efforts to obtain the information, or make the
   calculation, having been undertaken), that payment is instead to fall due
   at the end of that quarter.

Payments on account

21.6 Where the PCT and the contractor agree (but the PCT's agreement may
   be withdrawn where it is reasonable to do so and if it has given the
   contractor reasonable notice thereof), the PCT must pay to a contractor
   on account any amount that is –
   (a) the amount of, or a reasonable approximation of the amount of, a
        payment that is due to fall due pursuant to this SFE; or
   (b) an agreed percentage of the amount of, or a reasonable
        approximation of the amount of, a payment that is due to fall due
        pursuant to this SFE,
   and if that payment results in an overpayment in respect of the payment,
   paragraph 21.1 applies.

21.7 However, during the first quarter to which this SFE relates, if –
   (a) a PCT is unable to calculate a payment payable pursuant to this SFE
        that is due to fall due before the end of that quarter because it does
        not have the information or computer software it needs in order to
        calculate that payment (all reasonable efforts to obtain the
        information, or calculate the payment, having been undertaken); and
   (b) it cannot reach agreement with the contractor on a payment on
        account in respect of the payment pursuant to paragraph 21.6,
   it must nevertheless pay to the contractor on account a reasonable
   approximation of the amount of the payment, on or before the unrevised

due date for payment of that payment (i.e. before it is revised in accordance with paragraph 21.5). If that payment results in an overpayment in respect of the payment, paragraph 21.1 applies.

21.8 PCTs will not be able to calculate the correct amount of GP providers' Seniority Payments during the financial year 2004/05 because it will not be possible to calculate the correct value of the GP provider's Superannuable Income Fraction until –
(a) the Average Adjusted Superannuable Income for the financial year 2004/05 has been established; and
(b) the GP provider's own NHS superannuable profits from all sources for the financial year 2004/05, excluding –
(i) superannuable income which does not appear on his certificate submitted to the PCT in accordance with paragraph 22.10, and
(ii) any amount in respect of Seniority Payments,
have been established.
If a PCT cannot reach agreement with a contractor on a payment on account in respect of a Quarterly Seniority Payment pursuant to paragraph 21.6, it must nevertheless pay to the contractor on account a reasonable approximation of the Quarterly Seniority Payment, on or before the unrevised due date for payment of that payment (i.e. before it is revised in accordance with paragraph 21.4). If that payment results in an overpayment in respect of the Quarterly Seniority Payment, paragraph 21.1 applies.

Default contracts and payments to persons not able to enter into default contracts

21.9 If a contractor's GMS contract was agreed after 1 April 2004 but the contract takes effect for payment purposes on 1 April 2004, that contractor has received a payment under a default contract or pursuant to article 41(1) of the 2004 Order, and that payment could have been made –
(a) as a payment on account under the contractor's GMS contract pursuant to paragraph 21.6 or 21.7, it shall be treated as a payment on account pursuant to paragraph 21.6 or 21.7 (and for these purposes a payment of one-twelfth of a final global sum equivalent under a default contract or under article 41(1) of the 2004 Order shall be treated as a payment on account in respect of a Payable Global Sum Monthly Payment (GSMP)); and
(b) as a payment under the contractor's GMS contract pursuant to Part 4 or 5 of this SFE, it shall be treated as a payment under the contractor's GMS contract pursuant to Part 4 or 5 of this SFE,
and accordingly, any condition that attaches to such a payment by virtue of this SFE is attached to that payment.

21.10 In these circumstances, the payments that a contractor is entitled to receive under its GMS contract pursuant to this SFE that are or were due to fall due before the end of the first quarter are instead to fall due at the end of that quarter, unless –

(a) the GMS contract is agreed between 1 June 2004 and 1 September 2004, in which case they are instead to fall due at the end of the second quarter, as are all the payments that are or were due to fall due pursuant to this SFE in the second quarter;

(b) the GMS contract is agreed between 1 September and 1 December 2004, in which case they are instead to fall due at the end of the third quarter, as are all the payments that are or were due to fall due pursuant to this SFE in that quarter or in the second quarter; or

(c) the GMS contract is agreed between 1 December 2004 and the end of the financial year, in which case they are to fall due at the end of the financial year, as are all the other payments that are or were due to fall due pursuant to this SFE before the end of the financial year.

Payments to or in respect of suspended doctors whose suspension ceases

21.11 If the suspension of a GP from a medical practitioners list ceases, and –

(a) that GP enters into a GMS contract that takes effect for payment purposes on 1 April 2004, any payments that the GP received under a determination made under regulation 13(17) of the Performers List Regulations may be set off, equitably, against the payments that he is entitled to receive under his GMS contract pursuant to this SFE; or

(b) a contractor is entitled to any payments in respect of that GP pursuant to this SFE and a payment was made to the GP pursuant to a determination made under regulation 13(17) of the Performers List Regulations but the GP was not entitled to receive all or any part thereof, the amount to which the GP was not entitled may be set off, equitably, against any payment in respect of him pursuant to this SFE.

Effect on periodic payments of termination of a GMS contract

21.12 If a GMS contract under which a periodic payment is payable pursuant to this SFE is terminated before the date on which the payment falls due, a proportion of that payment is to fall due on the last day on which the contractor is under an obligation under its GMS contract to provide essential services. The amount of the periodic payment payable is to be adjusted by the fraction produced by dividing –

(a) the number of days during the period in respect of which the payment is payable for which the contractor was under an obligation under its GMS contract to provide essential services; by

(b) the total number of days in that period.

This is without prejudice to any arrangements for the recovery of money paid under the GMS contract that is recoverable as a result of the contract terminating or any breach thereof.

Time limitation for claiming payments

21.13 Payments under this SFE are only payable if claimed within 6 years of the date on which they could first have fallen due (albeit that the due date has changed pursuant to paragraph 21.4 or 21.5).

Dispute resolution procedures

21.14 Any dispute arising out of or in connection with this SFE between a PCT and a contractor (except one to which paragraph 19.4(a) applies) is to be resolved as a dispute arising out of or in connection with the contractor's GMS contract, i.e. in accordance with the NHS dispute resolution procedures or by the courts (see Part 7 of Schedule 6 to the 2004 Regulations).

21.15 The procedures require the contractor and the PCT to make every reasonable effort to communicate and co-operate with each other with a view to resolving the dispute between themselves before referring it for determination. Either the contractor or the PCT may, if it wishes to do so, invite the Local Medical Committee to participate in these discussions.

Protocol in respect of locum cover payments

21.16 Part 4 sets out a number of circumstances in which PCTs are obliged to pay a maximum amount of £948.33 for locum cover in respect of an absent performer. However, even where a PCT is not directed pursuant to this SFE to make payments in respect of such cover, it has powers to do so as a matter of discretion – and may also decide, as a matter of discretion, to make top-up payments in cases where the £948.33 maximum directed amount is payable.

21.17 As a supplementary measure, PCTs are directed to adopt a protocol, which they must take all reasonable steps to agree with any relevant Local Medical Committee, setting out in reasonable detail –

(a) how they are likely to exercise their discretionary powers to make payments (including top-up payments) in respect of locum cover, having regard to the budgetary targets they have set for themselves, where they are not obliged to make such payments;

(b) where they are obliged to make payments in respect of locum cover pursuant to Part 4, the circumstances in which they are likely to make payments in respect of locum cover of less than the maximum amount payable (e.g. to take account of less than full-time working);

(c) how they are likely to exercise their discretionary powers to make payments in respect of cover for absent GP performers, which is provided by nurses or other health care professionals; and

(d) how they are likely to exercise their discretionary powers to make payments to a partner or shareholder in a contractor, or an employee of a contractor, who is providing locum cover for an absent GP performer who is also a partner or shareholder in, or an employee of, the contractor.

Where a PCT departs from that protocol in any individual case and refuses an application for funding in respect of locum cover, this must be duly justified to the unsuccessful applicant.

Adjustment of Contractor Registered Populations

21.18 The starting point for the determination of a contractor's Contractor Registered Population is the number of patients recorded in the Exeter Registration System as being registered with the contractor, initially when its GMS contract takes effect and thereafter at the start of each quarter, when a new number must be established.

21.19 However, in respect of any quarter, this number may be adjusted as follows –

(a) if a contractor satisfies a PCT that a patient who registered with it before the start of a quarter was not included in the number of patients recorded in the Exeter Registration System as being registered with it at the start of that quarter, and the PCT received notification of the new registration within 48 hours of the start of that quarter, that patient –

(i) is to be treated as part of that contractor's Contractor Registered Population at the start of that quarter, and

(ii) is not to be treated as part of any other contractor's Contractor Registered Population at the start of that quarter (and the PCT must notify any other PCT that will need to adjust another contractor's Contractor Registered Population accordingly);

(b) if, included in the number of patients recorded in the Exeter Registration System as being registered with a contractor at the start of a quarter, there are patients who –

(i) transferred to another contractor in the quarter before the previous quarter (or earlier), but

(ii) notification of that fact was not received by the PCT until after the second day of the previous quarter,

those patients are not to be treated as part of the contractor's Contractor Registered Population at the start of that quarter; or

(c) if a patient is not recorded in the Exeter Registration System as being registered with a contractor at the start of a quarter, but that patient –

(i) had been removed from a contractor's patient list in error, and

(ii) was reinstated in the quarter before the previous quarter (or earlier),

that patient is to be treated as part of the contractor's Contractor Registered Population at the start of that quarter.

21.20 If a contractor wishes its Contractor Registered Population to be adjusted in accordance with paragraph 2.19, it must –

(a) within 10 days of receiving from the PCT a statement of its patient list size for a quarter, request in writing that the PCT makes the adjustment; and

(b) within 21 days of receiving that statement, provide the PCT with the evidence upon which it wishes to rely in order to obtain the adjustment,

and the PCT must seek to resolve the matter as soon as is practicable. If there is a dispute in connection with the adjustment, paragraphs 21.14 and 21.15 apply.

● Administrative removals

See also: Removals · Patient list

Guidance

2.47 Administrative removals are where groups or large numbers of patients are removed:

(i) for severe workload reasons, for example the departure of a GP who cannot be replaced in a two-handed practice. The removals are normally achieved by varying the contractor's area. In these cases, contractors would be required to discuss and agree this with the Primary Care Trust (PCT)

(ii) because a contractor stops holding a primary medical services contract.

2.48 The PCT must write to all affected patients with as much notice as is reasonably or practically possible, setting out the options available to them. It must ensure they can receive primary medical services, if need be by allocating them to lists of other providers, bearing in mind their best interests. Where the other providers are GMS contractors with closed lists, the PCT must comply with the assignment procedure.

Allocations (financial) to PCTs

Guidance

5.14 This section gives an overview of how allocations to Primary Care Trusts (PCTs) will work. It then describes:
   (i) Global sum and Minimum Income Practice Guarantee (MPIG) funds
   (ii) Out-of-hours funds
   (iii) Enhanced services funds
   (iv) Quality funds
   (v) PCT-administered funds
   (vi) Premises funds
   (vii) IT funds
   (viii) PMS funds.
   A summary timetable is provided at the end of the section.

How allocations to PCTs will work

5.15 Paragraph 5.35 of *Investing in General Practice* stated that GMS funds would be allocated as a single sum as part of an enlarged unified budget. In line with *Shifting the Balance of Power*, the Department is committed to allocating as much resource as possible to PCTs. Four funding elements will be held as central budgets:
   (i) £10 million for demand management: £5 million in 2004/05, and £5 million in 2005/06
   (ii) most of the Information Management and Technology (IM&T) funding which will be delivered in primary care through spend on the National Programme for IT
   (iii) personal administration and dispensing, which will continue to be non-cash limited for 2004/05
   (iv) recruitment and retention monies (which include golden hellos).
   All other primary medical services funds will be allocated to the NHS to manage locally.

5.16 The Health and Social Care Act 2003 brought GMS funding within the ambit of statutory provisions governing the allocation of the unified budget. This is in line with paragraph 7.59(vii) of *Investing in General Practice*. PCTs will receive cash-limited allocations rather than be reimbursed for the expenses they incur as a result of paying entitlements to contractors, dispensing and personal administration payments being the only exception. The majority of the funding that makes up the Gross Investment Guarantee (GIG) will be allocated to PCTs, which will receive notification of actual allocations for 2004/05 in January 2004. The allocations will identify notional amounts for each funding element, except for enhanced services, which will have a local funding floor that cannot be breached but can be exceeded. PCTs will need to manage risks in year arising from in-year population changes. This approach is consistent with the way in which unified budget allocations work.

5.17   The principle of contractor entitlement, combined with different levels of historic spend in PCTs for different funding streams, means that there can be no overall primary medical services allocation formula and target progression applied to the totality of those funds. Such an approach would not target resources with sufficient accuracy. For this reason a tailored approach will be taken to allocating each of the main funding sources.

5.18   The allocation method will achieve movement towards equity of funding whilst protecting historic levels of spend. In the particular, (i) global sum allocations, (ii) the Quality and Outcomes framework (QOF) disease prevalence adjustment and (iii) new premises funding will all target resources to relatively under-resourced areas. In this way primary care resource allocation will help address health inequalities. Equitable distribution of overall NHS resources will also be pursued by considering primary medical services allocations within the context of making unified budget allocations. At present the unified budget allocation formula takes account of GMS non-cash-limited (GMSNCL) spend when determining movement towards target allocations. Alternative ways of incorporating the new primary care funding arrangements will be considered as part of the next round of unified budget allocations.

5.19   Figure 14 summarises the main elements and their allocation method.

(i) Global sum and MPIG funds

5.20   Global sum and MPIG funds will be allocated to PCTs. Data to inform the allocations have been collected through Allocations Working Papers (AWP)(04–05)PCT05, AWP(04–05)PCT06, and AWP(04–05)PCT08. Data constraints mean that it has not been possible to calculate the exact amounts of contractor entitlements to inform allocations; to minimise financial risk for PCTs, the Department has developed as close a proxy as

Figure 14 **Allocation elements for primary medical services**

Global sum	MPIG correction factor	Enhanced services	QOF
Global sum allocation formula	Historic spend comparing GSE to global	Combination of UB formula and historic spend	Combination of costs of aspiration spend and NHS Bank risk management

PCO administered	IT	Out of Hours	Premises
Combination of historic spend and different formulae	Combination of UB formula, costs and central budget	Combination of UB formula and specific targeting	Combination of historic spend, planned spend and GS adjusted formula

Dispensing and PA	PMS allocation
Non-cash-limited in 2004/05	Combination of baseline and adapted methods for the 9 elements. Some of the elements will contain combined GMS and PMS funding

possible in the circumstances. The method for calculating actual global sums and MPIG is described in annex B.

5.21 PCTs should note that global sum and MPIG funding includes the staff element of GMS cash-limited resources that has already been allocated to PCTs as part of their unified budget. Data on cash-limited staff costs have been collected from PCTs through AWP(04–05)PCT06. Allocations to PCTs will take account of that resource.

5.22 PCTs will be notified before April 2004 of an additional allocation to fund an increase in the global sum price to support the increase in employer superannuation costs. The increase will reflect the rise in contributions from 7% to 14% and the 14% contribution in respect of the expected increase in net income. The Department will discuss the size of the increase, and the precise method for its delivery, with the GPC in January 2004.

A Allocations (financial) to PCTs
Guidance

(ii) Out-of-hours funds

5.23 When determining how to secure integrated out-of-hours services, PCTs will need to consider all the resources available to them both in the unified budget (e.g. resources used for emergency care networks) and elsewhere.

5.24 Additionally, they will have access to three specific sources of funding:
   (i)   allocations to PCTs from the Out of Hours Development Fund (OOHDF) are to be doubled from £45.6 million to £91.2 million per annum
   (ii) there is to be a further non-recurrent addition to the OOHDF of £28 million over 2 years to support areas facing the greatest challenges in developing out-of-hours services
   (iii) these resources will be supplemented by 6% of global sums (not global sums plus MPIGs) of contractors that opt out.

5.25 OOHDF allocations for 2004/05 were announced on 1 November 2003 (see http://www.out-of-hours.info). The 2004/05 method allocates the first £45.6 million on the basis of the current OOHDF and the additional £45.6 million on a weighted capitation basis. From 2005/06 the intention is that the whole of the allocation will be on a weighted capitation basis. The OOHDF will remain ring-fenced for use on out-of-hours primary medical services (however provided), but the detailed rules on its use contained in the Statement of Fees and Allowances will no longer apply.

5.26 The Department of Health is discussing with SHAs the best way to allocate the further £28 million (£14 million in 2004/05 and 2005/06). Details will be made available to PCTs in January 2004. These funds will also be ring-fenced for use on out-of-hours primary medical services.

(iii) Enhanced services funds

5.27 Most of the enhanced services funding has already been allocated to PCTs through HSC 2002/12 *PCT Revenue Resource Limits for 2003/04 to 2005/06*. This identified £315 million/£394 million/£460 million in the three successive financial years.

5.28 From 2004/05 there will be additional funding as the result of the transfer of existing non-cash-limited GMS payments to fund (i) intra partum care, (ii) intrauterine device fees, (iii) influenza immunisation payments, (iv) childhood vaccinations and immunisations target payments, and (v) part of minor surgery fees. This reflects the categorisation of these services as enhanced within new GMS. This money will be allocated on the basis of historical spend mapped through AWP(04–05)PCT08 to ensure that existing services are not destabilised.

5.29   Each PCT will receive a real rather than notional figure for enhanced services. PCTs should note that from 2004/05 a spending floor will be set for each PCT. This will replace the 2003/04 national floor mechanism. Planned spend against the local floor must be signed off by the PCT's Professional Executive Committee and discussed with the Local Medical Committee (LMC). Spend against the floor will be monitored by TSC on the basis of the definition described in chapter 2.

(iv) GMS quality funds

5.30   Chapter 3 explained how GMS contractors will receive four types of quality payment: (i) Quality Preparation (QPREP), (ii) Quality Information Preparation (QuIP), (iii) quality aspiration and (iv) quality achievement. These are all legal entitlements: in particular, PCTs must fund contractors fully for whatever level of points they achieve on the QOF scorecard. The Department is also introducing comparable quality incentives for PMS contractors; the way in which these will work will be set out in the December 2003 PMS guidance.

5.31   Allocations will be made on the following basis:
(i)   QuIP is an enhanced service funded from the unified allocation
(ii) funds for QPREP in 2004/05 will be included within the January 2004 allocations, on the basis of PCT registered populations collected from the Exeter registration system
(iii) funds for aspiration payments will be allocated to PCTs in April 2004 on the basis of the agreed Interim Aspiration Utility returns held on the Exeter payments system. From 2005/06 resources will be allocated on the new basis for calculating aspiration payments, once achievement payments have been confirmed by PCTs
(iv) the balance of quality funding to meet quality achievement for GMS will be allocated to the NHS Bank in April 2004, which will allocate the resource in year.

5.32   There is a cost to high quality primary care and higher than expected achievement against the QOF will require financial risk management across the NHS. PCTs should also note that high quality primary care, and in particular better chronic disease management, will over time help reduce avoidable A&E and outpatient attendances and hospital admissions, improve health outcomes and improve patient experience.

5.33   The Department's best current estimate is that the England GIG includes sufficient provision to support 74% and 85% achievement of points in 2004/05 and 2005/06 respectively for all contractors. This figure will change once allocations are made, and in particular, the MPIG requirement is known. Our current expectation is that these percentages are more likely to decrease than increase.

5.34   The Department has decided, in consultation with SHA Chief Executives, the NHS Confederation and the GPC, that the financial risks associated with quality achievement will be managed by the NHS through the NHS Bank, which will play a central role in monitoring and pooling resources. Given the devolution of the vast majority of NHS resources to PCTs under *Shifting the Balance of Power*, it makes sense to manage risk against that resource pot rather than the much smaller Department of Health central budgets.

5.35   Financial risk will be shared jointly between high achieving PCTs after utilising any agreed NHS Bank support. Any additional costs arising from more effective prescribing in line with the QOF clinical indicators will also need to be managed locally by PCTs. For the quality achievement risk sharing arrangements to work effectively, SHAs and the NHS Bank will need during spring 2004 to establish and agree arrangements. These will include:

(i)   monthly flows of financial information to assess current performance against the QOF and the projected out-turn position for the year-end. This will be supported, for GMS contractors and PMS contractors using the QOF unamended locally, by the QMAS system described in chapter 3. The system will go live by August 2004. Where PCTs have agreed local variations in PMS to the GMS QOF, they will need to make their own local risk management arrangements

(ii)   a further assessment of the likely out-turn position will need to be made towards the end of the financial year, following completion of the quality reviews described in chapter 3. If anticipated achievement is in line with the resource available, the role of the NHS Bank will be to facilitate the necessary resource allocation changes to ensure that at PCT level resource allocation equals anticipated expenditure

(iii)   any increase in achievement after this assessment has been made would need to be managed at a local level. This would be in addition to whatever risks SHAs may have signed up to accommodate as part of their agreements with the NHS Bank.

(v) PCT-administered funds

5.36   PCT-administered funds support a number of different entitlements, including (i) seniority, (ii) the retainer, returner, golden hello and flexible career schemes and (iii) locum allowances for maternity, paternity and adoptive leave, sickness, suspended doctors and prolonged study leave. They also include existing GMS resources under the Initial Practice Allowance for greenfield sites and a notional national amount of £8.5 million for new sabbatical schemes.

5.37   These resources will mainly be allocated on the basis of historic baselines. Guidance on establishing the baseline expenditure for GMS contractors was set out in AWP(04–05)PCT08. The precise methodology to be used will be explained as part of the main January allocations. The recruitment and retention funds, including for golden hellos, will be held as a central budget.

(vi) Premises funds

5.38   Allocations for premises costs will be based on three elements:
   (i)   existing spend. Allocations will cover a guaranteed baseline of current expenditure on: (a) rent payments (includes actual rent, cost rent, notional rent and LA economic rents), (b) business and water rates, (c) improvement grants, and (d) other existing premises expenditure. This information has been collected and verified with PCTs through AWP(04–05)PCT06 and AWP(04–05)PCT08
   (ii) agreed new premises developments. Allocations will include an additional element to meet the cost of new agreed premises developments (i.e. those ready for occupation, under construction and others contractually agreed by 30 September 2003 between the practice and the provider of the building/building works). The information to support the allocation is held by the Valuation Office Agency and NHS Estates databases of new developments, and is being validated through AWP(04–05)PCT11 and AWP(04–05)PCT15
   (iii) new premises development (including NHS LIFT) and premises flexibilities. A further element will based on the global sum allocation formula, adjusted to give greater weight to unavoidable costs of premises inflation. This will support the costs of the new premises flexibilities and new premises developments.

5.39   The first two elements will be allocated directly to individual PCTs as part of the main January 2004 allocation. The third will be allocated in January 2004 to a lead PCT in the SHA area to hold pending local agreement on the distribution of these funds to support government priorities and local priorities agreed with the SHA. This includes funding for PMS as well as GMS contractors.

5.40   The lead PCT will have two main functions:
   (i)   to act as the conduit for new premises funding to pass to other PCTs, and hold funds yet to be reallocated
   (ii) to advise PCTs as a group on primary care estate procurement, management and disposal.

5.41   SHAs should establish lead PCT arrangements now so that decisions can start being made on outstanding new premises developments as early as possible in January 2004.

(vii) Information technology funds

5.42   A significant part of the existing funding for GMS practices has already been allocated in the GMS cash-limited part of the unified budget. This covers the costs associated with part-reimbursement of the purchase, leasing, upgrades, and maintenance of computer systems in practices.

5.43   Guidance on identifying this expenditure for the January allocation was set out in AWP(04–05)PCT06. Additional funding of £20 million has also been allocated in 2003/04 on a weighted capitation basis to allow PCTs to meet their new obligations to fund 100% of the costs associated with minor upgrades and maintenance costs for all practices. This level of funding will be guaranteed in the allocation for 2004/05. The Department has also agreed that PCTs may be able to access additional funds for minor upgrades and maintenance where they can demonstrate central support has been insufficient in supplementing historical spending levels.

5.44   Most of the IT funding identified in the original envelope for spend in primary care will be held centrally by the National Programme for IT and used to support its work.

(viii) Personal Medical Services funds

5.45   From 2004/05 a single PMS allocation will be made alongside GMS funds as part of a combined primary medical services allocation. PMS funding will include existing PMS baseline spend plus a comparable uplift to that given for funding GMS practices. The way in which this is calculated in relation to the different funding elements will be set out in the December 2003 PMS guidance.

Appraisal and assessment

Regulations

68.   Appraisal and assessment

(1)   The contractor shall ensure that any medical practitioner performing services under the contract –
   (a) participates in the appraisal system provided by the PCT unless he participates in an appraisal system provided by another health service body or is an armed forces GP; and

(b) co-operates with an assessment by the NCAA when requested to do so by the PCT.

(2) The PCT shall provide an appraisal system for the purposes of sub-paragraph (1)(a) after consultation with the LMC (if any) for the area of the PCT and such other persons as appear to it to be appropriate.

(3) In sub-paragraph (1), "armed forces GP" means a medical practitioner who is employed on a contract of service by the Ministry of Defence, whether or not as a member of the United Kingdom Armed Forces of Her Majesty.

Standard Contract

367. The Contractor shall ensure that any medical practitioner performing services under the Contract –
367.1 participates in the appraisal system provided by the PCT, unless he participates in an appropriate appraisal system provided by another *health service body* or is an *armed forces GP*; and
367.2 co-operates with an assessment by the *NCAA* when requested to do so by the PCT.

368. The PCT shall provide an appraisal system for the purposes of clause 367.1 after consultation with the *Local Medical Committee* (if any) for the area of the PCT and such other persons as appear to it to be appropriate.

● Aspiration payments

See also: Achievement payments · Quality and outcome

Guidance

3.17 Aspiration payments provide in-year financial support against likely QOF achievement. This section sets out how aspiration payments will work in 2004/05 and 2005/06.

2004/05

3.18 Before aspiration payments are made, PCTs and practices must agree 2004/05 aspiration levels. An Excel spreadsheet called the Interim Aspiration Utility (IAU) has been developed to help contractors assess their likely level of quality achievement points. This was issued to PCTs by the National Programme for IT (NPfIT) in the first week of December 2003, with guidance notes. PCTs will have added practice identifiers and list sizes from the Exeter payment system and forwarded it to all their GMS contractors by Monday 15 December 2003.

3.19   To ensure that their first monthly aspiration payment can be made from the end of April 2004, contractors are advised to submit their completed IAU by 16 January 2004 to the PCT. PCTs will want to give their practices whatever help they require to complete their returns. Contractors that do not use the IAU should complete a hard-copy version and send this to their PCT. Whilst some PCTs have developed their own spreadsheets for calculating aspiration payments, there are good reasons why PCTs should only use the IAU to calculate aspiration points totals. It will ensure accuracy and national consistency. The completed IAUs will also be loaded onto the QMAS IT system in due course, to allow 2004/05 achievement to be compared with aspiration, and this system is only compatible with the IAU. PCTs that already have information on their contractors' aspirations should consider whether they have enough information to complete the IAU without re-sending it to their practices. However, they should discuss this with their contractors and offer them the opportunity to complete the IAU themselves should contractors so prefer.

3.20   The SFE contains a condition that the contractor's proposed aspiration level must be realistic. PCTs should bear in mind that, as a result of new contract QOF incentives, contractors will be taking major steps during 2004/05 to improve the quality of their services. When submitting their completed IAUs, contractors should include a brief covering explanation setting out why and how they think their aspiration level is achievable, for example through employing additional practice staff. This will normally be sufficient for the PCT to agree the aspiration level without the need for any further information to be sought from the contractor. PCTs should agree aspiration points with contractors by the end of February 2004.

3.21   If a contractor does not submit an aspiration claim it will not receive an aspiration payment. In these circumstances, the PCT may wish to confirm that the contractor does not wish to participate in the QOF. If the PCT and practice cannot agree an aspiration, either party has the right to invoke the formal pre-contract dispute resolution procedure. However, we advise PCTs and contractors not to go down this route; it is a disproportionately bureaucratic solution for what is basically an argument about marginal cash-flow. Instead, pending the outcome of the dispute, the practice would be awarded the level of aspiration that the PCT was prepared to agree or the lowest level of aspiration agreed between the PCT and its constituent practices, whichever is higher. This ensures that contractors will receive at least some aspiration payments from April. Once the dispute has ended and a final aspiration figure agreed, the PCT will need to pay any arrears that have accrued to the contractor, or recover any overpayment of aspiration.

3.22 Once the aspiration points are agreed, in line with the SFE, the PCT must pay the aspiration payment in monthly instalments, by the end of each month, starting from the end of April 2004. This will be done automatically, once the PCT has entered payment details on to the Exeter system. The payment will be calculated automatically by the IAU by:

(i) dividing the number of aspiration points by three to calculate the third on which the payment is based

(ii) multiplying the third by £75 to get the raw payment

(iii) adjusting the payment by the contractor's list size relative to the national average, as with QPREP and QuIP payments. In England the national average is currently 5891.

3.23 The 2004/05 aspiration payment will not be weighted by relative practice disease prevalence.

3.24 Pro-rata payments will be made to new contractors in year except where these arise from practice splits. Contracts that start at such a date that there is insufficient time to make a payment by the end of March 2005 will not receive an aspiration payment in advance of or after the achievement payment being made by the end of April 2005. If the contract comes to an end in year, and the contractor was receiving aspiration payments, then these are stopped on the date the contract ends. If the contract ends during a month, the practice receives a pro-rata payment in respect of the number of days the contract ran during that month. In the event of a practice merger, the monthly aspiration payments of the two practices are added together.

3.25 Figure 3 provides a worked example.

3.26 The flowchart in Figure 4 illustrates the complete aspiration process.

2005/06 aspiration payments

3.27 A different method for calculating aspiration payments will apply from 2005/06. This has been designed to meet three objectives:

(i) to enable contractors to receive a greater proportion of the quality money in-year, to improve their cash-flow, but without putting at risk PCT cash management requirements

(ii) to make the payment calculation automatic to remove the possibility of local dispute

(iii) to make the process of planning for quality improvement, through agreeing aspiration levels, simpler and less liable to distortion as a result of financial considerations.

> ### *Figure 3* **Worked example of 2004/05 aspiration payment**
>
> The PCT and contractor agree aspiration of 650 points.
>
> The contractor's registered list size is 7000 patients.
>
> The number of points is divided by three to arrive at the aspiration total
> 650/3 = 216.67
>
> The aspiration points total is multiplied by £75 to arrive at the raw
> aspiration payment:
>
> 216.67 × £75 = £16,250.00
>
> This payment is multiplied by the contractor's registered list size factor:
>
> (7000/5891) × £16,250.00 = 1.19 × £16,250.00 = £19,309.11
>
> **So the contractor's aspiration payment for 2004/05 is £19,309.11,
> payable in 12 monthly instalments of £1609.09.** (NB: In this and all
> other examples, although figures are rounded for presentation, they
> are not rounded within the calculation).

3.28 The new method of calculating aspiration payments will be as follows:
  (i) the aspiration payment for 2005/06 will be based on 60% of the
       achievement points that the contractor scored in 2004/05
  (ii) the pounds per point will be uprated to the 2005/06 level, i.e. £120
       for a contractor with an average list size and average prevalence. The
       2004/05 disease prevalence factors will be applied to this. The way in
       which disease prevalence will work is described in the next section of
       this chapter
  (iii) payments will be continue to be weighted by the contractor's relative
       list size
  (iv) where the contractor had not participated in the quality framework
       in 2004/05, or only participated to a very limited degree, its
       aspiration will be worked out using the process for 2004/05 (i.e. it
       will agree an aspiration total with the PCT and be paid a third of
       this, with no weighting by prevalence).

3.29 The new method from 2005/06 is illustrated in the worked example in
      Figure 5.

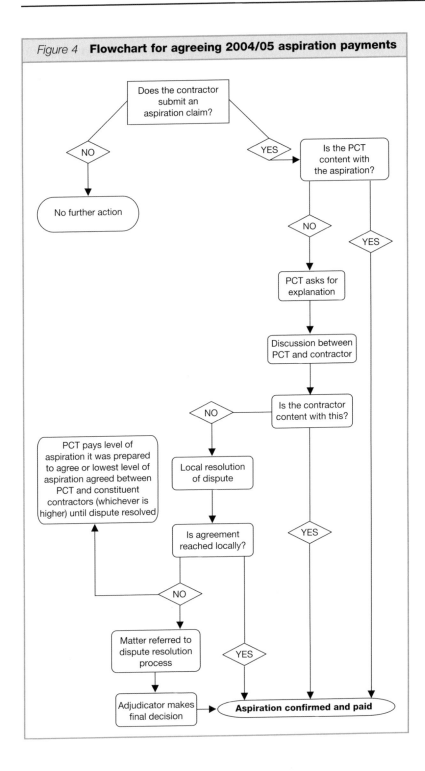

Figure 4 **Flowchart for agreeing 2004/05 aspiration payments**

Does the contractor submit an aspiration claim?

NO

No further action

YES

Is the PCT content with the aspiration?

NO

YES

PCT asks for explanation

Discussion between PCT and contractor

Is the contractor content with this?

NO

PCT pays level of aspiration it was prepared to agree or lowest level of aspiration agreed between PCT and constituent contractors (whichever is higher) until dispute resolved

Local resolution of dispute

Is agreement reached locally?

YES

NO

Matter referred to dispute resolution process

YES

Adjudicator makes final decision

Aspiration confirmed and paid

Figure 5 **Worked example of 2005/06 aspiration payment**

The figures in this example are based on the achievement of the hypothetical contractor in figure 10. Each QOF point is worth £120 in 2005/06.

The contractor's gross achievement payment for the QOF in 2004/05 is £56,561.79. To calculate the aspiration payment for 2005/06, the payment must be uprated to £120 per point and then 60% of the new figure found. This is represented by the following formula:

$$£56561.79 \times \frac{120}{75} \times \frac{60}{100} = £56,561.79 \times 1.6 \times 0.6 = £54,299.32$$

The contractor's aspiration payment for 2005/06 is £54,299.32 payable in 12 monthly instalments of £4524.94.

The formula works by adjusting the previous year's gross achievement payment, during the calculation of which clinical and additional services prevalence, and the contractor's relative list size have already been taken into account. There is therefore no need to readjust the 2005/06 aspiration figure to take these into account.

Assignment of patients to lists

Regulations

32. Assignment of patients to lists: open lists

(1) A PCT may, subject to paragraph 34, assign a new patient to a contractor whose list of patients is open.

(2) In this paragraph and in paragraphs 33 and 35 to 37, a "new" patient means a person who –
(a) is resident (whether or not temporarily) within the area of the PCT;
(b) has been refused inclusion in a list of patients of, or has not been accepted as a temporary resident by, a contractor whose premises are within such an area; and
(c) wishes to be included in the list of patients of a contractor whose practice premises are within that area.

33. Assignment of patients to lists: closed lists

(1)   A PCT may not assign a new patient to a contractor which has closed its list of patients except in the circumstances specified in sub-paragraph (2).

(2)   A PCT may, subject to paragraph 34, assign a new patient to a contractor whose practice premises are within the PCT's area and which has closed its list of patients, if –

(a) most or all of the providers of essential services (or their equivalent) whose practice premises are within the PCT's area have closed their lists of patients;

(b) the assessment panel has determined under paragraph 35(7) that patients may be assigned to the contractor in question, and that determination has not been overturned either by a determination of the Secretary of State under paragraph 36(13) or (where applicable) by a court; and

(c) the PCT has entered into discussions with the contractor in question regarding the assignment of a patient if such discussions are required under paragraph 37.

34. Factors relevant to assignments

In making an assignment to a contractor under paragraph 32 or 33, the PCT shall have regard to –

(a) the wishes and circumstances of the patient to be assigned;

(b) the distance between the patient's place of residence and the contractor's practice premises;

(c) whether, during the 6 months ending on the date on which the application for assignment is received by the PCT, the patient's name has been removed from the list of patients of any contractor in the area of the PCT under paragraph 20 or its equivalent provision in relation to a section 28C provider in the area of the PCT;

(d) whether the patient's name has been removed from the list of patients of any contractor in the area of the PCT under paragraph 21 or its equivalent provision in relation to a section 28C provider in the area of the PCT and, if so, whether the contractor has appropriate facilities to deal with such a patient;

(e) such other matters as the PCT considers to be relevant.

35. Assignments to closed lists: determinations of the assessment panel

(1)   This paragraph applies where most or all of the providers of essential services (or their equivalent) whose practice premises are within the area of a PCT have closed their lists of patients.

(2) If the PCT wishes to assign new patients to contractors which have closed their lists of patients, it must prepare a proposal to be considered by the assessment panel which must include details of those contractors to which the PCT wishes to assign patients.

(3) The PCT must ensure that the assessment panel is appointed to consider and determine its proposal made under sub-paragraph (2), and the composition of the assessment panel shall be as described in paragraph 31(5).

(4) The PCT shall notify in writing –
(a) the relevant SHA;
(b) contractors or section 28C providers whose practice premises are within the PCT's area which –
(i) have closed their list of patients, and
(ii) may, in the opinion of the PCT, be affected by the determination of the assessment panel; and
(c) the LMC (if any) for the area of the PCT,
that it has referred the matter to the assessment panel.

(5) In reaching its determination, the assessment panel shall have regard to relevant factors including –
(a) whether the PCT has attempted to secure the provision of essential services (or their equivalent) for new patients other than by means of their assignment to contractors with closed lists of patients; and
(b) the workload of those contractors likely to be affected by any decision to assign such patients to their list of patients.

(6) The assessment panel shall reach a determination within the period of 28 days beginning with the date on which the panel was appointed.

(7) The assessment panel shall determine whether the PCT may assign patients to contractors which have closed their lists of patients; and if it determines that the PCT may make such assignments, it shall also determine those contractors to which patients may be assigned.

(8) The assessment panel may determine that the PCT may assign patients to contractors other than those contractors specified by the PCT in its proposal under sub-paragraph (2), as long as the contractors were notified under sub-paragraph (4)(b).

(9) The assessment panel's determination shall include its comments on the matters specified in sub-paragraph (5), and shall be notified in writing to –
(a) the relevant SHA; and
(b) those contractors which were notified under sub-paragraph (4)(b).

36. Assignments to closed lists: NHS dispute resolution procedure relating to determinations of the assessment panel

(1) Where an assessment panel makes a determination under paragraph 35(7) that the PCT may assign new patients to contractors which have closed their lists of patients, any contractor specified in that determination may refer the matter to the Secretary of State to review the determination of the assessment panel.

(2) Where a matter is referred to the Secretary of State in accordance with sub-paragraph (1), it shall be reviewed in accordance with the procedure specified in the following sub-paragraphs.

(3) Where more than one contractor specified in the determination in accordance with paragraph 35(7) wishes to refer the matter for dispute resolution, those contractors may, if they all agree, refer the matter jointly, and in that case the Secretary of State shall review the matter in relation to those contractors together.

(4) Within the period of 7 days beginning with the date of the determination by the assessment panel in accordance with paragraph 35(7), the contractor (or contractors) shall send to the Secretary of State a written request for dispute resolution which shall include or be accompanied by –
(a) the names and addresses of the parties to the dispute;
(b) a copy of the contract (or contracts); and
(c) a brief statement describing the nature and circumstances of the dispute.

(5) Within the period of 7 days beginning with the date on which the matter was referred to him, the Secretary of State shall –
(a) give to the parties notice in writing that he is dealing with the matter; and
(b) include with the notice a written request to the parties to make in writing within a specified period any representations which they may wish to make about the dispute.

(6) The Secretary of State shall give, with the notice given under sub-paragraph (5), to the party other than the one which referred the matter to dispute resolution a copy of any document by which the dispute was referred to dispute resolution.

(7) The Secretary of State shall, upon receiving any representations from a party, give a copy of them to the other party, and shall in each case request (in writing) a party to which a copy of the representations is

given to make within a specified period any written observations which it wishes to make on those representations.

(8) For the purpose of assisting it in its consideration of the matter, the Secretary of State may –

(a) invite representatives of the parties to appear before him to make oral representations either together or, with the agreement of the parties, separately, and may in advance provide the parties with a list of matters or questions to which he wishes them to give special consideration; or

(b) consult other persons whose expertise he considers will assist him in his consideration of the dispute.

(9) Where the Secretary of State consults another person under sub-paragraph (8)(b), he shall notify the parties accordingly in writing and, where he considers that the interests of any party might be substantially affected by the result of the consultation, he shall give to the parties such opportunity as he considers reasonable in the circumstances to make observations on those results.

(10) In considering the dispute, the Secretary of State shall consider –

(a) any written representations made in response to a request under sub-paragraph (5)(b), but only if they are made within the specified period;

(b) any written observations made in response to a request under sub-paragraph (7), but only if they are made within the specified period;

(c) any oral representations made in response to an invitation under sub-paragraph (8)(a);

(d) the results of any consultation under sub-paragraph (8)(b); and

(e) any observations made in accordance with an opportunity given under sub-paragraph (9).

(11) Subject to the other provisions of this paragraph and to any agreement by the parties, the Secretary of State shall have wide discretion in determining the procedure of the dispute resolution to ensure the just, expeditious, economical and final determination of the dispute.

(12) In this paragraph, "specified period" means such period as the Secretary of State shall specify in the request, being not less than 1, nor more than 2, weeks beginning with the date on which the notice referred to is given, but the Secretary of State may, if the period for determination of the dispute has been extended in accordance with sub-paragraph (16), extend any such period (even after it has expired) and, where he does so, a reference in this paragraph to the specified period is to the period as so extended.

(13) Subject to sub-paragraph (16), within the period of 21 days beginning with the date on which the matter was referred to him, the Secretary of State shall determine whether the PCT may assign patients to contractors which have closed their lists of patients; and if he determines that the PCT may make such assignments, he shall also determine those contractors to which patients may be assigned.

(14) The Secretary of State may not determine that patients may be assigned to a contractor which was not specified in the determination of the assessment panel under paragraph 35(7).

(15) In the case of a matter referred jointly by contractors in accordance with sub-paragraph (3), the Secretary of State may determine that patients may be assigned to one, some or all of the contractors which referred the matter.

(16) The period of 21 days referred to in sub-paragraph (13) may be extended (even after it has expired) by a further specified number of days if an agreement to that effect is reached by –
(a) the Secretary of State;
(b) the PCT; and
(c) the contractor (or contractors) which referred the matter to dispute resolution.

(17) The Secretary of State shall record his determination, and the reasons for it, in writing and shall give notice of the determination (including the record of the reasons) to the parties.

37. Assignments to closed lists: assignments of patients by a PCT

(1) Before the PCT may assign a new patient to a contractor, it shall, subject to sub-paragraph (3), enter into discussions with that contractor regarding additional support that the PCT can offer the contractor, and the PCT shall use its best endeavours to provide appropriate support.

(2) In the discussions referred to in sub-paragraph (1), both parties shall use reasonable endeavours to reach agreement.

(3) The requirement in sub-paragraph (1) to enter into discussions applies –
(a) to the first assignment of a patient to a particular contractor; and
(b) to any subsequent assignment to that contractor to the extent that it is reasonable and appropriate having regard to the numbers of patients who have been or may be assigned to it and the period of time since the last discussions under sub-paragraph (1) took place.

Standard Contract

Assignment of patients to lists: open lists

253. The PCT may, subject to clause 257, assign a new patient to the Contractor whose list of patients is *open*.

254. In this clause, and in clauses 255 to 256 and clauses 258 to 267 a "new" patient means a person who –

254.1 is resident (whether or not temporarily) within the area of the PCT;

254.2 has been refused inclusion in a list of patients of, or has not been accepted as a *temporary resident* by a contractor whose premises are within such an area; and

254.3 wishes to be included in the list of patients of the Contractor whose *practice premises* are within that area.

Assignment of patients to lists: closed lists

255. The PCT may not assign a new patient to the Contractor where it has *closed* its list of patients except in the circumstances specified in clause 256.

256. The PCT may, subject to clause 267, assign a new patient to the Contractor when it has *closed* its list of patients if the Contractor's *practice premises* are within the PCT's area, and –

256.1 most or all of the providers of *essential services* (or their equivalent) whose *practice premises* are within the PCT's area have *closed* their lists of patients;

256.2 the *assessment panel* has determined under paragraph 35(7) of Schedule 6 to *the Regulations* that patients may be assigned to the Contractor, and that determination has not been overturned either by a determination of *the Secretary of State* under paragraph 36(13) of Schedule 6 *to the Regulations* or (where applicable) by a court; and

256.3 the PCT has entered into discussions with the Contractor in question regarding the assignment of a patient if such discussions are required under clause 264.

Factors relevant to assignments

257. In making an assignment to the Contractor under clauses 253 to 256 the PCT shall have regard to –

257.1 the wishes and circumstances of the patient to be assigned;

257.2 the distance between the patient's place of residence and the Contractor's *practice premises*;

257.3 whether, during the 6 months ending on the date on which the application for assignment is received by the PCT, the patient's name has been removed from the list of patients of any contractor in the area of the PCT under clauses 191 to 200 or the equivalent provision in relation to a *section 28C provider* in the area of the PCT;

257.4 whether the patient's name has been removed from the list of patients of any contractor in the area of the PCT under clauses 201 to 208 or the equivalent provision in relation to a *section 28C* provider in the area of the PCT and, if so, whether the Contractor has appropriate facilities to deal with such a patient;

257.5 such other matters as the PCT considers to be relevant.

Assignments to closed lists: determinations of the assessment panel

258. Clauses 259 to 261 apply where most or all of the providers of *essential services* (or their equivalent) whose *practice premises* are within the area of the PCT have *closed* their lists of patients and the PCT proposes to assign patients to contractors who have *closed* their lists (including the Contractor).

259. If the PCT wishes to assign new patients to the contractors specified in clause 258, it must prepare a proposal to be considered by the *assessment panel*, and the proposal must include details of those contractors to which the PCT wishes to assign new patients.

260. The PCT must ensure that the *assessment panel* is appointed to consider and determine its proposal made under clause 259, and the composition of the *assessment panel* shall be as described in clause 250.

261. The PCT shall notify in writing –

261.1 the *relevant SHA*;

261.2 contractors or *section 28C providers* whose *practice premises* are within the PCT's area which –

261.2.1 have *closed* their list of patients, and

261.2.2 may, in the opinion of the PCT, be affected by the determination of the *assessment panel*; and

261.3 the *Local Medical Committee* (if any) for the area of the PCT, that it has referred the matter to the *assessment panel*.

Assignments to closed lists: *NHS dispute resolution procedure* relating to determinations of the *assessment panel*

262. Where the *assessment panel* determines in accordance with paragraph 35(5) to (9) of Schedule 6 to *the Regulations* that the PCT may assign new patients to contractors which have *closed* their lists of patients, and the Contractor is specified in that determination, the Contractor may refer the matter to *the Secretary of State* to review the determination of the *assessment panel* pursuant to paragraph 36(2) to (17) of Schedule 6 to *the Regulations*.

263. Where, pursuant to clause 262, the Contractor wishes to refer the matter to *the Secretary of State* either by itself, or jointly with other contractors specified in the determination of the *assessment panel*, it must, either by itself or together with the other contractors, within the period of 7 days beginning with the date of the determination of the *assessment panel*, send to *the Secretary of State* a written request for dispute resolution which shall include or be accompanied by –
    263.1 the names and addresses of the parties to the dispute;
    263.2 a copy of the Contract (or contracts); and
    263.3 a brief statement describing the nature and circumstances of the dispute.

264. Where a matter is referred to the Secretary of State in accordance with paragraph 34 of Schedule 6 to *the Regulations*, it shall be reviewed in accordance with the procedure specified in that paragraph.

Assignments to closed lists: assignments of patients by the PCT

265. Before the PCT may assign a new patient to the Contractor where it has *closed* its list, it shall, subject to clause 267, enter into discussions with the Contractor regarding additional support that the PCT can offer the Contractor, and the PCT shall use its best endeavours to provide appropriate support.

266. In the discussions referred to in clause 265, both parties shall use reasonable endeavours to reach agreement.

267. The requirement in clause 256 to enter into discussions applies.

Guidance

2.39 Where a large number of contractors' lists are closed, it may not initially be possible for a patient to register with a practice. By establishing its own provision, the PCT is expected to prevent this from happening. However, this may not always prove possible, for example if, following recruitment exercises, there is insufficient supply of local GPs, or in a large rural PCT where the PCT provision is too far from the patient's home and there is no practical alternative provider to a contractor with the closed list. Given that the PCT is under a duty to ensure the provision of sufficient primary medical services to meet the reasonable needs of its population, it may in such instances need to assign patients to contractors with closed lists. In assigning patients to a practice the PCT must take the following into consideration:

(i) the patient's wishes and circumstances including the distance between the patient's home and the contractor's premises

(ii) the contractor's list status

(iii) whether during the previous 6 months the patient has been removed from the list of any contractor in the PCT's area, and whether the patient has been removed from a contractor's list because of violence.

Assignment procedure in relation to contractors with closed lists

2.40 The procedure for assigning patients to contractors with closed lists is in some respects the same as that for list closure. It is summarised in Table 3 (again, for a definitive statement of law, PCTs and contractors should read the Contract Regulations).

Table 3 **Assigning patients to contractors with closed lists**	
Stage	**Process**
1. Informal discussion	The PCT should carry out discussions with the contractor to achieve informal resolution
2. Assessment Panel determination	1. The PCT must prepare a proposal for consideration by the Assessment Panel which must include details of those contractors to which it wishes to assign patients
	2. The PCT should notify all the contractors in its area with closed lists, those contractors who may be affected by the Assessment Panel's determination, the SHA and the LMC
	Continued

Table 3 – continued	
Stage	**Process**
	3. In making its determination, the Assessment Panel should take into account whether the PCT has sought other ways of providing essential services for new patients other than assignment to closed lists, and the workload of those contractors with closed lists which may be subject to having patients assigned
	4. The Assessment Panel's determination must be made within 28 days of receiving the PCT proposal. It should be sent to the SHA and contractors with closed lists
	5. The Panel may set out the GMS contractors to which the PCT may assign patients
	6. Discussions between the PCT and contractor should happen the first time before assignment to that contractor occurs once the new arrangements are in force. Thereafter they must happen as appropriate given the frequency and volume of assignments
3. Fast track appeal to SHA	1. The PCT or contractor can appeal to the SHA under a fast-track process. The SHA is the formal arbiter when making binding decisions about patient assignments because local knowledge is essential
	2. Appeals must be initiated within 7 days of the date of the determination
	3. More than one contractor may appeal jointly to the SHA. Where that does happen, the SHA shall consider the appeal in respect of all the contractors as a whole
	4. The SHA shall write within seven days to the parties to the dispute notifying them of its appointment and in doing so give them the opportunity (within a given period of up to 2 weeks) to provide written representations. The SHA would copy these to the other parties inviting them to respond in writing, also within 2 weeks

Table 3 – continued	
Stage	**Process**
	5. In considering the appeal, the SHA may give the opportunity for oral representations to be made on behalf of the parties. It may also consult with experts (subject to any conflicts of interest) who may be able to help
	6. The SHA should make a determination within 21 days and send copies to the parties. This could be extended by mutual agreement of the parties and the SHA

2.41   PCTs should note that when these procedures take effect they will no longer be able to assign patients to contractors with closed lists without going through this formal procedure. This will require a change of behaviour for those PCTs that currently assign a large number of patients. PCTs:
   (i)   are expected to take steps to reduce patient assignments to contractors with closed lists, for example by establishing PCTMS services
   (ii) may also need to consider whether they will need to put proposals to assessment panels from 1 April 2004 to ensure that they can fulfil their duty to ensure that patients can access primary medical services, and may need to prepare such proposals by then
   (iii) should ensure that assessment panels are established to deal with forced assignments and list closures.

2.42   SHAs will need to establish the fast-track appeal procedure so that it can become operational from 1 April 2004.

Attendance to patients

Regulations

2.   Attendance to patients

(1)   The contractor shall take steps to ensure that any patient who –
   (a)   has not previously made an appointment; and
   (b)   attends at the practice premises during the normal hours for essential services,

is provided with such services by an appropriate health care professional during that surgery period except in the circumstances specified in sub-paragraph (2).

(2)   The circumstances referred to in sub-paragraph (1) are that –
    (a) it is more appropriate for the patient to be referred elsewhere for services under the Act; or
    (b) he is then offered an appointment to attend again within a time which is appropriate and reasonable having regard to all the circumstances and his health would not thereby be jeopardised.

3.   Attendance outside practice premises

(1)   In the case of a patient whose medical condition is such that in the reasonable opinion of the contractor –
    (a) attendance on the patient is required; and
    (b) it would be inappropriate for him to attend at the practice premises, the contractor shall provide services to that patient at whichever in its judgement is the most appropriate of the places set out in sub-paragraph (2).

(2)   The places referred to in sub-paragraph (1) are –
    (a) the place recorded in the patient's medical records as being his last home address;
    (b) such other place as the contractor has informed the patient and the PCT is the place where it has agreed to visit and treat the patient; or
    (c) some other place in the contractor's practice area.

(3)   Nothing in this paragraph prevents the contractor from –
    (a) arranging for the referral of a patient without first seeing the patient, in a case where the medical condition of that patient makes that course of action appropriate; or
    (b) visiting the patient in circumstances where this paragraph does not place it under an obligation to do so.

Standard Contract

Attendance at *practice premises*

29.   The Contractor shall take reasonable steps to ensure that any patient who has not previously made an appointment and attends at the *practice premises* during the *normal hours* for *essential services* is provided with such services by an appropriate *health care professional* during that surgery period except where:

29.1 it is more appropriate for the patient to be referred elsewhere for services under *the Act*; or

29.2 the patient is then offered an appointment to attend again within a time which is reasonable having regard to all the circumstances and his health would not thereby be jeopardised.

Attendance outside *practice premises*

30. In the case of a patient whose medical condition is such that in the reasonable opinion of the Contractor attendance on the patient is required and it would be inappropriate for the patient to attend at a place where services are provided in *normal hours* under the Contract, the Contractor shall provide services to that patient at whichever in its judgement is the most appropriate of the following places:

30.1 the place recorded in the patient's medical records as being his last home address;

30.2 such other place as the Contractor has informed the patient and the PCT is the place where it has agreed to visit and treat the patient;

30.3 some other place in the Contractor's *practice area*.

31. Nothing in this clause or clause 30 prevents the Contractor from:

31.1 arranging for the referral of a patient without first seeing the patient, in a case where the medical condition of that patient makes that course of action appropriate; or

31.2 visiting the patient in circumstances where this paragraph does not place it under an obligation to do so.

● Brownfield sites

See also: Premises

Guidance

2.16 The PCT has a range of options when making commissioning decisions about securing primary medical services in "brownfield" sites (i.e. pre-existing surgeries that were but are no longer delivering essential services, for example in the event of a single-handed GP retiring; or essential services in areas of historic under-provision). The options are to:

(i) seek to advertise a vacancy and enter into a GMS, PMS, or APMS contract, or

(ii) invite interest from existing primary medical services contractors, or

(iii) employ a GP using the PCTMS route.

Before making a decision the PCT is expected to consult with the LMC.

● Certificates

Regulations

21. Certificates

(1)   A contract must contain a term which has the effect of requiring the contractor to issue free of charge to a patient or his personal representatives any medical certificate of a description prescribed in column 1 of Schedule 4, which is reasonably required under or for the purposes of the enactments specified in relation to the certificate in column 2 of that Schedule, except where, for the condition to which the certificate relates, the patient –

(a) is being attended by a medical practitioner who is not –
   (i)   employed or engaged by the contractor,
   (ii) in the case of a contract with two or more individuals practising in partnership, one of those individuals; or
   (iii) in the case of a contract with a company limited by shares, one of the persons legally or beneficially owning shares in that company; or

(b) is not being treated by or under the supervision of a health care professional.

(2)   The exception in paragraph (1)(a) shall not apply where the certificate is issued pursuant to regulation 2(1)(b) of the Social Security (Medical Evidence) Regulations 1976 (which provides for the issue of a certificate in the form of a special statement by a doctor on the basis of a written report made by another doctor).

Standard Contract

470.   The Contractor shall issue free of charge to a patient or his personal representative any medical certificate of a description prescribed in column 1 of the table below which is reasonably required under or for the purposes of the enactments specified in relation to the certificate in column 2 of the table below, except where, for the condition to which the certificate relates, the patient –

470.1 is being attended by a medical practitioner who is not –
   470.1.1 employed or engaged by the Contractor,
   470.1.2 if this Contract is with a partnership, one of the partners, or
   470.1.3 if this Contract is with a company limited by shares, one of the persons legally or beneficially owning shares in the company; or

470.2 is not being treated by or under the supervision of a *health care professional.*

471. The exception in clause 470 shall not apply where the certificate is issued pursuant to regulation 2(1)(b) of the Social Security (Medical Evidence) Regulations 1976 (which provides for the issue of a certificate in the form of a special statement by a doctor on the basis of a written report made by another doctor).

List of prescribed medical certificates

Description of medical certificate	Enactment under or for the purpose of which certificate required
1. To support a claim or to obtain payment either personally or by proxy; to prove inability to work or incapacity for self-support for the purposes of an award by the Secretary of State; or to enable proxy to draw pensions etc.	Naval and Marine Pay and Pensions Act 1865 Air Force (Constitution) Act 1917 Pensions (Navy, Army, Air Force and Mercantile Marine) Act 1939 Personal Injuries (Emergency Provisions) Act 1939 Pensions (Mercantile Marine) Act 1942 Polish Resettlement Act 1947 Social Security Administration Act 1992 Social Security Contributions and Benefits Act 1992 Social Security Act 1998
2. To establish pregnancy for the purpose of obtaining welfare foods	Section 13 of the Social Security Act 1988 (schemes for distribution etc of welfare foods)
3. To secure registration of still-birth	Section 11 of the Births and Deaths Registration Act 1953 (special provision as to registration of still-birth)

Continued

List of prescribed medical certificates

Description of medical certificate	Enactment under or for the purpose of which certificate required
4. To enable payment to be made to an institution or other person in case of mental disorder of persons entitled to payment from public funds	Section 142 of the Mental Health Act 1983 (pay, pensions etc. of mentally disordered persons)
5. To establish unfitness for jury service	Juries Act 1974
6. To support late application . for reinstatement in civil employment or notification of non-availability to take up employment owing to sickness	Reserve Forces (Safeguarding of Employment) Act 1985
7. To enable a person to be registered as an absent voter on grounds of physical incapacity	Representation of the People Act 1983
8. To support applications for certificates conferring exemption from charges in respect of drugs, medicines and appliances	National Health Service Act 1977
9. To support a claim by or on behalf of a severely mentally impaired person for exemption from liability to pay the Council Tax or eligibility for a discount in respect of the amount of Council Tax payable	Local Government Finance Act 1992

Childhood immunisation – target payments

Statement of Financial Entitlement

8. Childhood Immunisations Scheme

8.1 Childhood Immunisation and Pre-school Booster Services are classified as Additional Services. If contractors are providing these services to patients registered with them, PCTs are to seek to agree a Childhood Immunisations Scheme plan with them, as part of their GMS contract. This plan will be the mechanism under which the payments set out in this Section will be payable.

Childhood Immunisations Scheme plans

8.2 Childhood Immunisations Scheme plans are to cover the matters set out in direction 6(2)(a) to (g) of the DES Directions.

Target payments in respect of 2-year-olds

8.3 PCTs must in respect of the financial year 2004/05 pay to a contractor under its GMS contract a Quarterly Two-Year-Olds Immunisation Payment ("Quarterly TYOIP") if it qualifies for that payment. A contractor qualifies for that payment if –

(a) as part of its GMS contract the contractor and the PCT have agreed a Childhood Immunisations Scheme plan; and

(b) on the first day of the quarter to which the payment relates, at least 70%, for the lower payment, or at least 90%, for the higher payment, of the children aged two (i.e. who have passed their second birthday but not yet their third) registered with the contractor have completed the recommended immunisation courses (i.e. those that have been recommended nationally and by the World Health Organisation) for protection against –

(i) diphtheria, tetanus, and poliomyelitis,

(ii) pertussis,

(iii) measles/mumps/rubella, and

(iv) *Haemophilus influenzae* type B (HiB).

Calculation of Quarterly Two-Year-Olds Immunisation Payment

8.4   PCTs will first need to determine the number of completed immunisation courses that are required over the four disease groups in paragraph 8.3(b) in order to meet either the 70% or 90% target. To do this the contractor will need to provide the PCT with the number of two-year-olds (A) whom it is under a contractual obligation to include in its Childhood Immunisations Scheme Register on the first day of the quarter in respect of which the contractor is seeking payment (the head count will in fact relate to children registered with the contractor at the start of the previous quarter), and then the PCT must make the following calculations –

   (a) $(0.7 \times A \times 4) = B^1$ (the number of completed immunisations needed to meet the 70% target); and

   (b) $(0.9 \times A \times 4) = B^2$ (the number of completed immunisations needed to meet the 90% target).

8.5   PCTs will then need to calculate which, if any, target was achieved. To do this, a PCT will also need from the contractor the sum of the total number of children aged two whom it is under a contractual obligation to include in its Childhood Immunisations Scheme Register and who have completed immunisations in each of the four groups ($C^{\Sigma 1-4}$). Only completed immunisation courses (whether or not carried out by the contractor) are to count towards the determination of whether or not the targets are achieved. No adjustment is to be made for exception reporting. A calculation is then to be made of whether or not the targets are achieved –

   (a) if $C^{\Sigma 1-4} \geq B^1$, then the 70% target is achieved; and

   (b) if $C^{\Sigma 1-4} \geq B^2$, then the 90% target is achieved.

8.6   Next the PCT will need to calculate the number of the completed immunisations that the contractor can use to count towards achievement of the targets (D). To do this, the contractor will need to provide the PCT with a breakdown of how many of the completed immunisation courses in each disease group were carried out by it, or by another GMS or PMS contractor, within the NHS.

8.7   Once the PCT has that information, D is to be calculated as follows –

$$\begin{array}{r} C^{\Sigma 1} - E^{\Sigma 1} \\ C^{\Sigma 2} - E^{\Sigma 2} \\ C^{\Sigma 3} - E^{\Sigma 3} \\ \underline{+\ C^{\Sigma 4} - E^{\Sigma 4}} \\ =\quad D \end{array}$$

For these purposes –

(a) $E^{\Sigma x}$ is the number of completed immunisations carried out other than by a GMS or PMS contractor for the NHS in each group (i.e. for Group 1, $E^{\Sigma 1}$); and

(b) in each case the sum of $C^{\Sigma x} - E^{\Sigma x}$ can never be greater than $C^{\Sigma x} \times 0.7$ or 0.9 (depending on which target achieved). Where it is, it is treated as the result of: $C^{\Sigma x} \times 0.7$ or as the case may be 0.9.

8.8 In the financial year 2004/05, the maximum amounts payable to a contractor will depend on the number of children aged two whom it is under a contractual obligation to include in its Childhood Immunisations Scheme Register on the first day of each quarter compared with the average UK number of such children per 5000 population, which is 59.25. The maximum amounts payable to the contractor (F) are therefore to be calculated as follows –

(a) where the 70% target is achieved: $F^1 = (A/59.25) \times £685.25$; and

(b) where the 90% target is achieved: $F^2 = (A/59.25) \times £2055.75$.

8.9 The Quarterly TYOIP payable to the contractor is thereafter calculated as a proportion of the maximum amounts payable as follows –

$$F^1 \text{ or } F^2 \times \frac{D}{B^1 \text{ or } B^2} = \text{Quarterly TYOIP}$$

8.10 The amount payable as a Quarterly TYOIP is to fall due on the last day of the quarter in respect of which the contractor is seeking payment (i.e. at the end of the quarter after the last quarter in which immunisations were carried out that count towards the targets). However, if the contractor delays providing the information the PCT needs to calculate its Quarterly TYOIP beyond the middle of the quarter, the amount is to fall due at the end of the next quarter. No Quarterly TYOIP is payable if the contractor provides the necessary information more than 4 months after the date to which the information relates.

Conditions attached to Quarterly Two-Year-Olds Immunisation Payments

8.11 Quarterly TYOIPs, or any part thereof, are only payable if the contractor satisfies the following conditions –

(a) the contractor must meet its obligations under its Childhood Immunisations Scheme plan;

(b) the contractor must make available to the PCT sufficient information to enable the PCT to calculate the contractor's Quarterly TYOIP. In particular, the contractor must supply the following figures –

(i) the number of 2-year-olds whom it is under a contractual obligation to include in its Childhood Immunisations Scheme Register on the first day of the quarter,

(ii) how many of those 2-year-olds have completed each of the recommended immunisation courses (i.e. that have been recommended nationally and by the World Health Organisation) for protection against the disease groups referred to in paragraph 8.3(b), and

       (iii) of those completed immunisation courses, how many were carried out by a GMS or PMS contractor within the NHS; and

    (c) all information supplied pursuant to or in accordance with this paragraph must be accurate.

8.12   If the contractor breaches any of these conditions, the PCT may, in appropriate circumstances, withhold payment of all or part of a Quarterly TYIOP that is otherwise payable.

Target payments in respect of five-year-olds

8.13   PCTs must in respect of the financial year 2004/05 pay to a contractor under its GMS contract a Quarterly Five-Year-Olds Immunisation Payment ("Quarterly FYOIP") if it qualifies for that payment. A contractor qualifies for that payment if –

    (a) as part of its GMS contract the contractor and the PCT have agreed a Childhood Immunisation Scheme plan; and

    (b) on the first day of the quarter to which the payment relates, at least 70%, for the lower payment, or at least 90%, for the higher payment, of the children aged five (i.e. who have passed their fifth birthday but not yet their sixth) registered with the contractor have received the recommended reinforcing doses (i.e. those that have been recommended nationally and by the World Health Organisation) for protection against diphtheria, tetanus, acellular pertussis and poliomyelitis.

Calculation of Quarterly Five-Year-Olds Immunisation Payment

8.14   PCTs will need to determine the number of completed immunisation courses that are required in order to meet either the 70% or the 90% target. To do this, the contractor will need to provide the PCT with the number of 5-year-olds (A) whom it is under a contractual obligation to include in its Childhood Immunisations Scheme Register on the first day of the quarter in respect of which the contractor is seeking payment (the head count will in fact relate to children registered with the contractor at the start of the previous quarter), and then the PCT must make the following calculations –

    (a) $(0.7 \times A) = B^1$ (the number of completed booster courses needed to meet the 70% target; and

(b) $(0.9 \times A) = B^2$ (the number of completed booster courses needed to meet the 90% target).

8.15 PCTs will then need to calculate which, if any, target was achieved. To do this, a PCT will also need from the contractor the sum of the total number of children aged five whom it is under a contractual obligation to include in its Childhood Immunisations Scheme Register and who have completed the booster courses required (C). Only completed booster courses (whether or not carried out by the contractor) are to count towards the determination of whether or not the target was achieved. No adjustment is to be made for exception reporting. A calculation is then to be made of whether or not the targets are achieved –
(a) if $C \geq B^1$, then the 70% target is achieved; and
(b) if $C \geq B^2$, then the 90% target is achieved.

8.16 Next the PCT will need to calculate the number of the completed booster courses that the contractor can use to count towards achievement of the targets (D), the initial value of which is (C) minus the number of children whose completed booster courses were not carried out by a GMS or PMS contractor within the NHS. To do this, the contractor will need to provide the PCT with a breakdown of how many of the completed booster courses were carried out by it, or by another GMS or PMS contractor, within the NHS.

8.17 If $D > B^1$ or B^2 (depending on the target achieved), then D is adjusted to equal the value of B^1 or B^2 as appropriate.

8.18 In the financial year 2004/05, the maximum amounts payable to a contractor will depend on the number of children aged five whom it is under a contractual obligation to include in its Childhood Immunisations Scheme Register on the first day of each quarter compared with the average UK number of such children per 5000 population, which is 61.45. The maximum amounts payable to the contractor (E) are therefore to be calculated as follows –
(a) where the 70% target is achieved: $E^1 = (A/61.45) \times £212.25$; or
(b) where the 90% target is achieved: $E^2 = (A/61.45) \times £636.75$.

8.19 The Quarterly FYOIP payable to the contractor is thereafter calculated as a proportion of the maximum amounts payable as follows –
$$\frac{E^1 \text{ or } E^2 \times D}{B^1 \text{ or } B^2} = \text{Quarterly FYOIP}$$

8.20 The amount payable as a Quarterly FYOIP is to fall due on the last day of the first month of the quarter in respect of which the contractor is seeking payment (i.e. at the end of the quarter after the last quarter in which booster courses were carried out that count towards the targets). However, if the contractor delays providing the information the PCT needs to calculate its Quarterly FYOIP beyond the middle of the quarter, the amount is to fall due at the end of the next quarter. No Quarterly FYOIP is payable if the contractor provides the necessary information more than 4 months after the date to which the information relates.

Conditions attached to Quarterly Five-Year-Olds Immunisation Payments

8.21 Quarterly FYOIPs, or any part thereof, are only payable if the contractor satisfies the following conditions –
  (a) the contractor must meet its obligations under its Childhood Immunisation Scheme plan;
  (b) the contractor must supply to the PCT with sufficient information to enable the PCT to calculate the contractor's Quarterly FYOIP. In particular, the contractor must supply the following figures –
    (i) the number of 5-year-olds whom it is under a contractual obligation to include in its Childhood Immunisations Scheme Register on the first day of each quarter,
    (ii) how many of those 5-year-olds have received the complete course of recommended reinforcing doses (i.e. that have been recommended nationally and by the World Health Organisation) for protection against diphtheria, tetanus, acellular pertussis and poliomyelitis, and
    (iii) of those completed courses, how many were carried out by a GMS or PMS contractor within the NHS; and
  (c) all information supplied pursuant to or in accordance with this paragraph must be accurate.

8.22 If the contractor breaches any of these conditions, the PCT may, in appropriate circumstances, withhold payment of all or part of a Quarterly FYOIP that is otherwise payable.

Clinical governance

Regulations

121. Clinical governance

(1) The contractor shall have an effective system of clinical governance.

(2) The contractor shall nominate a person who will have responsibility for ensuring the effective operation of the system of clinical governance.

(3)   The person nominated under sub-paragraph (2) shall be a person who performs or manages services under the contract.

(4)   In this paragraph "system of clinical governance" means a framework through which the contractor endeavours continuously to improve the quality of its services and safeguard high standards of care by creating an environment in which clinical excellence can flourish.

Standard Contract

487.   The Contractor shall have an effective *system of clinical governance*. The Contractor shall nominate a person who will have responsibility for ensuring the effective operation of the *system of clinical governance*. The person nominated shall be a person who performs or manages services under the Contract.

Clinical reports – NHS

Regulations

7.   Clinical reports

(1)   Where the contractor provides any clinical services, other than under a private arrangement, to a patient who is not on its list of patients, it shall, as soon as reasonably practicable, provide a clinical report relating to the consultation, and any treatment provided, to the PCT.

(2)   The PCT shall send any report received under sub-paragraph (1) –
        (a) to the person with whom the patient is registered for the provision of essential services or their equivalent; or
        (b) if the person referred to in paragraph (a) is not known to it, to the PCT in whose area the patient is resident.

Standard Contract

Clinical reports

38.   Where the Contractor provides any clinical services, other than under a private arrangement, to a patient who is not on its list of patients, it shall, as soon as reasonably practicable, provide a clinical report relating to the

consultation, and any treatment provided, to the PCT. The PCT shall send any report received to the person with whom the patient is registered for the provision of *essential services* or their equivalent or if that person is not known to the PCT, the PCT in whose area the patient is resident.

Closure of lists of patients

Regulations

29. Closure of lists of patients

(1) A contractor which wishes to close its list of patients shall notify the PCT in writing to that effect.

(2) Within a period of 7 days beginning with the date of receipt of the notification referred to in sub-paragraph (1), or, if that is not reasonably practicable, as soon as is practicable thereafter, the PCT shall enter into discussions with the contractor concerning the support which the PCT may give the contractor, or other changes which the PCT or the contractor may make, which would enable the contractor to keep its list of patients open.

(3) In the discussions referred to in sub-paragraph (2), both parties shall use reasonable endeavours to achieve the aim of keeping the contractor's list of patients open.

(4) The discussions mentioned in sub-paragraph (2) shall be completed within a period of 28 days beginning with the date of the PCT's receipt of the notification referred to in sub-paragraph (1), or within such longer period as the parties may agree.

(5) If, following the discussions mentioned in sub-paragraph (2), the PCT and the contractor reach agreement that the contractor's list of patients should remain open, the PCT shall send full details of the agreement in writing to the contractor.

(6) The PCT and the contractor shall comply with the terms of an agreement reached as mentioned in sub-paragraph (5).

(7) If, following the discussions mentioned in sub-paragraph (2) –
  (a) the PCT and the contractor reach agreement that the contractor's list of patients should close; or
  (b) the PCT and the contractor fail to reach agreement and the contractor still wishes to close its list of patients,
  the contractor shall send a closure notice to the PCT.

(8)   A closure notice shall be submitted in the form specified in Schedule 8, and shall include the following details which (in a case falling within sub-paragraph (7)(a)) have been agreed between the parties or (in a case falling within sub-paragraph (7)(b)) are proposed by the contractor –

    (a) the period of time (which may not exceed 12 months) for which the contractor's list of patients will be closed;

    (b) the current number of the contractor's registered patients;

    (c) the number of registered patients (lower than the current number of such patients, and expressed either in absolute terms or as a percentage of the number of such patients specified pursuant to paragraph (b)) which, if that number were reached, would trigger the re-opening of the contractor's list of patients;

    (d) the number of registered patients (expressed either in absolute terms or as a percentage of the number of such patients specified pursuant to paragraph (b)) which, if that number were reached, would trigger the re-closure of the contractor's list of patients; and

    (e) any withdrawal from or reduction in provision of any additional or enhanced services which had previously been provided under the contract.

(9)   The PCT shall forthwith acknowledge receipt of the closure notice in writing to the contractor.

(10)   Before the PCT reaches a decision as to whether to approve or reject the closure notice under sub-paragraph (12), the PCT and the contractor may enter into further discussions concerning the details of the closure notice referred to in sub-paragraph (8), with a view to reaching agreement; and, in particular, if the parties are unable to reach agreement regarding the period of time for which the contractor's list of patients will be closed, that period shall be 12 months.

(11)   A contractor may not withdraw a closure notice for a period of 3 months beginning with the date on which the PCT has received the notice, unless the PCT has agreed otherwise in writing.

(12)   Within a period of 14 days beginning with the date of receipt of the closure notice, the PCT shall –

    (a) approve the closure notice; or

    (b) reject the closure notice,

and shall notify the contractor of its decision in writing as soon as possible.

(13)   Approval of the closure notice under sub-paragraph (12)(a) includes approval of the details specified in accordance with sub-paragraph (8) (or, where those details are revised following discussions under sub-paragraph (10), approval of those details as so revised).

30. Approval of closure notice by the PCT

(1) If the PCT approves the closure notice in accordance with paragraph 29(12)(a), the contractor shall close its list of patients –
  (a) with effect from a date agreed between the PCT and the contractor; or
  (b) if no such agreement has been reached, with effect from the date on which the contractor receives notification of the PCT's decision to approve the closure notice.

(2) Subject to sub-paragraph (3), the contractor's list of patients shall remain closed for the period specified in the closure notice in accordance with paragraph 29(8)(a) (or, where the period of 12 months specified in paragraph 29(10) applies, for that period).

(3) The contractor's list of patients shall re-open before the expiry of the period mentioned in sub-paragraph (2) if –
  (a) the number of the contractor's registered patients falls to the number specified in the closure notice in accordance with paragraph 29(8)(c); or
  (b) the PCT and the contractor agree that the list of patients should re-open.

(4) If the contractor's list of patients has re-opened pursuant to sub-paragraph (3)(a), it shall nevertheless close again if, during the period specified in the closure notice in accordance with paragraph 29(8)(a) (or, where the period of 12 months specified in paragraph 29(10) applies, during that period) the number of the contractor's registered patients rises to the number specified in the closure notice in accordance with paragraph 29(8)(d).

(5) Except in cases where the contractor's list of patients is already open pursuant to sub-paragraph (3), the PCT shall notify the contractor in writing between seven and 14 days before the expiry of the period of closure specified in sub-paragraph (2), confirming the date on which the contractor's list of patients will re-open.

(6) Where the details specified in the closure notice in accordance with paragraph 29(8) have been revised following discussions under paragraph 29(10), references in this paragraph to details specified in the closure notice are references to those details as so revised.

31. Rejection of closure notice by the PCT

(1) This regulation applies where the PCT rejects the closure notice in accordance with paragraph 29(12)(b).

(2)   The contractor and the PCT may not refer the matter for determination in accordance with the NHS dispute resolution procedure (or, where applicable, commence court proceedings) until the assessment panel has given its determination in accordance with the following sub-paragraphs.

(3)   The PCT must ensure that the assessment panel is appointed as soon as is practicable to consider and determine whether the contractor should be permitted to close its list of patients, and if so, the terms on which it should be permitted to do so.

(4)   The PCT shall provide the assessment panel with such information as the assessment panel may reasonably require to enable it to reach a determination and shall include in such information any written observations received from the contractor.

(5)   The members of the assessment panel shall be –
(a) the Chief Executive of the PCT of which the assessment panel is a committee or sub-committee;
(b) a person representative of patients in an area other than that of the PCT which is a party to the contract; and
(c) a person representative of a Local Medical Committee which does not represent practitioners in the area of the PCT which is a party to the contract.

(6)   At least one member of the assessment panel shall visit the contractor before reaching a determination under sub-paragraph (7).

(7)   Within the period of 28 days beginning with the date on which the PCT rejected the closure notice, the assessment panel shall –
(a) approve the list closure; or
(b) reject the list closure,
and shall notify the PCT and the contractor of its determination in writing as soon as possible.

(8)   Where the assessment panel determines in accordance with sub-paragraph (7)(a) that the contractor's list of patients should close, it shall specify –
(a) a date from which the closure shall take effect, which must be within a period of 7 days beginning with the date of the assessment panel's determination; and
(b) those details specified in paragraph 29(8).

(9)   Where the assessment panel determines in accordance with sub-paragraph (7)(b) that the contractor's list of patients may not close, that list shall remain open, and the PCT and the contractor shall enter into discussions with a view to ensuring that the contractor receives support from the PCT which will enable it to continue to provide services safely and effectively.

(10) Where the assessment panel determines in accordance with sub-paragraph (7)(b) that the contractor's list of patients may not close, the contractor may not submit a further closure notice as described in paragraph 29 until –

(a) the expiry of a period of 3 months beginning with the date of the assessment panel's determination; or
(b) (if applicable) the final determination of the NHS dispute resolution procedure (or any court proceedings),

whichever is the later, unless there has been a change in the circumstances of the contractor which affects its ability to deliver services under the contract.

Standard Contract

Closure of lists of patients

229. Where the Contractor wishes to close its list of patients, it shall notify the PCT in writing to that effect.

230. Within a period of 7 days beginning with the date of receipt of the notification referred to in clause 229, or, if that is not reasonably practicable, as soon as is practicable thereafter, the PCT shall enter into discussions with the Contractor concerning the support which the PCT may give the Contractor, or other changes which the PCT or the Contractor may make, which would enable the Contractor to keep its list of patients *open*. In these discussions, both parties shall use reasonable endeavours to achieve the aim of keeping the Contractor's list of patients *open*.

231. The discussions referred to in clause 230 shall be completed within a period of 28 days beginning with the date of the PCT's receipt of the notification referred to in clause 229, or within such longer period as the parties may agree.

232. If, following the discussions referred to in clause 230, the PCT and the Contractor reach agreement that the Contractor's list of patients should remain *open*, the PCT shall send full details of the agreement in writing to the Contractor. The PCT and the Contractor shall comply with the terms of any agreement reached.

233. If, following the discussions referred to in clause 230-
233.1 the PCT and the Contractor reach agreement that the Contractor's list of patients should close; or

233.2 the PCT and the Contractor fail to reach agreement and the
Contractor still wishes to close its list of patients,
the Contractor shall send a closure notice to the PCT.

234. A closure notice shall be submitted in the form specified in Schedule 5 to
this Contract, and shall include the following details which (in a case
falling within clause 233.1) have been agreed between the parties or (in a
case falling within clause 233.2) are proposed by the Contractor –
234.1 the period of time (which may not exceed 12 months) for which
the Contractor's list of patients will be *closed*;
234.2 the current number of the Contractor's *registered patients*;
234.3 the number of *registered patients* (lower than the current number
of such patients, and expressed either in absolute terms or as a
percentage of the number of such patients specified pursuant to
clause 234.2) which, if that number were reached, would trigger the
re-opening of the Contractor's list of patients;
234.4 the number of *registered patients* (expressed either in absolute
terms or as a percentage of the number of such patients specified
pursuant to clause 243.2) which, if that number were reached,
would trigger the re-closure of the Contractor's list of patients; and
234.5 any withdrawal from or reduction in provision of any *additional* or
enhanced services which had previously been provided under the
Contract.

235. The PCT shall forthwith acknowledge receipt of the closure notice in
writing to the Contractor.

236. Before the PCT reaches a decision as to whether to approve or reject the
closure notice under clause 238, the PCT and the Contractor may enter
into further discussions concerning the details of the closure notice
referred to in clause 234, with a view to reaching agreement: and, in
particular, if the parties are unable to reach agreement regarding the
period of time for which the Contractor's list of patients will be *closed*,
that period shall be 12 months.

237. The Contractor may not withdraw a closure notice for a period of
3 months beginning with the date on which the PCT has received the
notice, unless the PCT has agreed otherwise in writing.

238. Within a period of 14 days beginning with the date of receipt of the
closure notice, the PCT shall approve or reject the closure notice and
shall notify the Contractor of its decision in writing as soon as possible.

239. Approval of the closure notice under clause 238 includes approval of the
details specified in accordance with clause 234 (or, where those details are
revised following discussions under clause 236, approval of those details
as so revised).

Closure of lists of patients
Standard Contract

Approval of closure notice by the PCT

240. If the PCT approves the closure notice in accordance with clause 238, the Contractor shall close its list of patients –
    240.1 with effect from a date agreed between the PCT and the Contractor; or
    240.2 if no such agreement has been reached, with effect from the date on which the Contractor receives notification of the PCT's decision to approve the closure notice.

241. Subject to clause 242, the Contractor's list of patients shall remain *closed* for the period specified in the closure notice in accordance with clause 234.1 (or, where the period of 12 months specified in clause 236 applies, for that period).

242. The Contractor's list of patients shall re-open before the expiry of the period referred to in clause 241 if –
    242.1 the number of the Contractor's *registered patients* falls to the number specified in the closure notice in accordance with clause 234.3; or
    242.2 the PCT and the Contractor agree that the list of patients should re-open.

243. If the Contractor's list of patients has re-opened pursuant to clause 242.1, it shall nevertheless close again if, during the period specified in the closure notice in accordance with 234.1 (or, where the period of 12 months specified in clause 236 applies, during that period) the number of the Contractor's *registered patients* rises to the number specified in the closure notice in accordance with clause 234.4.

244. Except in cases where the Contractor's list of patients is already open pursuant to clause 242, the PCT shall notify the Contractor in writing between 7 and 14 days before the expiry of the period of closure specified in clause 241, confirming the date on which the Contractor's list of patients will re-open.

245. Where the details specified in the closure notice in accordance with clause 234 have been revised following discussions under clause 236, references in this paragraph to details specified in the closure notice are references to those details as so revised.

Rejection of closure notice by the PCT

246. Clauses 247 to 251 apply where the PCT rejects the closure notice in accordance with clause 25.

247. The Contractor or the PCT shall not refer the matter for determination in accordance with the *NHS dispute resolution procedure* (or, where applicable, commence court proceedings) until the *assessment panel* has

given its determination in accordance with clauses 248 to 252 and paragraph 26(6) and (7) of Schedule 6 to *the Regulations*.

248. The PCT must ensure that the *assessment panel* is appointed as soon as is practicable to consider and determine whether the Contractor should be permitted to close its list of patients, and if so, the terms on which it should be permitted to do so.

249. The PCT shall provide the *assessment panel* with such information as the *assessment panel* may reasonably require to enable it to reach a determination and shall include in such information any written observations received from the Contractor.

250. The members of the *assessment panel* shall be –
    250.1 the Chief Executive of a PCT of which the *assessment panel* is a committee or sub-committee;
    250.2 a person representative of *patients* in an area other than that of the PCT; and
    250.3 a person representative of a *Local Medical Committee* which does not represent practitioners in the area of the PCT.

251. Where the *assessment panel* determines pursuant to paragraph 31(7)(a) of Schedule 6 to *the Regulations* that the Contractor's list of patients may close –
    251.1 that list shall close on the date specified by the *assessment panel* pursuant to paragraph 31(8)(a) of Schedule 6 to *the Regulations*; and
    251.2 that list shall re-open in accordance with the details specified by the *assessment panel* pursuant to paragraph 31(8)(b) of Schedule 6 to *the Regulations*.

252. Where the *assessment panel* determines pursuant to paragraph 31(7)(b) of Schedule 6 to *the Regulations* that the Contractor's list of patients may not close –
    252.1 that list shall remain *open*, and the PCT and the Contractor shall enter into discussions with a view to ensuring that the Contractor receives support from the PCT which will enable it to continue to provide services safely and effectively;
    252.2 the Contractor may not submit a further closure notice as described in clause 234 until –
        252.2.1 the expiry of a period of 3 months beginning with the date of the *assessment panel's* determination; or
        252.2.2 (if applicable) the final determination of the *NHS dispute resolution procedure* (or any court proceedings),
    whichever is the later, unless there has been a change in the circumstances of the Contractor which affects its ability to deliver services under the Contract.

Guidance

Factors to consider

2.36 PCTs and contractors should note that if a contractor's list is closed:
   (i) contractors must not accept new patients, except immediate family members of existing patients
   (ii) obligations in respect of immediately necessary and emergency treatment would continue
   (iii) PCTs can only assign patients to contractors with closed lists in line with the new procedures described in paragraphs 2.37 and 2.38
   (iv) given closed lists are designed to help the contractor manage workload, and the provision of more services would increase workload, the PCT may reasonably decide not to offer such contractors:
      (a) opted-out additional services for the patients of other practices, or
      (b) enhanced services for which the contractor does not have a preferential right, or
      (c) further essential services, for example those arising from greenfield or brownfield sites
   (v) contractors may wish to note that an increased proportion of funding under new GMS is capitation-based, compared to old GMS. Operating a closed list may therefore have a greater adverse effect on income.

(iv) The list closure procedure

2.37 Chapter 6 of *Investing in General Practice* describes the new list closure procedure. Table 2 provides a summary for ease of reference, updated to reflect the draft Contract Regulations. For a definitive statement of law PCTs and contractors must read the Contract Regulations.

2.38 Whilst PCTs and contractors are under an obligation to use their reasonable endeavours to avoid invoking the formal procedure, PCTs are nonetheless encouraged to work together to establish assessment panels by April 2004 in readiness for potential disputes over list closures or patient assignments. PCT Chief Executives should note that they cannot delegate their assessment panel role. SHAs are also encouraged to establish arrangements by April 2004 in readiness for taking on their appeal role.

Table 2 **List closure procedure**	
Stage	**Process**
1. Informal discussion	1. The contractor must write to the PCT if it wishes to close its list
	2. Normally within 7 days – or as soon as is practicable – the PCT should discuss with the contractor what can be done to keep the list open, e.g. by providing locum bank support (for which, to avoid unfairness to other contractors, the PCT may wish to charge), or commissioning enhanced services from other providers
	3. Discussions should be completed within 28 days of the notification
	4. If following these discussions both sides agree that the list should remain open, the PCT confirms this in writing
2. Formal closure notice	1. The contractor has to submit this if agreement is not reached, or if both sides agree the list should close. The Notice sets out the terms of the closure
	2. The contractor will not be able to withdraw a formal closure notice for 3 months starting from the date of receipt by the PCT, unless the PCT agrees otherwise. This rule is designed to discourage ill-considered, rash or otherwise inappropriate requests for list closure
	3. The Notice should include:
	(i) The proposed closure period; the default is 12 months
	(ii) The number of registered patients at the time
	(iii) The proposed percentage reduction in, or absolute number of, patients before the list closure would be suspended and the list would temporarily re-open. This can only happen once in a year except where agreed between the contractor and the PCT
	(iv) The proposed percentage increase in, or absolute number of, patients before such a

Continued

107

Table 2 – *continued*	
Stage	**Process**
	suspension is lifted. Again, this would only happen once a year unless agreed between the contractor and the PCT (v) Withdrawal from or amendment to the provision of any additional or enhanced services

3. PCT decision	1. The PCT should confirm receipt immediately in writing
	2. Further discussions may take place to resolve any differences of opinion or disputes about its content
	3. PCT decision must take place within 14 days from the date of the receipt of the formal closure notice
	4. If the PCT approves the closure notice:
	  (i) The contractor's list will close in accordance with the notice
	  (ii) Closure starts from the date that confirmation has been received by the contractor, unless otherwise agreed
	  (iii) The PCT must confirm its decision in writing
	  (iv) As the closure period draws to an end, the PCT is advised to write to the contractor giving notice that the list will re-open on a certain date

4. Assessment panel determination	1. If the PCT rejects the notice, this would lead to determination by an assessment panel. This is a new subcommittee of a different PCT, comprising a PCT Chief Executive from another PCT (to provide independence), a patient representative, and an LMC representative. (It will not include an SHA director as proposed in paragraph 6.17 of *Investing in General Practice* as this would prejudice the SHA's formal role in dispute resolution)

Table 2 – continued	
Stage	**Process**
	2. The PCT provides information to the panel which must include written observations received from the contractor
	3. The panel will be required to consider each rejected closure notice on its merits. This must be carried out in such a way that consistent standards are applied; practices should not be prejudiced according to whether they applied first or last for list closure in any particular area
	4. At least one of the panel members must have visited the contractor, who must comply with such requests, before the panel makes its decision
	5. The decision must take place within 28 days of the PCT rejecting the closure notice and the PCT and contractor must be informed in writing
	6. If the panel approves the notice, it must state a start date for closure within 7 days. It will also state the arrangements for re-opening the list
	7. If the panel rejects the closure notice, the list will remain open. The PCT should discuss further with the contractor whether any steps should be taken to enable it to continue to practise safely and effectively
	8. The contractor cannot seek to reapply for a closure notice within 3 months of the panel's determination
5. Formal appeal	1. Either the PCT or the contractor can appeal to the FHSAA (SHA) under the contract dispute resolution procedure described in chapter 6, but only following prior consideration of the assessment panel
	2. Throughout the process, lists remain open until otherwise determined

Commissioning routes

Guidance

2.4 Chapters 2 and 7 of *Investing in General Practice* envisaged four delivery routes for primary medical services: GMS, PMS, PCT direct provision, and alternative providers. These are shown in Table 1.

GMS contracts

2.5 Under GMS contracts, PCTs and contractors are bound by the GMS rules described in the Contract Regulations and will be using *The Standard GMS Contract* described in chapter 6. Primary medical services are described as general medical services only when they are delivered through a GMS contract. All GMS contracts must include essential services and will normally include additional services. GMS contracts can also cover enhanced services; alternatively, PCTs and GMS contractors can hold separate contracts for enhanced services.

Table 1 **Four contracting routes for primary medical services**

Contract	Providers
General medical services (GMS)	Practices with at least one GP provider (single-handers, partnerships, or a certain type of limited company described in chapter 6)
Personal medical services (PMS)	Practices (single-handers, partnerships, or a certain type of limited company described in chapter 6) Nurses and other clinicians PCTs
Alternative providers of medical services (APMS)	Commercial providers Voluntary sector Not-for-profit organisations NHS trusts and foundation trusts Other PCTs[14]
PCT medical services (PCTMS)	PCTs

PMS contracts

2.6   Separate PMS guidance is being issued by the Department in December
        2003. Under the new specialist PMS arrangements, contracts do not have
        to include the equivalent of GMS essential services. Under PMS, the PCT
        can be the contractor but this involves the SHA acting as the
        commissioner. The SHA commissioner role is increasingly anomalous
        given *Shifting the Balance of Power* and PCTs may wish over time to
        transfer such PMS contracts to PCTMS arrangements where the PCT is
        the direct provider.

Alternative providers

2.7   The Health and Social Care (Community Health and Standards) Act
        2003 allows a PCT in relation to primary medical services to make "such
        arrangements for their provision (whether within or outside its area) as it
        thinks fit (and may in particular make contractual arrangements with
        any person)". This power means that for the first time a PCT can, from
        April 2004, contract for delivery of primary medical services with a range
        of alternative providers: commercial providers, not-for-profit
        organisations, the voluntary sector, NHS trusts, NHS foundation trusts
        or other PCTs. The power will have particular use for contracting for
        out-of-hours and enhanced services but PCTs should note that primary
        legislation allows contracts with alternative providers to cover any or all
        aspects of primary medical services. These alternative providers could for
        example include voluntary sector providers of mental health, learning
        disability or drug misuse treatment services in primary care. Services
        delivered under contracts with alternative providers are described as
        alternative provider medical services, or APMS.

2.8   The December 2003 White Paper *Building the Best* set out the
        Department's intention to promote new entrants into primary care. To
        avoid conflicts of interest, alternative providers will be subject to
        appropriate market regulation including:
        (i) rules concerning cross-selling of services that they, or related
            companies, offer that are otherwise available on the NHS (e.g.
            encouraging patients to pay for flu jabs also provided by the provider

---

14   The primary legislation allows PCTs to make arrangements outside GMS or PMS with any type
of provider. This means that PCTs can contract with practices under the APMS arrangements,
although we expect that this is unlikely to be their preferred route given the GMS and PMS options.
If GMS contractors and PCTs sign separate enhanced services contracts rather than including them
as variations to GMS contracts, this is technically occurring under the legislation supporting the
APMS arrangements.

without making clear these are also available free of charge on the NHS), and

(ii) restrictions to prevent inappropriate decisions to prescribe certain drugs, or refer to specific providers, for commercial gain rather than purely clinical reasons.

PCT direct provision (PCT medical services or PCTMS)

2.9   From April 2004 PCTs will be able to employ health care professionals to provide primary medical services themselves; at present, they only have the power to employ them to support GMS and PMS providers, or when they are the PMS provider. This could be for provision of any or all aspects of primary medical services. Such arrangements are described as PCT Medical Services (PCTMS). As envisaged in chapter 2 of *Investing in General Practice*, this option will further enable PCTs to employ a range of full-time or part-time salaried staff and also support the creation of locum banks. It will also enable PCTs to act as the employer of practice managers to work across small practices where this and the funding arrangements are agreed locally. PCTs are encouraged to explore these options.

2.10   Where PCTs provide the equivalent of GMS essential services, patients will register with the PCT. PCTs are encouraged to develop a minimum level of such services by April 2004 as a way of avoiding the need to assign patients to GMS and PMS contractors with closed patient lists. As set out in paragraph 2.44 of *Investing in General Practice*, PCT provision should not exceed an appropriate volume and SHAs are expected to oversee this. If PCTs propose to become large-scale providers of primary medical services they are expected to discuss this first with their SHA. They are also expected to consult with LMCs.

Common principles

2.11   Common principles will apply across all four delivery routes to ensure minimum standards are met and encourage high quality care. Some of the standards will apply only to the delivery of essential services to registered patients. The range of standards may include:

(i) minimum legal requirements, such as having effective clinical governance systems in place; complying with the NHS complaints system, the new performer list arrangements, provider conditions and prescribing conditions; record keeping and providing information to the PCT; having suitable premises; producing patient leaflets; and complying where appropriate with the GMS rules about charging registered patients for delivering other services. Sale of goodwill will also be subject to restrictions and the way in which these will apply will be set out in separate regulations. These will be made before April 2004

(ii) arrangements to achieve comparable quality to the GMS quality and outcomes framework, where appropriate given the range of services being provided. Where PCTs and contractors propose different quality arrangements in relation to essential services these will need to be approved by PCT Medical Directors or SHA Directors of Public Health as being comparable to GMS standards. PCT quality visits, and CHAI assessment of primary care quality, will need to cover all primary care providers, not just GMS and PMS contractors

(iii) funding. Chapter 5 describes how PCTs will receive a combined allocation for primary medical services. They can choose to supplement this with resources from the unified budget should they so wish, just as they can similarly support GMS and PMS contractors

(iv) consultation. The PCT must involve and consult (in accordance with Section 11 of the 2001 Health and Social Care Act) local communities about the planning of the provision of services, the development and consideration of proposals for changes in the way those services are provided, and decisions affecting the operation of those services. The PCT must consult Patients' Forums and the LMC where appropriate.

2.12 Brief guidance on how these principles will apply in relation to different services in APMS and PCTMS, including the minimum requirements, will be published by February 2004 and the relevant Directions will be made before April 2004. The Department of Health advises PCTs to use relevant sections of *The Standard GMS Contract* as a reference source when drawing up contracts with alternative providers. PCTs may also wish to refer to standard commissioning guidance, as set out in the *Contractors' Companion*, published in September 2003, and accessible at http://www.doh.gov.uk/commissioning. Contracts with alternative providers for enhanced and out-of-hours services would normally be time-limited, for example for between 1 and 3 years.

Preferred provider status

2.13 Existing practices are protected by having preferred provider status for some services. Chapter 6 describes how existing GMS providers will have a right to a new GMS contract. Having a GMS contract confers the right and obligation to provide essential services; an expectation and a right to provide additional services; and a right to provide the access, quality information preparation and childhood vaccination and immunisation DESs. GMS and PMS contractors do not have preferred provider status for other enhanced services, or out-of-hours and additional services that other contractors have opted out of providing. Having a PMS contract

also confers the right to move to GMS, and GMS providers have a
reciprocal ability to agree, at any stage, PMS contracts with PCTs.

● Complaints

Regulations

92. Complaints procedure

(1) The contractor shall establish and operate a complaints procedure to deal
with any complaints in relation to any matter reasonably connected with
the provision of services under the contract which shall –

(a) until the coming into force of regulations in relation to complaints
about general medical services made under section 113 of the Health
and Social Care (Community Health and Standards) Act 2003
(complaints about health care) comply with the requirements in
paragraphs 93 to 96 and 98; and

(b) on the coming into force of such regulations, comply with those
regulations.

(2) The contractor shall take reasonable steps to ensure that patients are
aware of –

(a) the complaints procedure;

(b) the role of the PCT and other bodies in relation to complaints about
services under the contract; and

(c) their right to assistance with any complaint from independent
advocacy services provided under section 19A of the Act
(independent advocacy services).

(3) The contractor shall take reasonable steps to ensure that the complaints
procedure is accessible to all patients.

93. Making of complaints

A complaint may be made by or, with his consent, on behalf of a patient,
or former patient, who is receiving or has received services under the
contract, or –

(a) where the patient is a child –

(i) by either parent, or in the absence of both parents, the guardian
or other adult who has care of the child,

(ii) by a person duly authorised by a local authority to whose care
the child has been committed under the provisions of the
Children Act 1989; or

(iii) by a person duly authorised by a voluntary organisation by
which the child is being accommodated under the provisions of
that Act;

(b) where the patient is incapable of making a complaint, by a relative or
other adult who has an interest in his welfare.

94.   Where a patient has died a complaint may be made by a relative or other
adult person who had an interest in his welfare or, where the patient falls
within paragraph 93(a)(ii) or (iii), by the authority or voluntary
organisation.

95.   Period for making complaints

(1)   Subject to sub-paragraph (2), the period for making a complaint is –

(a) 6 months from the date on which the matter which is the subject of
the complaint occurred; or

(b) 6 months from the date on which the matter which is the subject of
the complaint comes to the complainant's notice provided that the
complaint is made no later than 12 months after the date on which
the matter which is the subject of the complaint occurred.

(2)   Where a complaint is not made during the period specified in sub-
paragraph (1), it shall be referred to the person nominated under
paragraph 96(2)(a) and if he is of the opinion that –

(a) having regard to all the circumstances of the case, it would have been
unreasonable for the complainant to make the complaint within that
period; and

(b) notwithstanding the time that has elapsed since the date on which the
matter which is the subject matter of the complaint occurred, it is
still possible to investigate the complaint properly,

the complaint shall be treated as if it had been received during the period
specified in sub-paragraph (1).

96.   Further requirements for complaints procedures

(1)   A complaints procedure shall also comply with the requirements set out
in sub-paragraphs (2) to (6).

(2)   The contractor must nominate –

(a) a person (who need not be connected with the contractor and who,
in the case of an individual, may be specified by his job title) to be
responsible for the operation of the complaints procedure and the
investigation of complaints; and

(b) a partner, or other senior person associated with the contractor, to be
responsible for the effective management of the complaints

procedure and for ensuring that action is taken in the light of the outcome of any investigation.

(3) All complaints must be –
  (a) either made or recorded in writing;
  (b) acknowledged in writing within the period of three working days beginning with the day on which the complaint was made or, where that is not possible, as soon as reasonably practicable; and
  (c) properly investigated.

(4) Within the period of 10 working days beginning with the day on which the complaint was received by the person specified under sub-paragraph (2)(a) or, where that is not possible, as soon as reasonably practicable, the complainant must be given a written summary of the investigation and its conclusions.

(5) Where the investigation of the complaint requires consideration of the patient's medical records, the person specified under sub-paragraph (2)(a) must inform the patient or person acting on his behalf if the investigation will involve disclosure of information contained in those records to a person other than the contractor or an employee of the contractor.

(6) The contractor must keep a record of all complaints and copies of all correspondence relating to complaints, but such records must be kept separate from patients' medical records.

97. Co-operation with investigations

(1) The contractor shall co-operate with –
  (a) any investigation of a complaint in relation to any matter reasonably connected with the provision of services under the contract undertaken by –
    (i) the PCT, and
    (ii) the Commission for Healthcare Audit and Inspection; and
  (b) any investigation of a complaint by an NHS body or local authority which relates to a patient or former patient of the contractor.

(2) In sub-paragraph (1) –
  "NHS body" means a PCT, (in England and Wales and Scotland) an NHS trust, an NHS foundation trust, a SHA, a Local Health Board, a Health Board, a Health and Social Services Board or a Health and Social Services Trust;
  "local authority" means –
  (a) any of the bodies listed in section 1 of the Local Authority Social Services Act 1970 (local authorities),
  (b) the Council of the Isles of Scilly, or

(c) a council constituted under section 2 of the Local Government etc., (Scotland) Act 1994 (constitution of councils).

(3) The co-operation required by sub-paragraph (1) includes –
(a) answering questions reasonably put to the contractor by the PCT;
(b) providing any information relating to the complaint reasonably required by the PCT; and
(c) attending any meeting to consider the complaint (if held at a reasonably accessible place and at a reasonable hour, and due notice has been given) if the contractor's presence at the meeting is reasonably required by the PCT.

98. Provision of information about complaints

The contractor shall inform the PCT, at such intervals as required, of the number of complaints it has received under the procedure established in accordance with this Part.

Standard Contract

Complaints procedure

499. The Contractor shall establish and operate a complaints procedure to deal with any complaints in relation to any matter reasonably connected with the provision of services under the Contract.

500. The complaints procedure referred to above shall –
500.1 until the coming into force of regulations in relation to complaints about general medical services made under section 113 of the Health and Social Care (Community Health and Standards) Act 2003 comply with the requirements in clauses 503 to 511 and 515; and
500.2 on the coming into force of such regulations, comply with those regulations.

501. The Contractor shall take reasonable steps to ensure that patients are aware of –
501.1 the complaints procedure;
501.2 the role of the PCT and other bodies in relation to complaints about services under the Contract, and
501.3 the right to assistance with any complaint from independent advocacy services provided under section 19A of *the Act*.

502. The Contractor shall take reasonable steps to ensure that the complaints procedure is accessible to all patients.

Making of complaints

503. A complaint may be made by or, with his consent, on behalf of a patient, or former patient, who is receiving or has received services under the Contract, or

503.1 where the patient is a child –

503.1.1 by either parent, or, in the absence of both parents, the guardian or other adult who has care of the child,

503.1.2 by a person duly authorised by a local authority to whose care the child has been committed under the provisions of the Children Act 1989; or

503.1.3 by a person duly authorised by a voluntary organisation by which the child is being accommodated under the provisions of that Act;

503.2 where the patient is incapable of making a complaint, by a relative or other adult who has an interest in his welfare.

504. Where a patient has died a complaint may be made by a relative or other adult person who had an interest in his welfare or, where the patient fell within clause 503.1.2 or 503.1.3, by the authority or voluntary organisation, as the case may be.

Period for making complaints

505. Subject to clause 506, the period for making a complaint is-

505.1 6 months from the date on which the matter which is the subject of the complaint occurred; or

505.2 6 months from the date on which the matter which is the subject of the complaint comes to the complainant's notice, provided that the complaint is made no later than 12 months after the date on which the matter which is the subject of the complaint occurred.

506. Where a complaint is not made during the period specified in clause 505, it shall be referred to the person specified in clause 507.1 who may, if he is of the opinion that –

506.1 having regard to all the circumstances of the case, it would have been unreasonable for the complainant to make the complaint within that period; and

506.2 notwithstanding the time that has elapsed since the date on which the matter which is the subject matter of the complaint occurred, it is still possible to investigate the complaint properly

treat the complaint as if it had been received during the period specified in clause 505.

Further requirements for complaints procedure

507. The Contractor shall nominate-
    507.1 a person (who need not be connected with the Contractor and who, in the case of an individual, may be specified by his job title) to be responsible for the operation of the complaints procedure and the investigation of complaints; and
    507.2 a partner, or other senior person associated with the Contractor, to be responsible for the effective management of the complaints procedure and for ensuring that action is taken in the light of the outcome of any investigation.

508. All complaints shall be –
    508.1 either made or recorded in writing,
    508.2 acknowledged in writing within the period of three working days beginning with the day on which the complaint was made or, where that is not possible, as soon as reasonably practicable; and
    508.3 properly investigated.

509. Within the period of 10 working days beginning with the day on which the complaint was received by the person specified under clause 507.1 or, where that is not possible, as soon as reasonably practicable, the complainant shall be given a written summary of the investigation and its conclusions.

510. Where the investigation of the complaint requires consideration of the patient's medical records, the person specified under clause 507.1 must inform the patient or person acting on his behalf if the investigation will involve disclosure of information contained in those records to a person other than the Contractor or an employee of the Contractor.

511. The Contractor shall keep a record of all complaints and copies of all correspondence relating to complaints, but such records must be kept separate from patients' medical records.

Co-operation with investigations

512. The Contractor shall co-operate with –
    512.1 any investigation of a complaint in relation to any matter reasonably connected with the provision of services under the Contract undertaken by the PCT and the Commission for Healthcare Audit and Inspection; and
    512.2 any investigation of a complaint by an NHS body or local authority which relates to a patient or former patient of the Contractor.

513.   In the previous clause –
    513.1   "NHS body" means a Primary Care Trust, (in England and Wales and Scotland) an NHS trust, an NHS foundation trust, a Strategic Health Authority, a Local Health Board, a *Health Board*, a *Health and Social Services Board* or a *Health and Social Services Trust*; and
    513.2   "local authority" means any of the bodies listed in section 1 of the Local Authority Social Services Act 1970, the Council of the Isles of Scilly or a council constituted under section 2 of the Local Government etc. (Scotland) Act 1994.

514.   In co-operating with any investigation, the Contractor shall, by way of example –
    514.1   answer questions reasonably put to the Contractor by the PCT;
    514.2   provide any information relating to the complaint reasonably required by the PCT; and
    514.3   attend any meeting to consider the complaint (if held at a reasonably accessible place and at a reasonable hour, and due notice has been given) if the Contractor's presence at the meeting is reasonably required by the PCT.

515.   The Contractor shall inform the PCT, at such intervals as required, of the number of complaints it has received under the procedure established in accordance with Part 23 of the Contract.

516.   Part 23 of this Contract shall survive the expiry or termination of the Contract insofar as it relates to any complaint or investigation reasonably connected with the provision of services under the contract before it terminated.[15]

Compliance with legislation and guidance

Regulations

125. Compliance with legislation and guidance

The contractor shall –
(a)   comply with all relevant legislation; and

---

15   This clause is not mandatory but it is recommended to ensure that the Contractor is still under an obligation to comply with the investigation of a complaint or with any relevant investigation where the Contract has terminated or expired.

(b) have regard to all relevant guidance issued by the PCT, the relevant
SHA or the Secretary of State.

Standard Contract

498. The Contractor shall comply with all relevant legislation and have regard
to all relevant guidance issued by the PCT, the *relevant Strategic Health
Authority* or *the Secretary of State.*

● Confidentiality of personal data

See also: Patient records

Regulations

75. Confidentiality of personal data

The contractor shall nominate a person with responsibility for practices
and procedures relating to the confidentiality of personal data held by it.

Standard Contract

436. The Contractor shall nominate a person with responsibility for practices
and procedures relating to the confidentiality of personal data held by it.

● Contract, the

Guidance

6.1 The old GMS was a set of statutory arrangements with individual GPs.
The Health and Social Care (Community Health and Standards) Act
2003 provides that new GMS:
(i) is a local contract between a PCT and a GMS contractor
(ii) is subject to a standard set of national rules and procedures. These
are contained in the GMS Contract Regulations and the Statement
of Financial Entitlements. Those documents flesh out and give effect

to the agreements described in *Investing in General Practice* and the supplementary letters which were subsequently endorsed by the GP ballot. They are being published in draft to accompany this guidance and the Regulations will be made and laid in Parliament in February 2004.

6.2   The national rules cover:
(i)   the different types of services to be provided (described in chapter 2)
(ii) the entitlement of contractors to different payments (described in chapters 2 to 5, and summarised in chapter 5)
(iii) other statutory requirements (described mainly in chapters 2 and 3)
(iv) how the contractual process works: who can be a contractor, the formal dispute resolution procedure where the PCT and contractor cannot reach local agreement, how contract conditions are enforced through breach and termination procedures, and the way in which contracts can be varied.

6.3   The Contract Regulations have in turn been translated into a standard NHS contract, *The Standard GMS Contract.* This document is being published in draft form in December 2004. PCTs and GMS contractors will want to use this. They should also note that the draft contract will be subject to marginal revision when the GMS Contract Regulations are finalised in February 2004. A revised version will be issued by the Department before the end of February 2004.

6.4   This chapter (6) explains how the contractual processes work. PCTs and contractors should note that, as is the case with other chapters, it is intended as guidance only; the chapter neither provides a detailed description of the Contract Regulations nor should be seen as a definitive statement of law. PCTs and contractors should therefore read this chapter in conjunction with the Regulations and standard contract.

● Contract – required terms

Regulations

11. Parties to the contract

A contract must specify –
(a) the names of the parties;
(b) in the case of a partnership –
    (i)   whether or not it is a limited partnership, and
    (ii) the names of the partners and, in the case of a limited partnership, their status as a general or limited partner; and

(c) in the case of each party, the address to which official correspondence and notices should be sent.

12. Health service contract

If the contractor is to be regarded as a health service body pursuant to regulation 10, the contract must state that it is an NHS contract.

13. Contracts with individuals practising in partnership

(1) Where the contract is with two or more individuals practising in partnership, the contract shall be treated as made with the partnership as it is from time to time constituted, and the contract shall make specific provision to this effect.

(2) Where the contract is with two or more individuals practising in partnership, the contractor must be required by the terms of the contract to ensure that any person who becomes a member of the partnership after the contract has come into force is bound automatically by the contract whether by virtue of a partnership deed or otherwise.

14. Duration

(1) Except in the circumstances specified in paragraph (2), a contract must provide for it to subsist until it is terminated in accordance with the terms of the contract or the general law.

(2) The circumstances referred to in paragraph (1) are that the PCT wishes to enter into a temporary contract for a period not exceeding 12 months for the provision of services to the former patients of a contractor, following the termination of that contractor's contract.

(3) Either party to a prospective contract to which paragraph (2) applies may, if it wishes to do so, invite the LMC for the area of the PCT to participate in the negotiations intending to lead to such a contract.

● Contract – services generally

Regulations

18. Services generally

(1) A contract must specify –
(a) the services to be provided;

(b) subject to paragraph (2), the address of each of the premises to be used by the contractor or any sub-contractor for the provision of such services;

(c) to whom such services are to be provided;

(d) the area as respects which persons resident in it will, subject to any other terms of the contract relating to patient registration, be entitled to –

    (i) register with the contractor, or

    (ii) seek acceptance by the contractor as a temporary resident; and

(e) whether, at the date on which the contract comes into force, the contractor's list of patients is open or closed.

(2) The premises referred to in paragraph (1)(b) do not include –

(a) the homes of patients; or

(b) any other premises where services are provided on an emergency basis.

(3) Where, on the date on which the contract is signed, the PCT is not satisfied that all or any of the premises specified in accordance with paragraph (1)(b) meet the requirements set out in paragraph 1 of Schedule 6, the contract must include a plan, drawn up jointly by the PCT and the contractor, which specifies –

(a) the steps to be taken by the contractor to bring the premises up to the relevant standard;

(b) any financial support that may be available from the PCT; and

(c) the timescale on which the steps referred to in sub-paragraph (a) will be taken.

(4) Where, in accordance with paragraph (1)(e), the contract specifies that the contractor's list of patients is closed, it must also specify in relation to that closure each of the items listed in paragraph 29(8)(a) to (d) of Schedule 6.

19.

(1) Except in the case of the services referred to in paragraph (2), the contract must state the period (if any) for which the services are to be provided.

(2) The services referred to in paragraph (1) are –

(a) essential services;

(b) additional services funded under the global sum; and

(c) out-of-hours services provided pursuant to regulations 30 and 31.

Contract holders

Regulations

4. Conditions relating solely to medical practitioners

(1) In the case of a contract to be entered into with a medical practitioner, that practitioner must be a general medical practitioner.

(2) In the case of a contract to be entered into with two or more individuals practising in partnership –
(a) at least one partner (who must not be a limited partner) must be a general medical practitioner; and
(b) any other partner who is a medical practitioner must –
(i) be a general medical practitioner, or
(ii) be employed by a PCT, a Local Health Board, (in England and Wales and Scotland) an NHS Trust, an NHS foundation trust, (in Scotland) a Health Board or (in Northern Ireland) a Health and Social Services Trust.

(3) In the case of a contract to be entered into with a company limited by shares –
(a) at least one share in the company must be legally and beneficially owned by a general medical practitioner; and
(b) any other share or shares in the company that are legally and beneficially owned by a medical practitioner must be so owned by –
(i) a general medical practitioner, or
(ii) a medical practitioner who is employed by a PCT, a Local Health Board, (in England and Wales and Scotland) an NHS Trust, an NHS foundation trust, (in Scotland) a Health Board or (in Northern Ireland) a Health and Social Services Trust.

5. General condition relating to all contracts

(1) It is a condition in the case of a contract to be entered into –
(a) with a medical practitioner, that the medical practitioner;
(b) with two or more individuals practising in partnership, that any individual or the partnership; and
(c) with a company limited by shares, that –
(i) the company,
(ii) any person legally and beneficially owning a share in the company, and
(iii) any director or secretary of the company,
must not fall within paragraph (2).

(2)   A person falls within this paragraph if –
(a) he or it is the subject of a national disqualification;
(b) subject to paragraph (3), he or it is disqualified or suspended (other than by an interim suspension order or direction pending an investigation) from practising by any licensing body anywhere in the world;
(c) within the period of 5 years prior to the signing of the contract or commencement of the contract, whichever is the earlier, he has been dismissed (otherwise than by reason of redundancy) from any employment by a health service body, unless he has subsequently been employed by that health service body or another health service body and paragraph (4) applies to him or that dismissal was the subject of a finding of unfair dismissal by any competent tribunal or court;
(d) within the period of 5 years prior to signing the contract or commencement of the contract, whichever is the earlier, he or it has been removed from, or refused admission to, a primary care list by reason of inefficiency, fraud or unsuitability (within the meaning of section 49F(2), (3) and (4) of the Act respectively) unless his name has subsequently been included in such a list;
(e) he has been convicted in the United Kingdom of murder;
(f) he has been convicted in the United Kingdom of a criminal offence other than murder, committed on or after 14 December 2001, and has been sentenced to a term of imprisonment of over 6 months;
(g) subject to paragraph (5) he has been convicted elsewhere of an offence –
   (i)   which would, if committed in England and Wales, constitute murder, or
   (ii) committed on or after 14 December 2001, which would if committed in England and Wales, constitute a criminal offence other than murder, and been sentenced to a term of imprisonment of over 6 months;
(h) he has been convicted of an offence referred to in Schedule 1 to the Children and Young Persons Act 1933 (offences against children and young persons with respect to which special provisions of this Act apply) or Schedule 1 to the Criminal Procedure (Scotland) Act 1995 (offences against children under the age of 17 years to which special provisions apply) committed on or after 1 March 2004;
(i) he or it has –
   (i)   been adjudged bankrupt or had sequestration of his estate awarded unless (in either case) he has been discharged or the bankruptcy order has been annulled,
   (ii) been made the subject of a bankruptcy restrictions order or an interim bankruptcy restrictions order under Schedule 4A to the

> Insolvency Act 1986 unless that order has ceased to have effect or has been annulled, or
>
> (iii) made a composition or arrangement with, or granted a trust deed for, his or its creditors unless he or it has been discharged in respect of it;

(j) an administrator, administrative receiver or receiver is appointed in respect of it;

(k) he has been –

> (i) removed from the office of charity trustee or trustee for a charity by an order made by the Charity Commissioners or the High Court on the grounds of any misconduct or mismanagement in the administration of the charity for which he was responsible or to which he was privy, or which he by his conduct contributed to or facilitated, or
>
> (ii) removed under section 7 of the Law Reform (Miscellaneous Provisions) (Scotland) Act 1990 (powers of the Court of Session to deal with management of charities), from being concerned in the management or control of any body; or

(l) he is subject to a disqualification order under the Company Directors Disqualification Act 1986, the Companies (Northern Ireland) Order 1986 or to an order made under section 429(2)(b) of the Insolvency Act 1986 (failure to pay under county court administration order).

(3) A person shall not fall within paragraph (2)(b) where the PCT is satisfied that the disqualification or suspension from practising is imposed by a licensing body outside the United Kingdom and it does not make the person unsuitable to be –

(a) a contractor;

(b) a partner, in the case of a contract with two or more individuals practising in partnership;

(c) in the case of a contract with a company limited by shares –

> (i) a person legally and beneficially holding a share in the company, or
>
> (ii) a director or secretary of the company,
>
> as the case may be.

(4) Where a person has been employed as a member of a health care profession any subsequent employment must also be as a member of that profession.

(5) A person shall not fall within paragraph (2)(g) where the PCT is satisfied that the conviction does not make the person unsuitable to be –

(a) a contractor;

(b) a partner, in the case of a contract with two or more individuals practising in partnership;

    (c) in the case of a contract with a company limited by shares –
        (i) a person legally and beneficially holding a share in the company, or
       (ii) a director or secretary of the company,
     as the case may be.

6. Reasons

(1) Where a PCT is of the view that the conditions in regulation 4 or 5 for entering into a contract are not met it shall notify in writing the person or persons intending to enter into the contract of its view and its reasons for that view and of his, its or their right of appeal under regulation 7.

(2) The PCT shall also notify in writing of its view and its reasons for that view, any person legally and beneficially owning a share in, or a director or secretary of, a company that is notified under paragraph (1) where its reason for the decision relates to that person or those persons.

7. Appeal

A person who has been served with a notice under regulation 6(1) may appeal to the FHSAA against the decision of the PCT that the conditions in regulation 4 or 5 are not met by giving notice in writing to the FHSAA within the period of 28 days beginning on the day that the PCT served its notice.

8. Prescribed period under section 28D(1)(bc) of the Act

The period prescribed for the purposes of section 28D(1)(bc) of the Act (persons with whom agreements may be made) is 6 months.

● Contract – NHS or private contract

Standard Contract

NHS contract[16]

13. The Contractor has [not] elected to be regarded as a *health service body* for the purposes of section 4 of the *1990 Act*. Accordingly, this Contract is [not] an *NHS contract*.[17]

Contract – non-survival of terms

Standard Contract

600. Unless expressly provided, no term of this Contract shall survive expiry or termination of this Contract. Express provision is made in relation to –
600.1 clauses 430 and 431 (patient records);
600.2 Part 18 (fees and charges), to the extent specified in clause 486;
600.3 Part 23 (complaints);
600.4 Part 24 (dispute resolution procedures);
600.5 clause 588 (notifications to the *Local Medical Committee*);
600.6 clauses 593 to 598 (consequences of termination); and
600.7 clauses 603 and 604 (governing law and jurisdiction).

Contract review and variations

See also: Contract sanctions · Contract terminations

Guidance

6.57 Chapter 7 of *Investing in General Practice* set out the principle of annual contract review. This is distinct from the quality review described in chapter 3, but it can be carried out at the same time if the contractor so wishes, to minimise disruption.

6.58 The contractor will be required to submit an annual return to the PCT on a standard *pro forma*. This *pro forma* will include a number of pieces of information pre-completed by the PCT, the accuracy of which the contractor should confirm. It will also include a declaration by the contractor that it is meeting all the statutory requirements under the

---

16 If the Contractor has elected to be regarded as a *health service* body for the purposes of section 4 of *the 1990 Act* pursuant to regulation 10 of *the Regulations*, then the Contract must state that it is an NHS *contract*: see regulation 12 of *the Regulations*.

17 Where the contract is an NHS *contract*, it is not enforceable in the courts but instead is subject to the dispute resolution procedures set out in clauses 522 to 527 of the Contract and paragraph 36 and Part 7 of Schedule 6 to *the Regulations*. Therefore, the Contract must specify whether or not the Contractor has elected to be regarded as a *health service body*, and if it has, the Contractor must indicate that the Contract is an NHS *contract*.

contract. The *pro forma* will be developed and introduced during 2004 by the Department and the NHS Confederation, and will be subject to consultation with the BMA.

6.59   *Investing in General Practice* also made clear that PCTs must not neglect the informal process of developing and maintaining, where appropriate, a sustained empathetic relationship with contractors, based on the principle of high trust and developing an understanding of the contractor's needs, pressures and aspirations, which may change in year.

6.60   Paragraph 7.25 of *Investing in General Practice* gave a commitment that the annual review would be strongly evidence-based. To support this commitment, the Department plans to develop in consultation with the BMA a contract information system for PCTs. The system might for example help PCTs to:

(i)   record basic data about contractors and aspects of the contractual process

(ii) support the completion of the annual contract review *pro forma* by contractors and inform discussions during the annual contract review

(iii) reduce to a minimum the need for PCTs to request information from the contractor in year. PCTs and contractors should also note that a code of practice on information requests will be produced in discussion with the GPC during spring 2004.

6.61   The information system specification has not been finalised but will draw on existing best practice in PCTs. At this stage there is no planned delivery date and the development of the QMAS and Exeter payment systems will take priority. PCTs will be encouraged to use this system but they will be free to make their own arrangements if they so wish.

6.62   PCTs would also be expected to share this information to inform national monitoring of the contract by the Department of Health, NHS Confederation, GPC and the TSC, and inform subsequent contract development. For example, if information were collected about the number of patient assignments, this could inform national consideration of whether the new arrangements are effective in achieving the aim of reducing the numbers of patients who were assigned.

Contract variations

6.63   Once a GMS contract has been agreed and signed it will be open to either party to seek to vary or amend the agreement. Any such variation or amendment must be agreed by both parties, other than variations made under the procedures for opting out of additional and out-of-hours services where special procedures apply. Save in certain limited cases (see paragraph 103 of Schedule 6) any variation or amendment will need to be set out in writing and signed by or on behalf of the PCT and contractor.

Variations without contractor consent

6.64 However, the PCT may vary the contract without the contractor's consent where it is reasonably satisfied that it is necessary to do so to comply with the NHS Act 1977 or any Regulations or Directions made under that Act. In these circumstances the PCT must notify the contractor in writing of the proposed variation and the date the variation is to take effect, which should where possible be at least 14 days after the date of the notification.

6.65 Such variations would only follow from the introduction of regulatory changes, for example following national negotiations. Where regulatory changes are made the Department will produce amendments to *The Standard GMS Contract* for PCTs and contractors to use. If the contractor is unhappy with a variation made in accordance with paragraph 9 it has a right of appeal to the FHSAA (SHA) through the dispute resolution procedures set out in section D of this chapter. However, contractors should note that such appeals will in all probability fail if (i) the regulations are not *ultra vires* and (ii) the PCT has used standard amendments produced by the Department of Health to *The Standard GMS Contract*. A matter referred for dispute under this provision shall not prevent the PCT implementing the variation from the stated date pending the decision of the adjudicator.

Contract sanctions

See also: Contract review and variations · Contract termination

Regulations

117. Contract sanctions

(1) In this paragraph and paragraph 118, "contract sanction" means –
   (a) termination of specified reciprocal obligations under the contract;
   (b) suspension of specified reciprocal obligations under the contract for a period of up to 6 months; or
   (c) withholding or deducting monies otherwise payable under the contract.

(2) Where the PCT is entitled to terminate the contract pursuant to paragraph 112, 113, 114 or 115(4) or (6) or paragraph 116, it may instead impose any of the contract sanctions if the PCT is reasonably satisfied that the contract sanction to be imposed is appropriate and proportionate to the circumstances giving rise to the PCT's entitlement to terminate the contract.

(3) The PCT shall not, under sub-paragraph (2), be entitled to impose any contract sanction that has the effect of terminating or suspending any obligation to provide, or any obligation that relates to, essential services.

(4) If the PCT decides to impose a contract sanction, it must notify the contractor of the contract sanction that it proposes to impose, the date upon which that sanction will be imposed and provide in that notice an explanation of the effect of the imposition of that sanction.

(5) Subject to paragraph 118, the PCT shall not impose the contract sanction until at least 28 days after it has served notice on the contractor pursuant to sub-paragraph (4) unless the PCT is satisfied that it is necessary to do so in order to –
(a) protect the safety of the contractor's patients; or
(b) protect itself from material financial loss.

(6) Where the PCT imposes a contract sanction, the PCT shall be entitled to charge the contractor the reasonable costs of additional administration that the PCT has incurred in order to impose, or as a result of imposing, the contract sanction.

118. Contract sanctions and the NHS dispute resolution procedure

(1) If there is a dispute between the PCT and the contractor in relation to a contract sanction that the PCT is proposing to impose, the PCT shall not, subject to sub-paragraph (4), impose the proposed contract sanction except in the circumstances specified in sub-paragraph (2)(a) or (b).

(2) If the contractor refers the dispute relating to the contract sanction to the NHS dispute resolution procedure within 28 days beginning on the date on which the PCT served notice on the contractor in accordance with paragraph 117(4) (or such longer period as may be agreed in writing with the PCT), and notifies the PCT in writing that it has done so, the PCT shall not impose the contract sanction unless –
(a) there has been a determination of the dispute pursuant to paragraph 102 and that determination permits the PCT to impose the contract sanction; or

(b) the contractor ceases to pursue the NHS dispute resolution procedure,
whichever is the sooner.

(3) If the contractor does not invoke the NHS dispute resolution procedure within the time specified in sub-paragraph (2), the PCT shall be entitled to impose the contract sanction forthwith.

(4) If the PCT is satisfied that it is necessary to impose the contract sanction before the NHS dispute resolution procedure is concluded in order to –
(a) protect the safety of the contractor's patients; or
(b) protect itself from material financial loss,
the PCT shall be entitled to impose the contract sanction forthwith, pending the outcome of that procedure.

Standard Contract

576. In clauses 577 to 585, 591and 592, "contract sanction" means –
576.1 termination of specified reciprocal obligations under the Contract;
576.2 suspension of specified reciprocal obligations under the Contract for a period of up to 6 months; or
576.3 withholding or deducting monies otherwise payable under the Contract.

577. Where the PCT is entitled to terminate the Contract pursuant to clauses 557, 558, 564, 568 and 570, it may instead impose any of the contract sanctions if the PCT is reasonably satisfied that the contract sanction to be imposed is appropriate and proportionate to the circumstances giving rise to the PCT's entitlement to terminate the Contract.

578. The PCT shall not, under clause 577, be entitled to impose any contract sanction that has the effect of terminating or suspending any obligation to provide, or any obligation that relates to, *essential services*.

579. If the PCT decides to impose a contract sanction, it must notify the Contractor of the contract sanction that it proposes to impose, the date upon which that sanction will be imposed and provide in that notice an explanation of the effect of the imposition of that sanction.

580. Subject to clauses 582 to 585, the PCT shall not impose the contract sanction until at least 28 days after it has served notice on the Contractor pursuant to clause 578 unless the PCT is satisfied that it is necessary to do so in order to protect the safety of the Contractor's patients, or protect itself from material financial loss.

581. Where the PCT imposes a contract sanction, the PCT shall be entitled to charge the Contractor the reasonable costs of additional administration

that the PCT has incurred in order to impose, or as a result of imposing, the contract sanction.

Contract sanctions and the *NHS dispute resolution procedure*

582. If there is a dispute between the PCT and the Contractor in relation to a contract sanction that the PCT is proposing to impose, the PCT shall not, subject to clause 585, impose the proposed contract sanction except in the circumstances specified in clause 583.1 or 583.2.

583. If the Contractor refers the dispute relating to the contract sanction to the *NHS dispute resolution procedure* within 28 days beginning on the date on which the PCT served notice on the Contractor in accordance with clause 579 (or such longer period as may be agreed in writing with the PCT), and notifies the PCT in writing that it has done so, the PCT shall not impose the contract sanction unless –
   583.1 there has been a determination of the dispute pursuant to paragraph 101 of Schedule 6 to *the Regulations* and that determination permits the PCT to impose the contract sanction; or
   583.2 the Contractor ceases to pursue the *NHS dispute resolution procedure*,
   whichever is the sooner.

584. If the Contractor does not invoke the *NHS dispute resolution procedure* within the time specified in clause 583, the PCT shall be entitled to impose the contract sanction forthwith.

585. If the PCT is satisfied that it is necessary to impose the contract sanction before *the NHS dispute resolution procedure* is concluded in order to protect the safety of the Contractor's patients or protect itself from material financial loss, the PCT shall be entitled to impose the contract sanction forthwith, pending the outcome of that procedure.

Guidance

6.55 Where a PCT is entitled to serve notice terminating a contract it may instead impose one of the other available contract sanctions (see paragraphs 116 and 117 of Schedule 6). These are:
   (i) termination of specified obligations under the contract
   (ii) suspension of specified obligations for a period of up to 6 months or
   (iii) withholding or deducting monies otherwise payable under the contract.

6.56 The PCT may not, however, terminate or suspend any obligation to provide, or any other obligation which relates to, essential services.

Contract termination

See also: Contract review and variation · Contract sanctions

Regulations

25. Arrangements on termination

A contract shall make suitable provision for arrangements on termination of a contract, including the consequences (whether financial or otherwise) of the contract ending.

107. Termination by agreement

The PCT and the contractor may agree in writing to terminate the contract, and if the parties so agree, they shall agree the date upon which that termination should take effect and any further terms upon which the contract should be terminated.

108. Termination by the contractor

(1) A contractor may terminate the contract by serving notice in writing on the PCT at any time.

(2) Where a contractor serves notice pursuant to sub-paragraph (1), the contract shall, subject to sub-paragraph (3), terminate 6 months after the date on which the notice is served ("the termination date"), save that if the termination date is not the last calendar day of a month, the contract shall instead terminate on the last calendar day of the month in which the termination date falls.

(3) Where the contractor is an individual medical practitioner, sub-paragraph (2) shall apply to the contractor, save that the reference to "6 months" shall instead be to "3 months".

(4) This paragraph and paragraph 109 are without prejudice to any other rights to terminate the contract that the contractor may have.

109. Late payment notices

(1) The contractor may give notice in writing (a "late payment notice") to the PCT if the Trust has failed to make any payments due to the contractor in accordance with a term of the contract that has the effect

specified in regulation 22, and the contractor shall specify in the late payment notice the payments that the Trust has failed to make in accordance with that regulation.

(2) Subject to sub-paragraph (3), the contractor may, at least 28 days after having served a late payment notice, terminate the contract by a further written notice if the PCT has still failed to make the payments due to the contractor, and that were specified in the late payment notice served on the PCT pursuant to sub-paragraph (1).

(3) If, following receipt of a late payment notice, the PCT refers the matter to the NHS dispute resolution procedure within 28 days of the date upon which it is served with the late payment notice, and it notifies the contractor in writing that it has done so within that period of time, the contractor may not terminate the contract pursuant to sub-paragraph (2) until –

(a) there has been a determination of the dispute pursuant to paragraph 102 and that determination permits the contractor to terminate the contract; or

(b) the PCT ceases to pursue the NHS dispute resolution procedure, whichever is the sooner.

110. Termination by the PCT: general

The PCT may only terminate the contract in accordance with the provisions in this Part.

111. Termination by the PCT for breach of conditions in regulation 4

(1) The PCT shall serve notice in writing on the contractor terminating the contract forthwith if the contractor is an individual medical practitioner and the medical practitioner no longer satisfies the condition specified in regulation 4(1).

(2) Where the contractor is –

(a) two or more persons practising in partnership, and the condition specified in regulation 4(2)(a) is no longer satisfied; or

(b) a company limited by shares, and the condition specified in regulation 4(3)(a) is no longer satisfied,

sub-paragraph (3) shall apply.

(3) Where sub-paragraph (2)(a) or (b) applies, the PCT shall –

(a) serve notice in writing on the contractor terminating the contract forthwith; or

(b) serve notice in writing on the contractor confirming that the PCT will allow the contract to continue, for a period specified by the PCT of up to 6 months (the "interim period"), during which time the PCT shall, with the consent of the contractor, employ or supply one or more general medical practitioners to the contractor for the interim period to assist the contractor in the provision of clinical services under the contract.

(4) Before deciding which of the options in sub-paragraph (3) to pursue, the PCT shall, whenever it is reasonably practicable to do so, consult the LMC (if any) for its area.

(5) If the contractor does not, pursuant to sub-paragraph (3)(b), consent to the PCT employing or supplying a general medical practitioner during the interim period, the PCT shall serve notice in writing on the contractor terminating the contract forthwith.

(6) If, at the end of the interim period, the contractor still falls within sub-paragraph (2)(a) or (b), the PCT shall serve notice in writing on the contractor terminating the contract forthwith.

112. Termination by the PCT for the provision of untrue etc. information

The PCT may serve notice in writing on the contractor terminating the contract forthwith, or from such date as may be specified in the notice if, after the contract has been entered into, it comes to the attention of the PCT that written information provided to the PCT by the contractor before the contract was entered into in relation to the conditions set out in regulations 4 and 5 (and compliance with those conditions) was, when given, untrue or inaccurate in a material respect.

113. Other grounds for termination by the PCT

(1) The PCT may serve notice in writing on the contractor terminating the contract forthwith, or from such date as may be specified in the notice if –
   (a) in the case of a contract with a medical practitioner, that medical practitioner;
   (b) in the case of a contract with two or more individuals practising in partnership, any individual or the partnership; and
   (c) in the case of a contract with a company limited by shares –
      (i) the company,
      (ii) any person legally and beneficially owning a share in the company, or
      (iii) any director or secretary of the company,
      falls within sub-paragraph (2) during the existence of the contract.

(2) A person falls within this sub-paragraph if –

    (a) it does not satisfy the conditions prescribed in section 28S(2)(b) or (3)(b) of the Act;

    (b) he or it is the subject of a national disqualification;

    (c) subject to sub-paragraph (3), he or it is disqualified or suspended (other than by an interim suspension order or direction pending an investigation or a suspension on the grounds of ill-health) from practising by any licensing body anywhere in the world;

    (d) subject to sub-paragraph (4), he has been dismissed (otherwise than by reason of redundancy) from any employment by a health service body unless before the PCT has served a notice terminating the contract pursuant to this paragraph, he is employed by the health service body that dismissed him or by another health service body;

    (e) he or it is removed from, or refused admission to, a primary care list by reason of inefficiency, fraud or unsuitability (within the meaning of section 49F(2), (3) and (4) of the Act respectively) unless his name has subsequently been included in such a list;

    (f) he has been convicted in the United Kingdom of murder;

    (g) he has been convicted in the United Kingdom of a criminal offence other than murder and has been sentenced to a term of imprisonment of over 6 months;

    (h) subject to sub-paragraph (5), he has been convicted elsewhere of an offence which would if committed in England and Wales –

        (i) constitute murder, or

        (ii) constitute a criminal offence other than murder and been sentenced to a term of imprisonment of over 6 months;

    (i) he has been convicted of an offence referred to in Schedule 1 to the Children and Young Persons Act 1933 (offences against children and young persons with respect to which special provisions of this Act apply) or Schedule 1 to the Criminal Procedure (Scotland) Act 1995 (offences against children under the age of 17 years to which special provisions apply);

    (j) he or it has –

        (i) been adjudged bankrupt or had sequestration of his estate awarded unless (in either case) he has been discharged or the bankruptcy order has been annulled,

        (ii) been made the subject of a bankruptcy restrictions order or an interim bankruptcy restrictions order under Schedule 4A to the Insolvency Act 1986, unless that order has ceased to have effect or has been annulled,

        (iii) made a composition or arrangement with, or granted a trust deed for, his or its creditors unless he or it has been discharged in respect of it, or

        (iv) been wound up under Part IV of the Insolvency Act 1986;

(k) there is –
  (i) an administrator, administrative receiver or receiver appointed in respect of it, or
  (ii) an administration order made in respect of it under Schedule B1 to the Insolvency Act 1986;

(l) that person is a partnership and –
  (i) a dissolution of the partnership is ordered by any competent court, tribunal or arbitrator, or
  (ii) an event happens that makes it unlawful for the business of the partnership to continue, or for members of the partnership to carry on in partnership;

(m) he has been –
  (i) removed from the office of charity trustee or trustee for a charity by an order made by the Charity Commissioners or the High Court on the grounds of any misconduct or mismanagement in the administration of the charity for which he was responsible or to which he was privy, or which he by his conduct contributed to or facilitated, or
  (ii) removed under section 7 of the Law Reform (Miscellaneous Provisions) (Scotland) Act 1990 (powers of the Court of Session to deal with management of charities), from being concerned in the management or control of any body;

(n) he is subject to a disqualification order under the Company Directors Disqualification Act 1986, the Companies (Northern Ireland) Order 1986 or to an order made under section 429(2)(b) of the Insolvency Act 1986 (failure to pay under county court administration order); or

(o) he has refused to comply with a request by the PCT for him to be medically examined on the grounds that it is concerned that he is incapable of adequately providing services under the contract and, in a case where the contract is with two or more individuals practising in partnership or with a company, the PCT is not satisfied that the contractor is taking adequate steps to deal with the matter.

(3) A PCT shall not terminate the contract pursuant to sub-paragraph (2)(c) where the PCT is satisfied that the disqualification or suspension imposed by a licensing body outside the United Kingdom does not make the person unsuitable to be –

(a) a contractor;

(b) a partner, in the case of a contract with two or more individuals practising in partnership; or

(c) in the case of a contract with a company limited by shares –
  (i) a person legally and beneficially holding a share in the company, or
  (ii) a director or secretary of the company,
  as the case may be.

(4)   A PCT shall not terminate the contract pursuant to sub-paragraph (2)(d) –
(a) until a period of at least 3 months has elapsed since the date of the dismissal of the person concerned; or
(b) if, during the period of time specified in paragraph (a), the person concerned brings proceedings in any competent tribunal or court in respect of his dismissal, until proceedings before that tribunal or court are concluded,
and the PCT may only terminate the contract at the end of the period specified in paragraph (b) if there is no finding of unfair dismissal at the end of those proceedings.

(5)   A PCT shall not terminate the contract pursuant to sub-paragraph (2)(h) where the PCT is satisfied that the conviction does not make the person unsuitable to be –
(a) a contractor;
(b) a partner, in the case of a contract with two or more individuals practising in partnership; or
(c) in the case of a contract with a company limited by shares –
(i) a person legally and beneficially holding a share in the company, or
(ii) a director or secretary of the company,
as the case may be.

114.   The PCT may serve notice in writing on the contractor terminating the contract forthwith or with effect from such date as may be specified in the notice if –
(a) the contractor has breached the contract and as a result of that breach, the safety of the contractor's patients is at serious risk if the contract is not terminated; or
(b) the contractor's financial situation is such that the PCT considers that the PCT is at risk of material financial loss.

115. Termination by the PCT: remedial notices and breach notices

(1)   Where a contractor has breached the contract other than as specified in paragraphs 111 to 114 and the breach is capable of remedy, the PCT shall, before taking any action it is otherwise entitled to take by virtue of the contract, serve a notice on the contractor requiring it to remedy the breach ("remedial notice").

(2)   A remedial notice shall specify –
(a) details of the breach;
(b) the steps the contractor must take to the satisfaction of the PCT in order to remedy the breach; and
(c) the period during which the steps must be taken ("the notice period").

(3) The notice period shall, unless the PCT is satisfied that a shorter period is necessary to –
(a) protect the safety of the contractor's patients; or
(b) protect itself from material financial loss,
be no less than 28 days from the date that notice is given.

(4) Where a PCT is satisfied that the contractor has not taken the required steps to remedy the breach by the end of the notice period, the PCT may terminate the contract with effect from such date as the PCT may specify in a further notice to the contractor.

(5) Where a contractor has breached the contract other than as specified in paragraphs 111 to 114 and the breach is not capable of remedy, the PCT may serve notice on the contractor requiring the contractor not to repeat the breach ("breach notice").

(6) If, following a breach notice or a remedial notice, the contractor –
(a) repeats the breach that was the subject of the breach notice or the remedial notice; or
(b) otherwise breaches the contract resulting in either a remedial notice or a further breach notice,
the PCT may serve notice on the contractor terminating the contract with effect from such date as may be specified in that notice.

(7) The PCT shall not exercise its right to terminate the contract under sub-paragraph (6) unless it is satisfied that the cumulative effect of the breaches is such that the PCT considers that to allow the contract to continue would be prejudicial to the efficiency of the services to be provided under the contract.

(8) If the contractor is in breach of any obligation and a breach notice or a remedial notice in respect of that default has been given to the contractor, the PCT may withhold or deduct monies which would otherwise be payable under the contract in respect of that obligation which is the subject of the default.

116. Termination by the PCT: additional provisions specific to contracts with two or more individuals practising in partnership and companies limited by shares

(1) Where the contractor is a company limited by shares, if the PCT becomes aware that the contractor is carrying on any business which the PCT considers to be detrimental to the contractor's performance of its obligations under the contract –
(a) the PCT shall be entitled to give notice to the contractor requiring that it ceases carrying on that business before the end of a period of

not less than 28 days beginning on the day on which the notice is given ("the notice period"); and

(b) if the contractor has not satisfied the PCT that it has ceased carrying on that business by the end of the notice period, the PCT may, by a further written notice, terminate the contract forthwith or from such date as may be specified in the notice.

(2) Where the contractor is two or more persons practising in partnership, the PCT shall be entitled to terminate the contract by notice in writing on such date as may be specified in that notice where one or more partners have left the practice during the existence of the contract if in its reasonable opinion, the PCT considers that the change in membership of the partnership is likely to have a serious adverse impact on the ability of the contractor or the PCT to perform its obligations under the contract.

(3) A notice given to the contractor pursuant to sub-paragraph (2) shall specify –

(a) the date upon which the contract is to be terminated; and

(b) the PCT's reasons for considering that the change in the membership of the partnership is likely to have a serious adverse impact on the ability of the contractor or the PCT to perform its obligations under the contract.

Paragraphs 117 and 118 – *See*: Contract sanctions

119. Termination and the NHS dispute resolution procedure

(1) Where the PCT is entitled to serve written notice on the contractor terminating the contract pursuant to paragraph 112, 113, 114, or 115(4) or (6), the PCT shall, in the notice served on the contractor pursuant to those provisions, specify a date on which the contract terminates that is not less than 28 days after the date on which the PCT has served that notice on the contractor unless sub-paragraph (2) applies.

(2) This sub-paragraph applies if the PCT is satisfied that a period less than 28 days is necessary in order to –

(a) protect the safety of the contractor's patients; or

(b) protect itself from material financial loss.

(3) In a case falling with sub-paragraph (1), where the exceptions in sub-paragraph (2) do not apply, where the contractor invokes the NHS dispute resolution procedure before the end of the period of notice referred to in sub-paragraph (1), and it notifies the PCT in writing that it has done so, the contract shall not terminate at the end of the notice

period but instead shall only terminate in the circumstances specified in sub-paragraph (4).

(4)   The contract shall only terminate if and when –
(a) there has been a determination of the dispute pursuant to paragraph 102 and that determination permits the PCT to terminate the contract; or
(b) the contractor ceases to pursue the NHS dispute resolution procedure,
whichever is the sooner.

(5)   If the PCT is satisfied that it is necessary to terminate the contract before the NHS dispute resolution procedure is concluded in order to –
(a) protect the safety of the contractor's patients; or
(b) protect itself from material financial loss,
sub-paragraphs (3) and (4) shall not apply and the PCT shall be entitled to confirm, by written notice to be served on the contractor, that the contract will nevertheless terminate at the end of the period of the notice it served pursuant to paragraph 112, 113(1), 114, 115(4) or (6) or 116.

120. Consultation with the Local Medical Committee

(1)   Whenever the PCT is considering –
(a) terminating the contract pursuant to paragraph 112, 113, 114, 115(4) or (6) or 116; or
(b) imposing a contract sanction,
it shall, whenever it is reasonably practicable to do so, consult the LMC (if any) for its area before it terminates the contract or imposes a contract sanction.

(2)   Whether or not the LMC has been consulted pursuant to sub-paragraph (1), whenever the PCT imposes a contract sanction on a contractor or terminates a contract pursuant to this Part, it shall, as soon as reasonably practicable, notify the LMC in writing of the contract sanction imposed or of the termination of the contract (as the case may be).

Standard Contract

Termination by agreement

542.   The PCT and the Contractor may agree in writing to terminate the Contract, and if the parties so agree, they shall agree the date upon which that termination will take effect and any further terms upon which the Contract should be terminated.

Termination by the Contractor

543. The Contractor may terminate the Contract by serving notice in writing on the PCT at any time.

544. [Where the Contractor serves notice pursuant to clause 542, the Contract shall terminate 6 months after the date on which the notice is served ("the termination date"), save that if the termination date is not the last calendar day of a month, the Contract shall instead terminate on the last calendar day of the month in which the termination date falls.][18]

545. [Where the Contractor serves notice pursuant to clause 543, the Contract shall terminate 3 months after the date on which the notice is served ("the termination date"), save that if the termination date is not the last calendar day of a month, the Contract shall instead terminate on the last calendar day of the month in which the termination date falls.][19]

546. The Contractor may give notice in writing ("late payment notice") to the PCT if the PCT has failed to make any payments due to the Contractor in accordance with Part 17 of this Contract. The Contractor shall specify in the late payment notice the payments that the PCT has failed to make in accordance with Part 17 of the Contract.

547. The Contractor may, at least 28 days after having served a late payment notice, terminate the contract by a further written notice if the PCT has still failed to make payments due to the Contractor, and that were specified in the late payment notice served on the PCT pursuant to clause 546.

548. If, following receipt of a late payment notice, the PCT refers the matter to the *NHS dispute resolution procedure* within 28 days of the date upon which it is served with the late payment notice, and it notifies the Contractor in writing that it has done so within that period of time, the Contractor may not terminate the Contract pursuant to clause 547 until –

548.1 there has been a determination of the dispute pursuant to paragraph 101 of Schedule 6 to *the Regulations*; or

548.2 the PCT ceases to pursue the *NHS dispute resolution procedure*, whichever is the sooner.

549. Clauses 543 to 548 are without prejudice to any other rights to terminate the Contract that the Contractor may have.

---

18   This clause should be included where the Contractor is a partnership or a limited company. Where the Contractor is an individual medical practitioner, this clause should be deleted.

19   This clause should be included where the Contractor is an individual medical practitioner. Where the Contractor is a partnership or a limited company, this clause should be deleted.

Termination by the PCT: general

550. The PCT may only terminate the Contract in accordance with the provisions of Part 25 of this Contract.

Termination by the PCT for breach of conditions in regulation 4 of *the Regulations*

551. The PCT shall serve notice in writing on the Contractor terminating the Contract forthwith if the Contractor is an individual medical practitioner, and the medical practitioner no longer satisfies the condition specified in regulation 4(1) of *the Regulations*.

552. Where the Contractor is –
    552.1 two or more persons practising in partnership, and the condition specified in regulation 4(2)(a) of *the Regulations* is no longer satisfied; or
    552.2 a company limited by shares, and the condition specified in regulation 4(3)(a) of *the Regulations* is no longer satisfied
    clause 553 shall apply.

553. Where clause 552.1 or 552.2 applies, the PCT shall –
    553.1 serve notice in writing on the Contractor terminating the Contract forthwith; or
    553.2 serve notice in writing on the Contractor confirming that the PCT will allow the Contract to continue, for a period specified by the PCT of up to 6 months (the "interim period"), during which time the PCT shall, with the consent of the Contractor, employ or supply one or more *general medical practitioners* to the Contractor for the interim period to assist the Contractor in the provision of clinical services under the Contract.

554. Before deciding which of the options in clause 553 to pursue, the PCT shall, whenever it is reasonably practicable to do so, consult the *Local Medical Committee* (if any) for its area.

555. If the Contractor does not, pursuant to clause 553.2, consent to the PCT employing or supplying a *general medical practitioner* during the interim period, the PCT shall serve notice in writing on the Contractor terminating the Contract forthwith.

556. If, at the end of the interim period, the Contractor still falls within clause 552.1 or 552.2, the PCT shall serve notice in writing on the Contractor terminating the Contract forthwith.

Termination by the PCT for provision of untrue etc. information

557.   The PCT may serve notice in writing on the Contractor terminating the contract forthwith, or from such date as may be specified in the notice if, after this Contract was entered into, it has come to the attention of the PCT that written information provided to the PCT by the Contractor before the contract was entered into in relation to the conditions set out in regulations 4 and 5 of *the Regulations* (and compliance with those conditions) was, when given, untrue or inaccurate in a material respect.

Other grounds for termination by the PCT

558.   The PCT may serve notice in writing on the Contractor terminating the Contract forthwith, or from such date as may be specified in the notice if –

558.1 in the case of a contract with a medical practitioner, that medical practitioner;

558.2 in the case of a contract with two or more individuals practising in partnership, any individual or the partnership; and

558.3 in the case of a contract with a company limited by shares, the company, any person legally and beneficially owning a share in the company, or any director or secretary of the company,

falls within clause 559 during the existence of the Contract.

559.   A person falls within this clause if –

559.1 it does not satisfy the conditions prescribed in section 28S(2)(b) or (3)(b) of *the Act*;

559.2 he or it is the subject of a *national disqualification*;

559.3 subject to clause 560, he or it is disqualified or suspended (other than by an interim suspension order or direction pending an investigation or a suspension on the grounds of ill-health) from practising by any *licensing body* anywhere in the world;

559.4 subject to clause 561, he has been dismissed (otherwise than by reason of redundancy) from any employment by a *health service body* unless before the PCT has served a notice terminating the Contract pursuant to this clause, he is employed by the *health service body* that dismissed him or by another *health service body*;

559.5 he or it is removed from, or refused admission to, a *primary care list* by reason of inefficiency, fraud or unsuitability (within the meaning of section 49F(2), (3) and (4) of *the Act* respectively) unless his or its name has subsequently been included in such a list;

559.6 he has been convicted in the United Kingdom of murder or an offence referred to in Schedule 1 to the Children and Young

Persons Act 1933 or Schedule 1 to the Criminal Procedure (Scotland) Act 1995;

559.7 he has been convicted in the United Kingdom of a criminal offence other than murder, and has been sentenced to a term of imprisonment of over 6 months;

559.8 subject to clause 563, he has been convicted elsewhere of an offence which would, if committed in England and Wales –

558.8.1 constitute murder, or

558.2.1 constitute a criminal offence other than murder, and been sentenced to a term of imprisonment of over 6 months;

559.9 he or it has –

559.9.1 been adjudged bankrupt or had sequestration of his estate awarded unless (in either case) he has been discharged or the bankruptcy order has been annulled;

559.9.2 been made the subject of a bankruptcy restrictions order or an interim bankruptcy restrictions order under Schedule 4A to the Insolvency Act 1986, unless that order has ceased to have effect or has been annulled;

559.9.3 made a composition or arrangement with, or granted a trust deed for, his or its creditors unless he or it has been discharged in respect of it;

559.9.4 been wound up under Part IV of the Insolvency Act 1986;

559.9.5 had an administrator, administrative receiver or receiver appointed in respect of it; or

559.9.6 had an administration order made in respect of it under Schedule B1 to the Insolvency Act 1986.

559.10 that person is a partnership and –

559.10.1 a dissolution of the partnership is ordered by any competent court, tribunal or arbitrator, or

559.10.2 an event happens that makes it unlawful for the business of the partnership to continue, or for members of the partnership to carry on in partnership together;

559.11 he has been –

559.11.1 removed from the office of charity trustee or trustee for a charity by an order made by the Charity Commissioners or the High Court on the grounds of any misconduct or mismanagement in the administration of the charity for which he was responsible or to which he was privy, or which he by his conduct contributed to or facilitated;

559.11.2 removed under section 7 of the Law Reform (Miscellaneous Provisions) (Scotland) Act 1990, from being concerned in the management or control of any body;

559.12 he is subject to a disqualification order under the Company Directors Disqualification Act 1986, the Companies (Northern Ireland) Order 1986 or to an order made under section 429(2)(b) of the Insolvency Act 1986;

559.13 he has refused to comply with a request by the PCT for him to be medically examined on the grounds that it is concerned that he is incapable of adequately providing services under the contract and, in a case where the contract is with two or more individuals practising in partnership or with a company, the PCT is not satisfied that the Contractor is taking adequate steps to deal with the matter.

560.   The PCT shall not terminate the Contract pursuant to clause 559.3 where the PCT is satisfied that the disqualification or suspension imposed by a *licensing body* outside the United Kingdom does not make the person unsuitable to be a contractor, a partner, a person legally and beneficially holding a share in the company, or a director or secretary of the company, as the case may be.

561.   The PCT shall not terminate the Contract pursuant to clause 559.4 until a period of at least 3 months has elapsed since the date of the dismissal of the person concerned; or if, during that period of time, the person concerned brings proceedings in any competent tribunal or court in respect of his dismissal, until proceedings before that tribunal or court are concluded. The PCT may only terminate the Contract in the latter situation if there is no finding of unfair dismissal at the end of those proceedings.

562.   [Where the PCT has entered into the Contract –
562.1 following a *default contract* with the Contractor; or
562.2 pursuant to an entitlement on the part of the Contractor under Part 2 of *the Transitional Order*, after 31 March 2004 other than following a *default contract*,
clause 558 shall apply as if it enabled the PCT to serve notice of termination on the Contractor on the grounds of a person falling within clause 559.4 at any time after 31 March 2004.][20]

563.   The PCT shall not terminate the Contract pursuant to clause 559.8 where the PCT is satisfied that the conviction does not make the person unsuitable to be a contractor, a partner, a person legally and beneficially holding a share in the company, or a director or secretary of the company, as the case may be.

20   This clause only needs to be included if the Contractor falls within 562.1 or 562.2. If not, this clause can be deleted.

Termination by the PCT for a serious breach

564. The PCT may serve notice in writing on the Contractor terminating the Contract forthwith or with effect from such date as may be specified in the notice if –
      564.1 the Contractor has breached the Contract and the PCT considers that as a result of that breach, the safety of the Contractor's patients is at serious risk if the Contract is not terminated; or
      564.2 the Contractor's financial situation is such that the PCT considers that the PCT is at risk of material financial loss.

Termination by the PCT: remedial notices and breach notices

565. Where the Contractor has breached the Contract other than as specified in clauses 551 to 564 and the breach is capable of remedy, the PCT shall, before taking any action it is otherwise entitled to take by virtue of the Contract, serve a notice on the Contractor requiring it to remedy the breach ("remedial notice").

566. A remedial notice shall specify –
      566.1 details of the breach;
      566.2 the steps the Contractor must take to the satisfaction of the PCT in order to remedy the breach; and
      566.3 the period during which the steps must be taken ("the notice period").

567. The notice period shall, unless the PCT is satisfied that a shorter period is necessary to protect the safety of the Contractor's patients or protect itself from material financial loss, be no less than 28 days from the date that notice is given.

568. Where the PCT is satisfied that the Contractor has not taken the required steps to remedy the breach by the end of the notice period, the PCT may terminate the Contract with effect from such date as the PCT may specify in a further notice to the Contractor.

569. Where the Contractor has breached the Contract other than as specified in clauses 551 to 564 and the breach is not capable of remedy, the PCT may serve notice on the Contractor requiring it not to repeat the breach ("breach notice").

570. If, following a breach notice or a remedial notice, the Contractor –
      570.1 repeats the breach that was the subject of the breach notice or the remedial notice; or
      570.2 otherwise breaches the Contract resulting in either a remedial notice or a further breach notice,

the PCT may serve notice on the Contractor terminating the Contract with effect from such date as may be specified in that notice.

571. The PCT shall not exercise its right to terminate the Contract under the previous clause unless it is satisfied that the cumulative effect of the breaches is such that it would be prejudicial to the efficiency of the services to be provided under the Contract to allow the Contract to continue.

572. If the Contractor is in breach of any obligation and a breach notice or a remedial notice in respect of that default has been given to the Contractor, the PCT may withhold or deduct monies which would otherwise be payable under the Contract in respect of that obligation which is the subject of the default.

Termination by the PCT: additional provisions specific to Contracts with companies limited by shares[21]

573. If the PCT becomes aware that the Contractor is carrying on any business which the PCT considers to be detrimental to the Contractor's performance of its obligations under the Contract –
    573.1 the PCT shall be entitled to give notice to the Contractor requiring that it ceases carrying on that business before the end of a period of not less than 28 days beginning on the day on which the notice is given ("the notice period"); and
    573.2 if the Contractor has not satisfied the PCT that it has ceased carrying on that business by the end of the notice period, the PCT may, by a further written notice, terminate the Contract forthwith or from such date as may be specified in the notice.

Termination by the PCT: additional provisions specific to Contracts with two or more individuals practising in partnership[22]

574. Where the Contractor is two or more persons practising in partnership, the PCT shall be entitled to terminate the Contract by notice in writing on such date as may be specified in that notice where one or more partners have left the practice during the existence of the Contract if in

---

21 If the Contractor is not a company limited by shares, this clause should be deleted.

22 If the Contractor is not two or more individuals practising in partnership, this clause should be deleted.

its reasonable opinion, the PCT considers that the change in membership
of the partnership is likely to have a serious adverse impact on the ability
of the Contractor or the PCT to perform its obligations under the
Contract.

575. A notice given to the Contractor pursuant to clause 574 shall specify –
      575.1 the date upon which the Contract is to be terminated; and
      575.2 the PCT's reasons for considering that the change in the
            membership of the partnership is likely to have a serious adverse
            impact on the ability of the Contractor or the PCT to perform its
            obligations under the Contract.

Termination and the *NHS dispute resolution procedure*

586. Where the PCT is entitled to serve written notice on the Contractor
      terminating the contract pursuant to clauses 557, 558, 564, 568 or 570,
      the PCT shall, in the notice served on the Contractor pursuant to those
      clauses, specify a date on which the Contract terminates that is not less
      than 28 days after the date on which the PCT has served that notice on
      the Contractor unless clause 587 applies.

587. This clause applies if the PCT is satisfied that a period less than 28 days is
      necessary in order to protect the safety of the Contractor's patients or
      protect itself from material financial loss.

588. In a case falling within clause 586 where the exception in clause 587 does
      not apply, where the Contractor invokes the *NHS dispute resolution
      procedure* before the end of the period of notice referred to in clause 586,
      and it notifies the PCT in writing that it has done so, the Contract shall
      not terminate at the end of the notice period but instead shall only
      terminate in the circumstances specified in clause 589.

589. The Contract shall only terminate pursuant to this clause if and when
      there has been a determination of the dispute pursuant to paragraph 101
      of Schedule 6 to *the Regulations* and that determination permits the PCT
      to terminate the Contract or the Contractor ceases to pursue the *NHS
      dispute resolution procedure*, whichever is the sooner.

590. If the PCT is satisfied that it is necessary to terminate the Contract before
      the *NHS dispute resolution procedure* is concluded in order to protect the
      safety of the Contractor's patients or protect itself from material financial
      loss, clauses 588 and 589 shall not apply and the PCT shall be entitled to
      confirm by written notice to be served on the Contractor, that the
      Contract will nevertheless terminate at the end of the period of the
      notice it served pursuant to clauses 557, 558, 564, 568 or 570.

Contract termination
Standard Contract

Consultation with the *Local Medical Committee*

591. Whenever the PCT is considering terminating the Contract pursuant to clauses 557, 558, 564, 568, 570, 573 or 574 or imposing a contract sanction, it shall, whenever it is reasonably practicable to do so, consult the *Local Medical Committee* (if any) for its area before it terminates the Contract or imposes a contract sanction.

592. Whether or not the *Local Medical Committee* has been consulted pursuant to clause 591, whenever the PCT imposes a contract sanction on the Contractor or terminates the Contract pursuant to this Part, it shall, as soon as reasonably practicable, notify the *Local Medical Committee* in writing of the contract sanction imposed or of the termination of the Contract (as the case may be). The obligation to notify the *Local Medical Committee* of the matters set out in this clause shall survive the termination of the Contract.

Consequences of termination[23]

593. The termination of the Contract, for whatever reason, is without prejudice to the accrued rights of either party under the Contract.

594. On the termination of the Contract for any reason, the Contractor shall –
     594.1 subject to the requirements of this clause, cease performing any work or carrying out any obligations under the Contract;
     594.2 co-operate with the PCT to enable any outstanding matters under the Contract to be dealt with or concluded in a satisfactory manner;
     594.3 co-operate with the PCT to enable the Contractor's patients to be transferred to one or more other contractors or providers of *essential services* (or their equivalent), which shall include –
          594.3.1 providing reasonable information about individual patients, and
          594.3.2 delivering patient records
          to such other appropriate person or persons as the PCT specifies.
     594.4 deliver up to the PCT all property belonging to the PCT including all documents, forms, computer hardware and software, drugs, appliances or medical equipment which may be in the Contractor's possession or control;

---

23 The parties are required to make suitable provision for arrangements on the termination of the Contract, including the consequences (whether financially or otherwise) of the Contract ending, subject to any specific requirements of *the Regulations*: see paragraph 116 of Schedule 6 to *the Regulations*. Subject to this requirement, the parties could draft their own provisions dealing with the consequences of termination.

595. Subject to clauses 596 to 598, the PCT's obligation to make payments to the Contractor in accordance with the Contract shall cease on the date of termination of the Contract.

596. On termination of the Contract or termination of any obligations under the Contract for any reason, the PCT shall perform a reconciliation of the payments made by the PCT to the Contractor and the value of the work undertaken by the Contractor under the Contract. The PCT shall serve the Contractor with written details of the reconciliation as soon as reasonably practicable, and in any event no later than 28 days after the termination of the Contract.

597. If the Contractor disputes the accuracy of the reconciliation, the Contractor may refer the dispute to the *NHS dispute resolution procedure* in accordance with the terms of the Contract within 28 days beginning on the date on which the PCT served the Contractor with written details of the reconciliation. The parties shall be bound by the determination of the dispute.

598. Each party shall pay the other any monies due within 3 months of the date on which the PCT served the Contractor with written details of the reconciliation, or the conclusion of the *NHS dispute resolution procedure,* as the case may be.

599. The obligations contained in clauses 593 to 598 shall continue to apply notwithstanding the termination of the Contract.

Guidance

6.40 Provision for the termination of GMS contracts is set out in part 8 of Schedule 6 to the GMS Regulations. A PCT may serve notice terminating the contract immediately if the contractor no longer satisfies the contractor conditions. See paragraphs 109 to 112 of Schedule 6 of the GMS Regulations.

6.41 In operating this provision the PCT should note that:
(i) where the contractor holding a GMS contract changes so that it no longer includes a medical practitioner who is on the General Practitioner Register, the PCT will need to review the viability of the contract
(ii) where the medical practitioner was a sole practitioner the PCT must issue a notice terminating the contract forthwith – there is no longer anyone with whom the PCT is in contract
(iii) where the medical practitioner was part of a partnership, for example with a nurse and/or a practice manager, the PCT may issue

a notice terminating the contract forthwith. However, where the loss of the medical practitioner was sudden and there had been no reasonable opportunity for the remaining partners to regularise their affairs the PCT may decide to allow the contract to continue for up to 6 months. This will either allow the PCT to bring matters to an orderly conclusion or allow the remaining partners to recruit a suitable medical practitioner. In reaching such a decision the PCT is recommended to take into account the best interests of the contractor's patients.

6.42   If it exercises its discretion in this the PCT ought to:
(i)   consult with the LMC immediately
(ii) appoint one or more suitable medical practitioners to support the practice under its powers to provide support and assistance (the PCT may charge for this service)
(iii) complete all processes within a period of no more than 6 months
(iv) terminate the contract after 6 months if the contractor still does not include a medical practitioner whose name is included in the General Practitioner Register (or a practitioner who is suitably experienced).

6.43   Although in most circumstances a GMS contract cannot be terminated simply because there is a change in the structure of the partnership (for example the acquisition or loss of partners) the PCT does have the ability to terminate a contract following such changes in two specific circumstances:
(i)   if the PCT considers, in its reasonable opinion, that the change in the partnership is such that it is likely to have a serious impact on the ability of the contractor or the PCT to perform its obligations under the contract it may serve notice terminating the contract forthwith or from such other date as it might indicate. Any such notice should specify why the PCT has chosen this course of action and should, where practical, follow consultation with the LMC (or a notification to the LMC where this is not practical)
(ii) a change in the structure of the partnership might be sudden and/or acrimonious. In these circumstances (which include a two-partner practice splitting and not indicating which partner should continue with the contract) the PCT may be unable to determine which of the remaining partners has the right to retain the GMS contract. It would be unreasonable for the PCT to be involved in any practice dispute, or to take sides. In these circumstances the PCT may serve notice terminating the contract forthwith or from such other date as

it might indicate. Any such notice should specify why the PCT has
chosen this course of action and should, where practical, follow
consultation with the LMC (or a notification to the LMC where this
is not practical).

6.44 Where a PCT takes such action it will need to take steps to secure the
provision of patient services. It is normally expected that in these
circumstances the PCT will wish to enter into short-term temporary
contracts (for no more than 12 months) with any of the parties to the old
GMS contract who wish to continue to provide GMS services and who
meet the GMS provider conditions. The PCT could make alternative
arrangements if for example the temporary contracts required the
provision of new practice premises, or if the granting of temporary
contracts would otherwise be to the detriment of NHS efficiency.

6.45 It is similarly envisaged that at the end of temporary contracts, the
temporary contractor(s) would normally be offered a permanent
contract or, where they agree, be allowed to continue to provide services
under a wider GMS contract with other persons, for example by
merging with a neighbouring practice.

6.46 PCTs should:
(i) consult with the LMC before refusing the holder of a temporary
contract a permanent contract
(ii) ensure patient representatives are appraised of all decisions to
terminate a contract in these circumstances, and to ensure that
individual patients are aware of the choices available to them.

6.47 Notwithstanding the above paragraphs, a PCT may serve notice in
writing terminating a contract immediately, or from such other date as
may be specified if:
(i) the PCT considers that the contractor has breached the contract and
as a result of that breach the safety of the contractor's patients is at
serious risk
(ii) if the contractor's financial situation is such that the PCT considers
that the PCT is at risk of material financial loss.

6.48 Contractors must provide 6 months notice before they withdraw from
the contract, although this is reduced to 3 months in the case of a single-
handed practitioner. By mutual agreement these periods can be changed.
The different treatment of single-handers reflects the fact it is easier to
find alternative provision for a small contractor than if a large contractor
stops providing services.

● Contractor budgets

Guidance

5.47   PCTs are responsible for calculating contractor budgets. PCT Directors of
Finance should oversee this important, time-critical and time-consuming
task. This section describes:
(i)   timetable
(ii) indicative contractor budgets
(iii) contractor global sums and MPIGs.
Each is considered in turn.

(i) Timetable

5.48   PCTs should already have put in place arrangements to enable them to
construct and share indicative budgets for all their contractors by the end
of the first week in February 2004. Delivery against this deadline is
essential to allow all GMS contracts and budgets to be negotiated and
provisionally agreed by the end of February 2004. In turn, that date is
necessary to allow time for any fine tuning and further consideration
within contractor partnerships and by contractor accountants, so that
contracts can be finalised and signed by the end of March 2004. PCTs are
also responsible for ensuring that the first payments under the new GMS
contract are made by the end of April 2004. SHAs will have an important
performance-management role in ensuring these deadlines are achieved
for all GMS contractors in every PCT. The performance-management
process is described further in chapter 7.

5.49   If provisional agreement has not been reached by the end of February
2004, PCTs will need to offer the default contract, described in chapter 6,
to GMS contractors as a potential alternative. This is needed so that
contractors can continue to provide and their patients receive primary
medical services. The default contract will be less flexible than the new
GMS contract. To ensure that there is no unfairness to contractors, PCTs
will need to have undertaken the necessary steps to calculate and agree
contractor budgets for new GMS contracts within the timetable outlined
in this section. SHAs will need to ensure that the only reasons why
default contracts are offered are either (i) disputes between the PCT and
the contractor, or (ii) insufficient engagement from the
contractor – rather than insufficient action by PCTs.

5.50   The Exeter payments system is being revised to provide payment
calculations and payment facilities from April 2004. This will provide the

basis for calculating actual practice budgets backdated to April 2004, and for monthly financial monitoring. It will include a facility to enable PCTs to calculate automatically the monthly and annual budgets for all contractors. The revised system will reduce the work that PCTs need to undertake to finalise the calculations, and give contractors confidence that the figures are accurate. The GPC is being fully consulted on the changes. PCTs will be notified of the changes by the end of February 2004.

5.51   PCTs should use the revised Exeter payments system to:
(i)   calculate actual global sums and MPIG
(ii) discuss and agree these with contractors as quickly as possible and by no later than the end of May 2004
(iii) ensure that revised payments (including payment of arrears if the indicative budget was too low, or clawbacks if the indicative budget was too high) can be made by no later than the end of June 2004.

5.52   Thereafter PCTs should use the payments system to produce, send to and agree with contractors revised budgets in the event of any contract variations, or otherwise quarterly. They should also amend any over- or under-payments as necessary.

(ii) Indicative contractor budgets

5.53   The timing of the changes to the Exeter system means that PCTs will need to calculate indicative rather than actual budgets prior to agreeing and signing their GMS contracts by 31 March 2004. To help PCTs before the revised Exeter system goes live, the Department is distributing in December 2003 an Indicative Contractor Budget Spreadsheet (ICBS). The spreadsheet is accompanied by guidance notes explaining how it should be completed, and these are attached at annex C. When PCTs use the spreadsheet, they should derive payments from the different SFE entitlements and then reconcile them with the January 2004 allocation, rather than the other way round. The spreadsheet also profiles estimated contractor income month by month.

5.54   PCTs should start completing the spreadsheet for all contractors in advance of allocations being made by the end of January 2004. They already have most of the necessary data as a result of (i) completing the various AWP exercises set out in this chapter, and (ii) their preliminary discussions with contractors about what services they are planning to provide. When PCTs have completed the spreadsheet, they should share this with the contractor by the end of the first week in February 2004. They should also, at the same time, share with contractors the global sum and MPIG spreadsheets that show their weightings for each of the different global sum indices. PCTs should be as open as possible in discussing the basis of the calculations, to build confidence that the interim figures are accurate on the basis of the available data.

5.55   Local negotiations on the contract can then be finalised during February 2004. There should be no reason for disagreements about the indicative budget to prevent both sides signing GMS contracts because the figures will be indicative. Signing up to contracts does not mean that the PCT and contractor have agreed the actual global sum and MPIG, which the contractor would be able to dispute subsequently when it is known. This is considered further in the section on pre-contract disputes in chapter 6. Once agreement has been reached on either the GMS contract or the default contract, PCTs should ensure that all contractors get paid by the end of April 2004.

(iii) Contractor global sums and correction factors

5.56   The global sum and MPIG are key elements of contractor budgets. The January allocation to PCTs will include initial estimates of global sums, global sum equivalents and MPIGs for all contractors. The Department of Health is calculating global sum estimates using data collected directly from the 2003 Exeter Attribution Data Set (ADS), and estimates of annual global sum equivalents have been collected from PCTs through AWP(04–05)PCT07, with Exeter payment information used as a guide. This has taken into account: (i) converting the cash information onto a resource basis taking account of opening and closing debtors and creditors; (ii) practice splits and mergers; and (iii) GP vacancies at contractor level (rather than more widely across the PCT). The Department will then use these two data sets to estimate correction factors.

5.57   PCTs must turn the Department's estimates into indicative amounts for contractors. They should read annex B carefully and understand how the global sum and MPIG are calculated. They should then use the ICBS to make a number of adjustments, in line with the guidance in the first part of annex C.

5.58   PCTs and contractors should note that the end of January 2004 indicative global sum and MPIG amounts will vary from the actual amount that contractors are entitled to from 1 April 2004 because:
(i)   indicative practice lists will be based on the ADS from April 2003, whereas final payments will be based on lists at April 2004
(ii)   the MPIG will be adjusted to reflect changes in the list size between the collection period at April 2004
(iii) the temporary patients adjustments will be based on 1 year of data in the indicative budget but will be a 5 year average in the actual global sum payments. The method is set out in annex B

(iv) any agreed staff vacancy or staff funding adjustment to the MPIG will not be included.

5.59 The steps in the global sum and correction factor payments will be automated after April 2004. However, before payments are made, PCTs will still need to input changes on a regular basis through their links to the Exeter system to:
(i) take account of contractor movement between GMS and PMS
(ii) confirm that contractor registered populations are accurate
(iii) reflect new opt-outs, or resumption of providing additional services that contractors had temporarily opted out of providing
(iv) take account of contract terminations, withholding of monies (as described in chapter 6), contractor splits and mergers
(v) record, for annual revision of the Temporary Patients Adjustment, the number of clinical records sent to them by contractors providing services to temporary patients for their onward distribution by PCTs to the contractors with whom the patients are registered.

5.60 Contractors should also note that the global sum contractor weighting is a measure of need and unavoidable cost relative to other contractors. Changes to the patient characteristics and patient list size of other contractors may result in a contractor's weighting going up or down when the recalculation of the weightings takes place. Quarterly recalculation will minimise sharp adjustments; the extent of change is likely to be marginal.

E. FINANCIAL MONITORING AND MANAGEMENT

5.61 This section considers financial monitoring and PCT cash and resource management.

(i) Monitoring

5.62 National and local financial monitoring arrangements need to improve to support the new GMS financial arrangements. PCTs will need to provide the Department of Health with sufficient information not just to monitor expenditure against the resource limit but also to support the monitoring of the GIG and the local enhanced services floor. New arrangements will deliver all requirements through a single reporting system and PCTs will be required to hold information on expenditure at a sufficiently detailed level to meet the new reporting requirements.

5.63 PCT financial reporting will feed into national monitoring undertaken by the joint DH/NHSC/GPC Technical Steering Committee (TSC). The TSC will:
(i) source and review data for the financial allocation formula

(ii) monitor outcome against the Gross Investment Guarantee described in paragraphs 5.3 to 5.6, which replaces the old GMS concept of IANI

(iii) monitor and forecast total earnings, GP net incomes and expenses (which includes PMS and salaried doctors)

(iv) monitor outcome against the local PCT-level enhanced services floor in line with the definition in chapter 2 and monitor overall expenditure on enhanced services

(v) monitor dispensing and quality payments

(vi) adjust the proposed pensions dynamising factor to take account of the shift from full-time to part-time working.

The TSC will also undertake a continuous workload survey and monitor skill mix.

5.64 Annex D describes how PCT financial reporting arrangements will need to change, including details of the required information for the new FIS 4 returns. A line-by-line explanation of the data requirements will be provided in conjunction with the detailed guidance on 2004/05 FIMS monitoring to be issued early in 2004. It is anticipated that similar lines of reporting will be required for PMS and guidance will follow separately.

5.65 PCTs will need to ensure that their ledger systems are suitably reconfigured in order to generate the relevant information.

(ii) PCT cash and resource management

5.66 The new GMS contract will require PCTs to change their cash and resource management arrangements. As section C of this chapter described, funds for primary medical services will now be allocated as a resource allocation together with a cash-financing requirement within which PCTs have a statutory obligation to contain spending. PCTs are advised to draw up indicative resource management plans in January and revise these in year. They will need to consider with particular care the financial management of quality achievement payments and the NHS Bank risk-sharing arrangements with SHAs described in paragraphs 5.32 to 5.35.

5.67 PCTs will also need to review treasury management processes to ensure that they can maintain effective in-year control over the requisitioning and reporting of cash payments. The new contract will change both the timing and the level of in-year cash payments to contractors. In addition, it will be necessary to manage the transition from the old payments regime to one that underpins the new contract. PCTs will need to:

(i) provide a robust estimate of year-end non-cash-limited creditors for the 2003/04 year-end

(ii) benchmark this creditors figure against previous years

(iii) ensure that accruals are adequate as the year-end creditor assessment will inform the maximum additional cash-limit that can be drawn down, subject to the level of year-end creditors in 2004/05

(iv) seek to ensure that all claims for activities prior to April 2004 are received by 30 September 2004

(v) manage any excess creditors from within existing resource and cash allocations available in 2004/05.

Contractor entitlements

Guidance

5.7 This section:
(i) describes arrangements for making outstanding Red Book payments
(ii) summarises the Statement of Financial Entitlements (SFE)
(iii) describes general conditions attached to SFE payments.

5.8 GMS GPs were entitled to a number of payments under the old Red Book arrangements that come to an end on 31 March 2004. The principle of entitlement continues in new GMS, but on the basis of a contractor practice rather than an individual GP. The new SFE gives contractors certainty about the minimum level of key resources they will receive that year. PCTs will have no discretion over (i) whether to make most SFE payments (an obvious exception being the Prolonged Study Leave payments which require PCT approval) or (ii) the value of those payments. Discretionary funds will also be available to practices, for example those that successfully compete for provision of enhanced services. Contractors will also be entitled to receive pensions entitlements under separate pensions regulations.

(i) Completing final payments under the Red Book

5.9 PCTs will want to encourage GMS GPs to submit by the end of March 2004 all claims for services undertaken in the financial year 2003/04 and prior years. This will enable prompt payment by PCTs, and will improve contractors' cash-flow.

5.10 When completing their 2003/04 Statutory Accounts PCTs should make adequate year-end provision for sums outstanding to practices for services provided before 1 April 2004. This will have implications for in-year cash and resource management and is considered further in paragraph 5.67. Any understatement of year-end creditors will need to be managed in 2004/05 by the PCT. There will be no additional resource cover from the Department.

(ii) SFE entitlements

5.11 PCTs and contractors are encouraged to read the draft SFE issued with this guidance. The final version will be laid for Parliamentary approval in February 2004. The first SFE covers 2004/05 only and a revised SFE for subsequent years will be published, following consultation, before April 2005. We anticipate that this will include a schedule of payments to be revised annually, to avoid the need for updating the whole SFE each year thereafter.

5.12 There are 17 different types of entitlement. The global sum and MPIG are described in annex B. Table 14 summarises the entitlements.

Table 14 **Contractor entitlements**

Entitlement	Description of key aspects
1. **Global sum** See annex B of the guidance, and Part 1 of the SFE	1. New entitlement that subsumes 27 existing payments (three for temporary patients) relating to running costs of the practice 2. Based on the global sum allocation formula that reflects patient need and contractor costs 3. Price is an average of £50 per registered patient. This price will increase to reflect the increase in employer superannuation contributions from 7% to 14% and the expected increase in net contractor income 4. An off-formula London weighting of £2.18 per registered patient, rather than weighted population, for contractors in PCTs in the five London SHA areas 5. An off-formula Temporary Patients Adjustment, calculated on a rolling 5 year historic average 6. Calculated quarterly, paid by end of each month

Table 14 – continued	
Entitlement	**Description of key aspects**
2. **MPIG** See annex B of the guidance and Part 1 of the SFE	1. Based on comparison on 1 April 2004 of initial global sum (adjusted for historic opt-outs) with uplifted historic income from relevant fees and allowances between 1 July 2002 and 30 June 2003 2. Adjusted for GP vacancies, practice mergers and splits, and also changes in list size between 1 July 2003 and 31 March 2004 3. Fixed amount, but uplifted in line with the global sum uplift 4. Paid to qualifying contractors in addition to the monthly global sum
3. **Quality preparation (QPREP)** See chapter 3 of the guidance and Part 2 of the SFE	1. £3250 for a contractor with average national list size of registered patients, for practice to decide how to support preparation required for implementing contract 2. 2004/05 is the second and final year of QPREP 3. Paid as a lump sum in April 2004 subject to agreeing aspiration points
4. **Quality aspiration** See chapter 3 of the guidance and Part 2 of the SFE	1. For 2004/05, one-third of anticipated achievement points agreed with PCT, at £75 per point for a contractor with average national list size of registered patients 2. New method from 2005/06 based on 60% of previous year achievement points, up-rated to 2005/06 price and adjusted for prevalence 3. Paid at end of every month
5. **Quality achievement** See chapter 3 of the guidance and Part 2 of the SFE	1. Achievement payment is the difference between the total QOF entitlement and aspiration payments made 2. Total QOF entitlement is the achievement points multiplied by £75 per point in 2004/05 for a contractor with average national list size

Continued

Table 14 – continued	
Entitlement	Description of key aspects
	3. For each disease area, pounds per point are multiplied by the Adjusted Disease Prevalence Factor to reflect differential workload
	4. For the additional services domain, pounds per point are adjusted to reflect the relative contractor target population
	5. 2004/05 achievement paid as a lump sum by end of April 2005
6. **DES – Quality Information Preparation (QuIP)** See chapter 3 of the guidance and Part 3 of the SFE	1. Must be offered by PCTs to all contractors that agree a QuIP plan. For 2003/04 this must be by January 2004
	2. Provides a contribution to the costs of summarising and maintaining summaries of patient records
	3. Price must be between £1000 and £5000 per contractor with an average national list size of patients
	4. 2004/05 QuIP must be paid by end of April 2004 for plans agreed on or before 1 April. For plans agreed after 1 April, payment is made when the next global sum monthly payment falls due
	5. 2004/05 is second and final year of QuIP
7. **DES – Improved Access Scheme (IAS)** See Part 3 of the SFE	1. Must be offered to all contractors which agree with the PCT a plan for delivering improved access in line with England primary care access targets
	2. 2003/04 price depends on existing access payments such that the total payment is at least £5000 for a contractor with average national list size of registered patients
	3. 2004/05 price is £5160 for a contractor with average national list size of registered patients
	4. For 2004/05 scheme, following PCT agreement of the plan, half (implementation payments) must be paid with the next

Table 14 – continued	
Entitlement	**Description of key aspects**
	monthly global sum payment. The other half (reward payments) must be paid by the end of April 2005 if the PCT is satisfied that the plan has been achieved
	5. IAS is a three-year scheme ending in 2005/06. Access achievement is rewarded separately through the QOF 50 points access bonus
8. **DES – childhood vaccinations and immunisations (CVI)** See Part 3 of the SFE	1. From April 2004, PCTs must offer CVI DES to all contractors which do not opt out of providing the vaccinations and immunisation additional service
	2. Existing arrangements are rolled forward from the Red Book. For achieving the 70% and 90% targets for both 2 and 5 year olds average payments of £897 and £2691 will be paid per quarter These amounts are adjusted by determining the proportion of children immunised against those on the Childhood Vaccinations and Immunisations Register and comparing this with the average number of children per 5000 population
	3. Informed dissent does not apply
	4. Payments are made quarterly
9. **Locum payments** See Part 4 of the SFE	Existing Red Book arrangements are simplified for locum cover for GP partners for: (a) sickness leave (b) adoptive leave (c) paternity leave (d) maternity leave (e) suspended doctors (f) prolonged study leave
	PCTs must develop local policies on paying locum reimbursement and seek to agree these with LMCs. The policies must include how less

Continued

Table 14 – continued	
Entitlement	Description of key aspects

than full-working commitment would be treated, using the salaried GP employment contract hours as a guide

Link to years of service ends but list size criteria remain

Maximum amount payable is £948.33 per week for a full-time GP

Payments must be made within 14 days of claims being submitted

10. Seniority payments
See Part 4 of the SFE

1. The new payments scale in the 2003/04 scheme is further enhanced in 2004/05
2. Entitlement will be based on superannuable earnings of GP providers. PCTs and contractors will need to agree notional superannuable earnings during February 2004 to produce an indicative seniority payment. This will subsequently be adjusted upwards or downwards once year-end certificates of superannuable earnings have been agreed in the following year
3. The delayed retirement scheme (DRS) ends from 31 March 2004. If a GP's seniority entitlement in each year from 2004/05 is less than the sum of the old seniority amount in 2002/03 and DRS income in 2003/04, the difference is made up
4. Payments must be made by the end of each month

11. Golden Hello Scheme
See Part 4 of the SFE

1. The existing scheme is rolled forward from the Red Book
2. Working commitment is determined by the proportion of hours worked compared with the 37.5 hours specified in the model contract for salaried GPs
3. Eligible GPs are entitled to submit applications for payments of between £5000 and £12,000 according to PCT area. The

Table 14 – continued	
Entitlement	**Description of key aspects**
	differing amounts reflect differential levels of comparative under-doctoring
	4. The scheme will be reviewed and is expected to change in 2005/06
12. Returner Scheme See Part 4 of the SFE	1. The existing scheme will be rolled forward from the Red Book
	2. Contractors receive a single lump sum payment of £1050 for each eligible doctor
	3. Payments are due on the last day of the month in which the doctor joins the scheme (for doctors entering the scheme before 1 April 2004 payment is due at the end of the month in which the anniversary of the doctor joining the scheme falls)
13. Flexible Career Scheme (FCS) See Part 4 of the SFE	1. The existing scheme is rolled forward from the Red Book
	2. If the FCS GP started before January 2004, reimbursement of eligible costs is made at 50% reimbursement for years 1 and 2, then 25% in year 3, then 10% in year 4. Otherwise reimbursement is at 50% for year 1, then 25% for year 2, then 10%
	3. FCS Doctor payments are due on the last day of the month in which the doctor's qualifying date falls. Quarterly payments are due on the last day of the month following the quarter in respect of which the quarterly return is made
14. Retainer Scheme See Part 4 of the SFE	1. PCTs must pay to contractors £57.33 for each full session undertaken by a member of the Doctors' Retainer Scheme up to four sessions a week provided that the sessions have been arranged with the Director of Postgraduate GP Education
	2. Payments must be made by the end of the month in which the sessions were worked

Continued

Table 14 – continued	
Entitlement	**Description of key aspects**
15. **Dispensing** See Part 4 of the SFE	1. The existing arrangements are rolled forward from the Red Book 2. Fees are up-rated by 5.4% to reflect the transfer of dispensers' salary costs
16. **Existing premises costs** See chapter 4 of the guidance, Part 5 of the SFE and separate Directions	Existing payments for premises are brought forward from the Red Book to reflect the new GMS funding arrangements
17. **IT minor upgrades and maintenance** See chapter 4 of the guidance and Part 5 of the SFE	1. PCTs must pay to contractors all reasonable costs of contractors in respect of IT maintenance and minor upgrades 2. Major upgrades are subject to business case approval by the PCT

(iii) Conditions attached to SFE payments

5.13   Specific conditions are attached to each entitlement and these are described in the SFE. A broad summary is:
(i)   contractors must make available to the PCT any information which the PCT does not have and needs
(ii) information supplied by the contractor must be accurate to the best of its knowledge. This includes information used for capitation-based payments on the size of the contractor's registered patient list held by the Exeter payments system. Contractors must ensure that they provide full, accurate and timely information to registration systems and will as a result be co-operating with list cleaning exercises undertaken by PCTs
(iii) sums are generally payable only in respect of the duration of the contract, so if a contract starts or ends in year the full annual payment is reduced according to the number of days for which the contract has run

(iv) breach of the SFE conditions is treated as a breach of contract and is subject to the rules set out in chapter 6

(v) PCTs and contractors are obliged to co-operate with investigations by authorities such as auditors and counter-fraud services.

Contractor – form and conditions

Guidance

6.22 This section sets out who can be a GMS provider, the constitution of a GMS provider, and conditions that need to be met by GMS providers. Full details of the conditions applying to GMS providers are set out in Regulations 4 and 5 of the GMS Regulations. The conditions apply to individuals, partnerships and contractor bodies. They cover such areas as qualifications, career, employment status, criminal history, and financial status. These conditions are intended to prevent unsuitable individuals such as murderers or undischarged bankrupts from contracting to provide GMS and have been based on the conditions that apply to PCT board members and the new primary care performers' list.

6.23 A contract may only be entered into with a contractor which satisfies the conditions set out in section 28S of the Health and Social Care (Community Health and Standards) Act 2003 and regulations 4 and 5 of the GMS Contract Regulations. After the contract has been entered into the GMS contractor is responsible for ensuring compliance with the conditions set out in regulations 4 and 5 of the GMS Contract Regulations. The contractor can be made up of individual providers who do not have to perform clinical services under that contract, although many will do that as well. However, the provider conditions in no way operate as a substitute, in whole or in part, to those set out in the Primary Care Performer List Regulations which apply in full to all GPs performing clinical services under the GMS contract.

WHO CAN BE A GMS PROVIDER?

6.24 The contract provides considerable new flexibility about how GMS providers are constituted. GMS contracts may be entered into with any of the following:

(i) single-handed GPs

(ii) partnerships that include at least one GP

(iii) certain types of company limited by shares, similar to the existing PMS Qualifying Body option.

It will be possible in GMS, as it is in PMS, for there to be a nurse-managed (or therapist-managed) service.

Single-handed GPs

6.25　Where a GMS contract is made with an individual medical practitioner, that practitioner's name must be included in the General Practitioner Register set up under the General and Specialist Medical Practice (Education, Training and Qualifications) Order 2003. It is possible that the GMS Contract Regulations and this guidance may come into operation before the coming into force of this Order. In this case the condition may be treated as being satisfied if the medical practitioner is suitably experienced within the meaning of section 31(2) of the 1977 NHS Act, section 21 of the 1978 NHS (Scotland) Act, or Article 8(2) of the Health and Personal Social Services (Northern Ireland) Order 1978.

Partnerships

6.26　Where the contract is with one or more individuals practising in partnership at least one of the partners must be a medical practitioner whose name is included in the GP register (or is suitably experienced). Other individual partners can be other health professionals, including practice nurses, dentists, consultants together with other persons such as practice managers, who could be offered partnership shares and help deliver enhanced services in a primary care setting. Contractors will want to consider whether they want to take advantage of this new flexibility before signing GMS contracts or thereafter, and when bidding for enhanced services. The definition of a NHS employee is described in annex F.

6.27　The GMS contract can be continued with the partnership "as it is from time to time constituted". This delivers the concept of a rolling contract set out in Chapter 7 of *Investing in General Practice*. Routine changes in the partnership will not therefore affect the contract. However, if in the reasonable opinion of the PCT, the change in membership of the partnership is likely to have a serious adverse impact on the ability of the contractor or the PCT to perform its obligations, the PCT may serve notice terminating the contract. The contract requires the PCT to be given a written notice of any changes (see paragraphs 85 and 105 of Schedule 6 to the GMS Regulations). Where there is a change in the partnership the GMS contract may need to be varied to reflect the change in contractor status. Provisions covering a change in a partnership or change in status from individual medical practitioner to partnership and vice versa can be found at paragraphs 103 to 105 of Schedule 6.

Companies limited by shares

6.28 This is a similar concept to the qualifying body provided for in Section 28D of the 1977 Act. The ownership rules for GMS companies are that:
   (i) all shares in such a company must be legally and beneficially owned by a person who could lawfully enter into a GMS contract as an individual or as part of a partnership
   (ii) at least one share must be legally and beneficially owned by a medical practitioner whose name is included in the GP Register (or is suitably experienced)
   (iii) any other shares owned by a medical practitioner must be so owned by a medical practitioner whose name is included in the GP Register or who is employed by a PCT, a Local Health Board, a NHS trust (including an NHS Trust in Scotland), a NHS foundation trust, a Health Board, or a Health and Social Services Trust

6.29 The contract will require that the GMS provider inform the PCT immediately if there is any change in the ownership of the shares or any other event occurs that would prevent the company from continuing its business.

CONDITIONS RELATING TO ALL GMS CONTRACTS

6.30 A GMS contract cannot be entered into if the provider conditions are not satisfied, so PCTs should ensure that any potential GMS contractor confirms in writing that it satisfies all of these conditions. Contractors are encouraged to write to the PCT to confirm this at the same time as they apply for Health Service Body status, that is by 13 February 2004. The new contractual arrangements are intended to be a high trust system. PCTs should therefore consider carefully whether they require any additional information to support this statement. Where the individual is a GP, PCTs will already have received much of this information in response to enquiries made under the Primary Care Performers' List Regulations.

6.31 Where a PCT is of the view that the conditions for entering into a contract are not met it should notify in writing the person or persons intending to enter into the contract of its views. Where the prospective contractor is a company limited by shares, the PCT should at the same time inform any shareholder, director or company secretary where that person is the subject of the PCT's decision because it is him or her that has failed to meet the conditions. Any person refused a contract on these grounds may appeal to the Family Health Service Appeals Authority (FHSAA) concerning the PCT decision that the provider conditions have not been met by writing to the FHSAA within 28 days beginning on the day that the PCT served notice. These appeals are to the independent FHSAA. Notices of appeal should be sent to:

FHSAA
30 Victoria Avenue
Harrogate HG1 5PR.
The chairman of the FHSAA is Mr Paul Kelly.

6.32   GMS contractors must give notice to the PCT in writing that any new partner joining the partnership after the GMS contract has been signed meets these conditions. Again it is for the PCT to decide the extent to which it seeks to verify this statement. The PCT may serve notice terminating the contract immediately if any of these conditions is broken. This is also described in paragraph 6.37.

Core and normal hours

Regulations

20.   A contract must contain a term which requires the contractor in core hours –
(a) to provide –
(i)   essential services, and
(ii) additional services funded under the global sum,
at such times, within core hours, as are appropriate to meet the reasonable needs of its patients; and
(b) to have in place arrangements for its patients to access such services throughout the core hours in case of emergency.

Guidance

2.20   The Contract Regulations define:
(i)   core hours. These are Monday to Friday, 8 a.m. to 6.30 p.m., except Good Friday, Christmas Day and Bank Holidays. It is the responsibility of the contractor to ensure (and, if need be, fund cover for) the provision of essential services during these core hours. PCTs can provide and fund alternative cover at their discretion

(ii) normal surgery hours. The Contract Regulations state that these must be "to the extent necessary to meet reasonable need". Normal hours may be different for different services. Normal hours do not have to be within core hours; a contractor might propose for example that existing surgery hours are changed and daytime sessions substituted for early morning, evening or weekend surgeries. Alternatively, the contractor may propose to provide such surgeries in addition to their existing surgery hours, in which case these could be funded through enhanced services. PCTs and contractors may wish to discuss normal hours as contracts are finalised during February 2004, and as part of the annual review process described in chapter 6.

To reflect the move to a practice-based contract, the old GMS obligation on any individual full-time GP to be available for face-to-face consultations for 26 hours a week will end from 1 April 2004.

Criminal record checks – enhanced

Guidance

4.6   From 1 April 2004, applicants for inclusion in PCT medical performer lists must provide an enhanced criminal record certificate (ECRC). The PCT will only get a copy of the ECRC (the original will go to the doctor) when it countersigns the doctor's application to the Criminal Records Bureau (CRB), and only if the information is required to assess the suitability of an individual for a post. There is a £29 fee payable to the Bureau; the cost should be borne by the PCT, not by the practitioner. A PCT has to register with the Bureau in order to be entitled to countersign an application, and therefore receive a copy of the enhanced certificate. In return the PCT is required to adhere to a strict "Code of Practice". The Code of Practice is available from the CRB or via its website at http://www.crb.gov.uk. PCTs should register now if they have not already done so. There is a registration fee, currently £300, which also covers registration of the lead counter-signatory for applications. For each additional counter-signatory to be included within the registered body a further fee, currently £5, has to be paid.

4.7   The CRB is not a source of data about overseas offences and convictions, although they may hold very limited data about some countries. If so, the data will be limited to whatever data from overseas are held on the Police

National Computer. The CRB may, however, be able to advise PCTs on how they might themselves go about trying to check details of convictions outside the UK.

4.8 For the time being, PCTs should not generally attempt to obtain certificates from doctors who are already listed and who have not already provided certificates. They should only ask listed performers to provide a certificate where information comes to their attention that throws into doubt the openness of the declaration a performer had previously provided.

Default contract

Guidance

6.5 If agreement is not reached and new GMS contracts are not signed by PCTs and contractors by 31 March 2004, no payments can be made to GPs and services cannot be provided to patients. GMS GPs would also lose their transitional rights to a new GMS contract (unless there are exceptional circumstances or where the PCT incorrectly refuses to offer a new GMS contract). For these reasons the Department of Health, the NHS Confederation and the GPC advise that PCTs and GMS providers should all sign GMS contracts before 31 March 2004. It is important to note, however, that this does not mean that PCTs cannot offer GMS contracts after this date should they so wish.

6.6 The default contract will be available to allow payments to continue until a new GMS contract is signed. It will also need to be agreed to and signed by both parties. The default contract is being developed by the Department and the NHS Confederation in consultation with the GPC, and will be published by 13 February 2004. The principle underlying its development is that its terms are black and white and not open to discussion. It will be based on *The Standard GMS Contract* but will not offer the same flexibility to either party and will be a short-term contract of fixed duration. We do not envisage that the default contract will need to be used other than in exceptional cases.

● Disease prevalence

See also: Quality and outcomes

Guidance

3.30   The joint letter of 30 May 2003 from Dr John Chisholm and Mike Farrar
made clear that quality payments would be adjusted by practice disease
prevalence, as recorded by QOF data and relative to national prevalence.
This will apply to QOF achievement payments, and from 2005/06,
aspiration payments. The aim of the prevalence adjustment to QOF
clinical domain payments factors is to deliver a more equitable
distribution of quality rewards in the light of the different workloads that
contractors will face in delivering the same number of quality points. It
will target resources effectively at areas where both morbidity and
contractor achievement are greatest and thereby help tackle health
inequalities.

3.31   In developing the prevalence adjustment methodology, the following
requirements were borne in mind:
(i)   the need to provide adequate income protection to those with lowest
prevalence, such as university practices
(ii) the need to deliver appropriate rewards for those contractors with
the highest prevalence
(iii) the need to ensure that the quality and outcomes framework delivers
the agreed overall levels of funding
(iv) the need to develop a sound method based on the best available
research evidence. A research study was undertaken by the Office of
National Statistics and is attached at annex A.

3.32   Applying the raw prevalence data, without an adjustment, would lead to
a very significant redistribution of quality resources away from practices
with the lowest prevalence to those with the highest. This would not be
fair given that it would seriously destabilise those contractors with the
lowest relative prevalence. Nor would it be an intellectually sound
approach because even practices with low prevalence have significant
fixed costs in identifying morbidity and establishing quality systems, and
the relationship between workload and prevalence is not a linear
correlation. For these reasons the raw factor will be subject to an
adjustment to reduce variation and relatively protect the losers, whilst at
the same time providing fair rewards to those who have the highest
prevalence.

Prevalence factor methodology

3.33   The calculation involves three steps:
   (i)   the calculation of the contractor's raw practice disease prevalence. A
         separate factor will be calculated for each disease area
   (ii) making an adjustment to give an adjusted disease prevalence factor
         (ADPF). This is necessary to avoid a radical and unjustified
         redistribution of quality resources from those with lowest prevalence
         to those with highest
   (iii) using the ADPF to adjust the pounds per point in each disease area.

3.34   The raw contractor disease prevalence is calculated by dividing the
       number of patients on the relevant disease register by the number of
       patients on the registered list. This will be the most up-to-date list size
       held by the revised Exeter payments system.

3.35   The adjusted contractor disease factor is determined by:
   (i)   calculating the national range of raw contractor disease prevalence in
         England and applying a 5% cut-off at the bottom of the range.
         Contractors below this will be treated as having the same prevalence
         as the cut-off point. This recognises the fixed costs of providing care
         and provides a measure of financial protection for those with very
         low prevalence. There will not, however, be a cut-off at the top of the
         distribution, so as to recognise and reward those with the highest
         prevalence
   (ii) once the cut-off has been applied, making a square root
         transformation of all the contractor prevalence figures. This means
         that the prevalence distribution will be compressed to within a
         narrower range. It will prevent financial destabilisation of those with
         the lowest prevalence and reflects the workload consequences of
         participation in the clinical domain in practices with the lowest
         prevalence
   (iii) after the transformation, re-basing the contractor figures around the
         new national mean to give the ADPF. For example, an ADPF of 1.2
         indicates a 20% greater prevalence than the mean, in the adjusted
         distribution. The re-basing ensures that the average contractor
         receives £75 per point, after adjustment.
       The factor adjusts the contractor's average pound per point for each
       disease, rather than the contractor's points score. It does not adjust
       payments in the other domains.

Prevalence data collection

3.36   The ADPF is a measure of relative recorded disease prevalence within
       individual countries. Disease register information will be extracted from

the clinical systems of all contractors at the same time, through automated links, and aggregated by the new Quality Management and Analysis System (QMAS) to calculate the national recorded prevalence for each disease area. Contractors will know approximately what their prevalence will be from the reports available on QMAS throughout the year.

3.37   From 2005, 14 February will be National Prevalence Day. This is as late in the financial year as possible whilst enabling prompt payment of achievement rewards by the end of April. Contractors that are not using the QMAS system will have to send each PCT details of their disease prevalence for each of the QOF disease areas they are working towards for the prevalence data collection. They will need to send to the PCT (i) the number of patients on the disease register for each disease area and (ii) the total number of registered patients, as measured on 14 February. This is information that practices should already have, given being able to produce a disease register is the first indicator in each clinical area.

3.38   Contractors will be asked to submit this data by 21 February from 2005. Those that do not submit by 14 March, but are participating in the QOF, will be treated as having the lowest national contractor prevalence (see above for more details) when their achievement payment is calculated. They will not be included in the national calculation of contractor prevalence factors. Contractors that are not working towards the QOF clinical domain, or are not working towards certain of the disease areas, will not be included in the prevalence collection as appropriate. PCTs should remind contractors of the approaching data collection and confirm which disease areas the contractor plans to achieve against.

Dispensing

Regulations

47.   Provision of dispensing services

(1)   Without prejudice to any separate right one or more medical practitioners may have under regulation 20 of the Pharmaceutical Regulations (arrangements for provision of pharmaceutical services by doctors), a contractor may provide dispensing services to its registered patients under the contract only if it is authorised or required to do so by the PCT in accordance with the following provisions of this paragraph or paragraph 49.

(2) A PCT may authorise or require a contractor to provide dispensing services to a registered patient only if that patient –
(a) satisfies one of the conditions in sub-paragraph (3); and
(b) has requested the contractor in writing to provide him with dispensing services.

(3) The conditions referred to in sub-paragraph (2)(a) are that the patient –
(a) satisfies the PCT that he would have serious difficulty in obtaining any necessary drugs, medicines or appliances from a pharmacy by reason of distance or inadequacy of means of communication; or
(b) is resident in a controlled locality at a distance of more than 1.6 kilometres from any pharmacy, and both the conditions in sub-paragraph (4) are satisfied in his case.

(4) The conditions referred to in sub-paragraph (3)(b) are that –
(a) the contractor has been granted consent to dispense under paragraph 48 in respect of –
(i) the area in which the patient resides, and
(ii) the contract under which the patient receives primary medical services; and
(b) any conditions imposed in connection with that grant under regulation 12(15) or 13(13)(b) of the Pharmaceutical Regulations as they apply pursuant to paragraph 48(5) or (6) are such as to permit dispensing services to be provided under this paragraph by that contractor to the patient.

(5) If a contractor which has been requested to provide dispensing services by a patient who satisfies one of the conditions in sub-paragraph (3) –
(a) applies to the PCT for the right to provide dispensing services to that patient, and sends with its application the patient's request to the contractor, the PCT shall grant its application; or
(b) does not so apply, within the period of 30 days beginning with the date on which the patient made that request, a PCT may, subject to sub-paragraph (7), require the contractor to provide dispensing services to that patient, and shall give the contractor notice in writing to that effect.

(6) An application granted by a PCT under sub-paragraph (5)(a) shall, with effect from the date of the patient's request to the contractor, enable that contractor to provide dispensing services to that patient, so long as the contract remains in effect.

(7) A PCT shall not, under sub-paragraph (5)(b), require a contractor to provide dispensing services to a patient if the contractor satisfies the PCT that –
(a) it does not normally provide dispensing services under the contract; or

(b) in the case of a patient to whom sub-paragraph (3)(b) applies, the patient would not have serious difficulty by reason of distance or inadequacy of means of communication in obtaining drugs, medicines or appliances from a pharmacy.

(8)   A PCT shall give the contractor reasonable notice –

    (a) that it requires it to provide dispensing services to a registered patient in accordance with the contract; or

    (b) that, subject to sub-paragraph (9), where a patient no longer satisfies the requirements of sub-paragraph (3), the contractor shall discontinue the provision of dispensing services to that patient.

(9)   A notice under sub-paragraph (8)(b) –

    (a) shall be subject to any postponement or termination of arrangements to provide dispensing services under this paragraph in accordance with conditions imposed under regulation 12(15) or 13(13) of the Pharmaceutical Regulations as they apply pursuant to paragraph 48(5) or (6); and

    (b) shall not be given –

       (i) pending the outcome of the resolution of any dispute concerning the decision by a PCT to postpone the making or termination of arrangements to provide dispensing services under this paragraph in accordance with conditions referred to in paragraph (a); or

      (ii) during the period for bringing an appeal, or pending the determination of any appeal, referred to in regulation 9(10) of the Pharmaceutical Regulations (determination of whether an area is a controlled locality).

(10)   A contractor which has been granted the right under this paragraph to provide dispensing services to some or all of its registered patients may provide any necessary dispensing services to a person whom that contractor has accepted as a temporary resident.

(11)   In this paragraph, "controlled locality" and "pharmacy" have the same meanings as in the Pharmaceutical Regulations.

48. Consent to dispense

(1)   A contractor which wishes to be granted the right under paragraph 47 to secure the provision of dispensing services to some or all of its registered patients may apply to the PCT in writing for consent to dispense, specifying –

    (a) the area; and

    (b) the contract,

in relation to which it wishes the consent to dispense to be granted.

(2) An application under sub-paragraph (1) shall be determined by the PCT in accordance with regulations 12 and 13 of the Pharmaceutical Regulations (as modified in accordance with sub-paragraphs (5) and (6)), as though it were an application under regulation 21 of those Regulations.

(3) Consent to dispense, in relation to the specified contract, shall have effect from its final grant but shall cease to have effect if –
 (a) no dispensing services have been provided under that contract within 12 months from the final grant of the consent to dispense; or
 (b) more than 12 months has elapsed since the last provision of dispensing services under that contract pursuant to the grant of consent.

(4) In sub-paragraph (3), "final grant" shall be construed in accordance with regulation 12(16) of the Pharmaceutical Regulations.

(5) Regulation 12 of the Pharmaceutical Regulations shall apply as if modified as follows –
 (a) all references to provisions being "subject to regulation 6A" were omitted;
 (b) for all references to regulation 21, there were substituted references to this paragraph;
 (c) in paragraph (14), the reference to "regulation 4(4)" were omitted; and
 (d) in paragraph (15) –
  (i) for "regulation 20" there were substituted a reference to paragraph 47, and
  (ii) for the reference to "provision by a doctor of pharmaceutical services" there were substituted a reference to provision by a contractor of dispensing services.

(6) Regulation 13 of the Pharmaceutical Regulations shall apply as if modified as follows –
 (a) in paragraph (2), for "regulation 20" there were substituted a reference to paragraph 47; and
 (b) in paragraph (13)(b) –
  (i) for "regulation 20" there were substituted a reference to paragraph 47, and
  (ii) for the reference to "provision by a doctor of pharmaceutical services" there were substituted a reference to provision by a contractor of dispensing services.

49. Contractors who previously provided dispensing services under pilot schemes or section 28C arrangements

(1) This paragraph applies where, immediately before the commencement of the contract –

(a) one of the persons specified in sub-paragraph (2), was a pilot doctor in the area of the PCT; or

(b) the contractor was providing primary medical services in the area of the PCT in accordance with section 28C arrangements,

and the requirements in sub-paragraph (3) are met.

(2) The persons referred to in sub-paragraph (1) are –

(a) the contractor;

(b) in the case of a contract with two or more individuals practising in partnership, one or more of those individuals; or

(c) in the case of a contract with a company, one or more of the legal and beneficial shareholders in that company.

(3) The requirements referred to in sub-paragraph (1) are that –

(a) the pilot doctor, or, as the case may be, the contractor was, immediately before the commencement of the contract, providing dispensing services to some or all of his or its patients under the pilot scheme or in accordance with the section 28C arrangements; and

(b) the contractor has notified the PCT before entering into the contract that it intends to provide dispensing services under it.

(4) In a case to which this paragraph applies, the contractor shall be regarded –

(a) as being authorised or required under paragraph 47 to provide dispensing services under the contract to any patient –

(i) to whom, immediately before commencement of the contract, it or, as the case may be, the pilot doctor, provided dispensing services under the pilot scheme or section 28C arrangement, and

(ii) who wishes the contractor to continue to provide him with such services; and

(b) subject to sub-paragraph (5), as having been granted consent to dispense in relation to the contract under paragraph 48 in relation to the area for which it or, as the case may be, the pilot doctor, had such consent under the pilot scheme or section 28C arrangement.

(5) Paragraph 48(3) shall apply in relation to a contract to which this paragraph applies as if the references to the final grant of the consent to dispense were references to the date of commencement of the contract.

(6) In this paragraph "pilot doctor" means a medical practitioner who performs personal medical services in connection with a pilot scheme.

50. Terms relating to the provision of dispensing services

(1) A contractor which has been granted the right to provide dispensing services under paragraph 47 or 49 shall ensure that dispensing services are provided in accordance with the following sub-paragraphs.

(2) Subject to sub-paragraphs (3) and (4), a contractor providing dispensing services shall –

    (a) record an order for the provision of any drugs, medicines or appliances which are needed for the treatment of the patient on a prescription form completed in accordance with paragraph 39(3);

    (b) provide those drugs, medicines or appliances in a suitable container;

    (c) provide for the patient a drug or medicine specified in any directions given by the Secretary of State under section 28U of the Act (GMS contracts: prescription of drugs etc.) as being a drug or medicine which can only be ordered for specified patients and specified purposes only if –

        (i) that patient is a person of the specified description, and

        (ii) the drug or medicine is supplied for that patient only for the specified purpose; and

    (d) provide for the patient a restricted availability appliance only if the patient is a person, or it is for a purpose, specified in the Drug Tariff.

(3) Sub-paragraph (2) does not apply to drugs, medicines or appliances ordered on a prescription form by an independent nurse prescriber.

(4) Where a patient presents an order on a prescription form for drugs, medicines or appliances signed by an independent nurse prescriber, or an order for a restricted availability appliance signed by and endorsed on its face with the reference "SLS" by an independent nurse prescriber, to a contractor who may provide dispensing services, the contractor may provide to the patient such of the drugs, medicines or appliances so ordered as it supplies in the normal course of its practice.

(5) Drugs, medicines or appliances provided under sub-paragraph (4) shall be provided in a suitable container.

(6) A contractor providing dispensing services shall not provide for a patient a drug or medicine specified in any directions given by the Secretary of State under section 28U of the Act as being drugs or medicines which may not be ordered for patients in the provision of medical services under the contract, except that, where it has ordered a drug or medicine which has an appropriate non-proprietary name either by the name or by its formula, it may provide a drug or medicine which has the same specification notwithstanding that it is a drug or medicine specified in such directions (but, in the case of a drug or medicine which combines more than one drug, only if the combination has an appropriate non-proprietary name).

(7) Subject to sub-paragraph (9), nothing in this paragraph shall prevent a contractor providing a Scheduled drug or a restricted availability appliance in the course of treating a patient under a private arrangement.

(8)   A contractor providing dispensing services shall comply with paragraph
11B of Schedule 2 to the Pharmaceutical Regulations [90], as if modified
as follows –
(a) for "paragraph 11(a)", substitute "sub-paragraph (3)(a)";
(b) for "paragraph 11A(2)", substitute "sub-paragraph (5)";
(c) for "a doctor who is authorised or required by the Health Authority
or PCT under regulation 20 to provide drugs and appliances to a
patient", substitute "a contractor providing dispensing services to a
patient"; and
(d) for "doctor", substitute "medical practitioner".

(9)   The provisions of regulation 24 (fees and charges) apply in respect of the
provision of any drugs, medicines or appliances by a contractor
providing dispensing services as they apply in respect of prescriptions for
drugs, medicines or appliances.

(10)   A contractor who is entitled to provide dispensing services may, with the
consent of the patient, order a drug, medicine or appliance for a patient
on a prescription form or a repeatable prescription, rather than
providing it itself.

51.   Dispensing contractor list

(1)   Where the contractor is authorised or required by the PCT under
paragraph 47 or 49 to provide dispensing services to its patients and is
actually doing so, the PCT shall include –
(a) the contractor's name; and
(b) the address of the practice premises from which it is authorised or
required to dispense,
on a list of such contractors (to be called the dispensing contractors list)
which it shall prepare, maintain and publish.

(2)   The PCT shall remove the name of the contractor from the list referred
to in sub-paragraph (1) where –
(a) the contractor's consent to dispense ceases to have effect pursuant to
paragraph 48(3); or
(b) the contractor ceases to provide dispensing services to its patients for
any other reason.

52.   Provision of drugs, medicines and appliances for immediate treatment or personal administration

(1)   Subject to sub-paragraph (2), a contractor –
(a) shall provide to a patient any drug, medicine or appliance, not being
a Scheduled drug, where such provision is needed for the immediate

treatment of that patient before a provision can otherwise be obtained; and

(b) may provide to a patient any drug, medicine or appliance, not being a Scheduled drug, which he personally administers or applies to that patient,

but shall, in either case, provide a restricted availability appliance only if it is for a person or a purpose specified in the Drug Tariff.

(2) Nothing in sub-paragraph (1) authorises a person to supply any drug or medicine to a patient otherwise than in accordance with Part 3 of the Medicines Act 1968 or any regulations or orders made thereunder.

Statement of Financial Entitlement

18. DISPENSING

18.1 Some contractors are authorised or required to provide dispensing services to specific patients. The arrangements for this are set out in Part 3 of Schedule 6 to the 2004 Regulations.

Costs in respect of which reimbursement is payable

18.2 Where drugs and appliances are provided by a medical practitioner –
(a) in accordance with the terms relating to the provision of dispensing services set out in paragraph 50 in Part 3 of Schedule 6 to the 2004 Regulations (or related transitional arrangements); or
(b) either for immediate treatment or for personal administration, in accordance with paragraph 52 in Part 3 of Schedule 6 to the 2004 Regulations,
then subject to the following provisions of this Section, the PCT must pay to the contractor under its GMS contract the payments listed in paragraph 18.3, as calculated in accordance with this Section.

18.3 The payable payments in relation to the provision of drugs and appliances are –
(a) the basic price of the drug or appliance, which is the price as defined in Part II, Clauses 8 and 11, of the Drug Tariff, less a discount calculated in accordance with Part 1 of Annex I;
(b) an on-cost allowance of 10.5% of the basic price of the drug or appliance before the deduction of the discount referred to in sub-paragraph (a);
(c) a container allowance of 3.8 pence per prescription;
(d) the appropriate dispensing fee, as set out in Part 2 of Annex I (in respect of contractors authorised or required to provide dispensing

services in accordance with Part 3 of Schedule 6 to the 2004 Regulations) or Part 3 of Annex I (in respect of all other contractors);

(e) unless the contractor is registered with Customs and Excise for VAT purposes, an allowance to cover the VAT payable on the purchase of drugs, appliances and containers. The allowance is to be calculated as a percentage of –

    (i) the basic price of the drug or appliance before the deduction of the discount referred to in sub-paragraph (a), and

    (ii) the container allowance referred to in sub-paragraph (c),

and for these purposes, the rate payable shall be equivalent to the percentage rate of VAT in force on the first day of the quarter in which the items were dispensed; and

(f) exceptional expenses, as provided for in Part II, clause 12, of the Drug Tariff.

Personally administered drugs and appliances, and those used for diagnosis

18.4 A contractor who is providing services under a GMS contract may, whether or not the contractor is authorised or required to provide dispensing services to specific patients, be entitled to the payments listed in paragraph 18.3. This applies only in relation to the following products–

(a) vaccines, anaesthetics and injections;

(b) the following diagnostic reagents: Dick Test; Schick Test; Protein Sensitisation Test Solutions; and Tuberculin Tests (i.e. Koch Test, Mantoux Test, Patch Test and Diagnostic Jelly);

(c) intrauterine contraceptive devices (including drug-releasing IUCDs, contraceptive caps and diaphragms);

(d) pessaries which are appliances; and

(e) sutures (including skin closure strips).

18.5 In respect of these products, subject to the provisions of this Section, the PCT must pay to all contractors under their GMS contracts the payments listed in paragraph 18.3, as calculated in accordance with this Section – if the products are provided in accordance with paragraph 52(1)(a) or (b) in Part 3 of Schedule 6 to the 2004 Regulations.

Products not covered by this Section

18.6 No payments are payable under this Section in respect of the following products (which are centrally supplied vaccines): HiB (*Haemophilus influenzae* type B); MMR (Measles, Mumps and Rubella); BCG (Bacillus Calmette–Guérin); Diphtheria Vaccine Adsorbed (Child); Low dose

Diphtheria vaccine for adults (adsorbed); D/T (Diphtheria/Tetanus); D/T/P (Diphtheria/Tetanus/ Pertussis); D/T/P-HiB (Diphtheria/Tetanus/ Pertussis and *Haemophilus influenzae* type B combined product for administration as one injection); Td ampoule presentation (Tetanus combined with Diphtheria Vaccine for adults); Pertussis; oral Polio; inactivated Polio; Tuberculin Purified Protein Derivative; Meningococcal C conjugate vaccine (for children under five and persons entering the first year of higher education); and Menigococcal A and C polysaccharide vaccine (for persons entering the first year of higher education).

18.7   If a medical practitioner issues a prescription for a drug or appliance instead of supplying it himself, no payments are payable in respect of that drug or appliance under this Section.

Oxygen and oxygen therapy equipment

18.8   The payments listed in paragraph 18.3 do not apply in respect of the supply of oxygen and oxygen therapy equipment. These are covered by separate arrangements set out in Part 4 of Annex I.

Deductions in respect of charges

18.9   Payment in respect of prescriptions shall be subject to any deduction required to be made under the National Health Service (Charges for Drugs and Appliances) Regulations 2000[24] in respect of charges required to be made and recovered by the dispensing practitioner.

Contractors unable to obtain discounts

18.10   If a contractor satisfies the PCT that, by reason of the remoteness of the contractor's practice premises, the contractor is unable to obtain any discount on the basic price of drugs and appliances for which a payment is payable by the PCT under this section (and the PCT must consult the LMC, if there is one, before being so satisfied), the PCT must approve an exemption for that contractor from the application of the discount scale. The exemption shall be granted for a period of up to 1 year, and may be renewed thereafter for further periods, each not exceeding 1 year, if the contractor is able to satisfy the PCT that it is still unable to obtain any discount on the basic price of drugs and appliances for which a payment is payable under this section.

---

24   S.I. 2000620 as amended by 2000/122, 2001/746 and 2887, 2002/548 and 2352 and 2003/699, 585, 1084 and 3189.

18.11   Where a PCT approves such an exemption, it must inform the
        Prescription Pricing Authority (PPA) of the exemption and of the period
        for which it is to apply.

Contractors that are to receive special payments

18.12   If a contractor satisfies the PCT that –
        (a) by reason of the remoteness of the contractor's practice premises or
            the small quantities of drugs and appliances that the contractor
            needs to buy, the contractor has had to pay more than the basic price
            for drugs and appliances it orders; and
        (b) its payments under paragraph 18.3(a) should be calculated at special
            payment levels rather than basic price levels,
        (and the PCT must consult the LMC, if there is one, before being so
        satisfied), the PCT must agree to reimburse the contractor on the basis of
        the special payment levels, instead of the basic price levels, of the drugs
        and appliances it supplies, as set out in the table below.

Where on average the price paid by the contractor (excluding VAT) has been:	Special payment price level
In excess of 5% and up to 10% over the basic price	5% over the basic price
In excess of 10% and up to 15% over the basic price	10% over the basic price
In excess of 15% and up to 20% over the basic price	15% over the basic price
In excess of 20% over the basic price	20% over the basic price

18.13   However –
        (a) the VAT allowance (see paragraph 18.3(f)) shall be calculated on the
            basis of the basic price; and
        (b) the on-cost allowance (see paragraph 18.3(b)) shall be calculated on
            the basis of the basic price (with no discount deducted).

18.14   Agreement to reimburse on the basis of special payment levels shall be
        granted for a period of up to 1 year, and may be renewed thereafter if the
        contractor is still able to satisfy the PCT that its payments under
        paragraph 18.3(a) should be calculated at special payments levels rather
        than basic price levels.

Preconditions before payments under this Section are payable

18.15   The payments listed in paragraph 18.3 are only payable if the contractor has –

(a) noted, counted and sent all the prescriptions in respect of drugs or appliances in respect of which it wishes to claim reimbursement to the PPA, Bridge House, 152 Pilgrim Street, Newcastle-upon-Tyne NE1 6SN, not later than the 5th of the month following the month to which the prescriptions relate; and

(b) included all the claims under cover of a single claim form, and divided all the prescriptions into two bundles (for the calculation of the dispensing fee), and –

   (i)   one of these two bundles must be of prescription forms in respect of which no charge is payable, because –

   (aa)   the patient is entitled to an exemption,

   (bb)   the drugs or appliances were no-charge contraceptives, or

   (cc)   the drugs or appliances were personally administered items, and are in the list in paragraph 18.4, and

   (ii)   the other of these two bundles must be of prescription forms in respect of which a charge is payable, whether or not the charge has been collected (if the prescription form is for more than one item, at least one of which is chargeable, it should be included in this bundle),

   and if the claim is in respect of the following high-volume personally administered vaccines – influenza, typhoid, hepatitis A, hepatitis B, pneumococcal, and meningococcal – it must be made in the form of bulk entries on the claim form.

Payment arrangements

18.16   Where a contractor has satisfied the conditions in paragraph 18.15, the PCT must pay to the contractor under its GMS contract –

(a) on the first day of the month after the month on which the contractor submitted its claim to the PPA, an amount that represents 80% of the amount that the PCT reasonably estimates is likely to be due to the contractor in respect of the claim, once the PPA has certified the amount due in respect of the claim (having taken into account the charges that are required to be made and recovered), although the PCT may pay less than 80% if the contractor's claims each month in respect of prescriptions vary significantly; and

(b) on the first day of the second month after the month on which the contractor submitted its claim to the PPA, the balance of the amount due in respect of the claim, having had that amount certified by the PPA, and taking into account –

(i) the charges that are required to be made and recovered, and

(ii) the amount already paid out in respect of the claim pursuant to sub-paragraph (a).

Accounting obligations

18.17 It is a condition of the payments payable under this section that the payments are only payable under this section if the contractor ensures that –

(a) its actual expenditure on drugs and appliances (i.e. the amount it pays its suppliers) is shown "gross" on its practice accounts, and

(b) its payments from PCTs pursuant to this section, and collected from patients in accordance with the National Health Service (Charges for Drugs and Appliances) Regulations 2000, are brought "gross" into its contractor accounts as "income".

Standard Contract

Provision of dispensing services

304. Without prejudice to any separate right one or more medical practitioners may have under regulations 20 of the *Pharmaceutical Regulations*, *the* Contractor may provide *dispensing services* to its *registered patients* under the Contract only if it is authorised or required to do so by the PCT in accordance with clauses 305 to 314 and clauses 321 to 325.

305. The PCT may authorise or require the Contractor to provide *dispensing services* to a *registered patient* only if that *patient* –

305.1 satisfies one of the conditions in clause 306; and

305.2 has requested the Contractor in writing to provide him with *dispensing services*.

306. The conditions referred to in clause 305.1 are that the patient –

306.1 satisfies the PCT that he would have serious difficulty in obtaining any necessary drugs, medicines or appliances from a pharmacy by reason of distance or inadequacy of means of communication; or

306.2 is resident in a controlled locality at a distance of more than 1.6 kilometres from any pharmacy, and both the conditions in clause 307 are satisfied in his case.

307. The conditions referred to in clause 306.2 are that –

307.1 the Contractor has been granted consent to dispense under clauses 315 to 320 in respect of –

307.1.1 the area in which the patient resides, and

307.1.2 the contract under which the patient receives primary
medical services; and

307.2 any conditions imposed in connection with that grant under
regulation 12(15) or 13(13) of the *Pharmaceutical Regulations* as
they apply pursuant to clauses 319 or 320 are such as to permit
dispensing services to be provided under clauses 304 to 314 by the
Contractor to the patient.

308. If the Contractor has been requested to provide *dispensing services* by a
patient who satisfies one of the conditions in clause 306, and the
Contractor –

308.1 applies to the PCT for the right to provide dispensing services to
that patient, and sends with its application the patient's request to
the Contractor, the PCT shall grant its application; or

308.2 does not so apply within the period of 30 days beginning with the
date on which the patient made that request, the PCT may, subject
to clause 310, require the Contractor to provide dispensing services
to that patient, and shall give the Contractor notice in writing to
that effect.

309. An application granted by the PCT under clause 308.1 shall, with effect
from the date of the patient's request to the Contractor, enable the
Contractor to provide *dispensing services* to that patient, so long as the
Contract remains in effect.

310. The PCT shall not, under clause 308.2, require the Contractor to
provide *dispensing services* to a patient if the Contractor satisfies the
PCT that –

310.1 it does not normally provide *dispensing services* under the
Contract; or

310.2 in the case of a patient to whom clause 306.2 applies, the patient
would not have serious difficulty by reason of distance or
inadequacy of means of communication in obtaining drugs,
medicines or appliances from a pharmacy.

311. The PCT shall give the Contractor reasonable notice –

311.1 that it requires it to provide *dispensing services* to a *registered
patient* in accordance with the Contract; or

311.2 that, subject to clause 312 where a patient no longer satisfies the
requirements of clause 306, the Contractor shall discontinue the
provision of *dispensing services* to that patient.

312. A notice under clause 311 –

312.1 shall be subject to any postponement or termination of
arrangements to provide *dispensing services* under clauses 304 to
314 in accordance with conditions imposed under regulation

12(15) or 13(13) of the *Pharmaceutical Regulations* as they apply pursuant to clauses 319 or 320; and

312.2 shall not be given –

    312.2.1 pending the outcome of the resolution of any dispute concerning the decision by the PCT to postpone the making or termination of arrangements to provide *dispensing services* under clauses 304 to 314 in accordance with conditions referred to in clause312.2.1; or

    312.2.2 during the period for bringing an appeal, or pending the determination of any appeal, referred to in regulation 9(10) of the *Pharmaceutical Regulations* (determination of whether an area is a controlled locality).

313. If the Contractor has been granted the right under clauses 304 to 312 to provide *dispensing services* to some or all of its *registered patients*, it may provide any necessary *dispensing services* to a person whom the Contractor has accepted as a *temporary resident*.

314. In clauses 304 to 312, "controlled locality" and "pharmacy" have the same meanings as in the *Pharmaceutical Regulations*.

Consent to dispense

315. If the Contractor wishes to be granted the right under clauses 304 to 314 to secure the provision of *dispensing services* to some or all of its *registered patients*, it may apply to the PCT in writing for consent to dispense, specifying –

315.1 the area; and

315.2 the contract,

in relation to which it wishes the consent to dispense to be granted.

316. An application under clause 315 shall be determined by the PCT in accordance with regulations 12 and 13 of the *Pharmaceutical Regulations* (as modified in accordance with clauses 319 and 320), as though it were an application under regulation 21 of those Regulations.

317. Consent to dispense, in relation to the Contract, shall have effect from its final grant but shall cease to have effect if –

317.1 no *dispensing services* have been provided under the Contract within 12 months from the final grant of the consent to dispense; or

317.2 more than 12 months has elapsed since the last provision of *dispensing services* under the Contract pursuant to the grant of consent.

318. In clause 317, "final grant" shall be construed in accordance with regulation 12(16) of the *Pharmaceutical Regulations*.

319. Regulation 12 of the *Pharmaceutical Regulations* shall apply as if modified as follows –
    319.1 all references to provisions being "subject to regulation 6A" were omitted;
    319.2 for all references to regulation 21, there were substituted references to clauses 315 to 320;
    319.3 in paragraph (14), the reference to "regulation 4(4)" were omitted; and
    319.4 in paragraph (15), for "regulation 20" there were substituted a reference to clauses 304 to 314 above, and for the reference to "provision by a doctor of pharmaceutical services" there were substituted a reference to provision by the Contractor of *dispensing services*.

320. Regulation 13 of the *Pharmaceutical Regulations* shall apply as if modified as follows –
    320.1 in paragraph (2), for "regulation 20" there were substituted a reference to clauses 304 to 314 above; and
    320.2 in paragraph (13)(b), for "regulation 20" there were substituted a reference to clauses 304 to 314 above, and for the reference to "provision by a doctor of pharmaceutical services" there were substituted a reference to provision by the Contractor of *dispensing services*.

Contractors who previously provided *dispensing services* under a *pilot scheme* or *section 28C arrangements*

321. Clauses 324 and 325 apply where, immediately before the commencement of the Contract –
    321.1 one of the persons specified in clause 322, was a *pilot doctor* in the area of the PCT; or
    321.2 the Contractor was providing primary medical services in the area of the PCT in accordance with *section 28C arrangements*,
    and the requirements of clause 323 are met.

322. The persons referred to in clause 321 are –
    322.1 the Contractor;
    322.2 if the Contract is with a partnership, one or more of the partners;
    322.3 if the Contract is with a company, one or more of the legal and beneficial shareholders in that company.

323. The requirements referred to in clause 321 are that –
    323.1 the *pilot doctor*, or, as the case may be, the Contractor was, immediately before the commencement of the Contract, providing

dispensing services to some or all of his or its patients under the *pilot scheme* or in accordance with *section 28C arrangements*; and

323.2. the Contractor has notified the PCT before entering into the Contract that it intends to provide *dispensing services* under it.

324. In a case falling within clause 321, the Contractor shall be regarded –

324.1 as being authorised or required under clauses 304 to 314 to provide *dispensing services* under the Contract to any patient –

324.1.1 to whom, immediately before commencement of the Contract, it or, as the case may be, the *pilot doctor*, provided *dispensing services* under the *pilot scheme* or *section 28C arrangements*, and

324.1.2 who wishes the Contractor to continue to provide him with such services; and

324.2 subject to clause 325, as having been granted consent to dispense in relation to the Contract under clauses 315 to 320 in relation to the area for which it or, as the case may be, the *pilot doctor*, had such consent under the *pilot scheme* or *section 28C arrangements*.

325. Where clauses 321 to 324 apply, clause 317 shall apply to the Contract as if the references to the final grant of the consent to dispense were references to the date of the commencement of the Contract.

Terms relating to the provision of *dispensing services*

326. Where the Contractor which has been granted the right to provide *dispensing services* under clauses 304 to 314 or clauses 321 to 325, it shall ensure that *dispensing services* are provided in accordance with clauses 327 to 335.

327. Subject to clauses 328 and 329, the Contractor providing *dispensing services* shall –

327.1 record an order for the provision of any drugs, medicines or appliances which are needed for the treatment of the patient on a *prescription form* completed in accordance with clause 272;

327.2 provide those drugs, medicines or appliances in a suitable container;

327.3 provide for the patient a drug or medicine specified in any directions given by *the Secretary of State* under section 28U of *the Act* as being a drug or medicine which can only be ordered for specified patients and specified purposes only if –

327.3.1 that patient is a person of the specified description, and

327.3.2 the drug or medicine is supplied for that patient only for the specified purpose; and

327.4 provide for the *patient* a *restricted availability appliance* only if the patient is a person, or it is for a purpose, specified in the *Drug Tariff*.

328. Clause 327 does not apply to drugs, medicines or appliances ordered on a *prescription form* by an *independent nurse prescriber*.

329. Where a patient presents an order on a *prescription form* for drugs, medicines or appliances signed by an *independent nurse prescriber*, or an order for a *restricted availability appliance* signed by and endorsed on its face with the reference "SLS" by an *independent nurse prescriber*, to a Contractor who may provide *dispensing services*, the Contractor may provide to the patient such of the drugs, medicines or appliances so ordered as it supplies in the normal course of its practice.

330. Drugs, medicines or appliances provided under clause 329 shall be provided in a suitable container.

331. If the Contractor is providing *dispensing services*, it shall not provide for a patient a drug or medicine specified in any directions given by *the Secretary of State* under section 28U of *the Act* as being drugs or medicines which may not be ordered for patients in the provision of medical services under the Contract, except that, where it has ordered a drug or medicine which has an appropriate non-proprietary name either by the name or by its formula, it may provide a drug or medicine which has the same specification notwithstanding that it is a drug or medicine specified in such directions (but, in the case of a drug or medicine which combines more than one drug, only if the combination has an appropriate non-proprietary name).

332. Subject to clause 334, nothing in clauses 326 to 331, 333 and 335 shall prevent a medical practitioner providing a *Scheduled drug* or a *restricted availability appliance* in the course of treating a patient under a private arrangement.

333. If the Contractor is providing *dispensing services*, it shall comply with paragraph 11B of Schedule 2 to the *Pharmaceutical Regulations*, modified as follows –
    333.1 for "paragraph 11(a)", substitute "sub-paragraph (3)(a)";
    333.2 for "paragraph 11A(2)", substitute "sub-paragraph (5)";
    333.3 for "a doctor who is authorised or required by the Health Authority or PCT under regulation 20 to provide drugs and appliances to a patient", substitute "a Contractor providing dispensing services to a patient"; and
    333.4 for "doctor", substitute "medical practitioner".

334. The provisions of Part 18 apply in respect of the provision of any drugs, medicines or appliances by the Contractor if it is providing *dispensing services* as they apply in respect of prescriptions for drugs, medicines or appliances.

335. If the Contractor is entitled to provide *dispensing services*, it may, with the consent of the patient, order a drug, medicine or appliance for a patient on a *prescription form* or a *repeatable prescription*, rather than providing it itself.

Dispensing contractor list

336. If the Contractor is authorised or required by the PCT under clauses 304 to 314 or clauses 321 to 325 to provide *dispensing services* to its patients and is actually doing so, the PCT shall include –
336.1 the Contractor's name; and
336.2 the address of the *practice premises* from which it is authorised or required to dispense
on a list of such contractors (to be called the dispensing contractors list) which the PCT shall prepare, maintain and publish.

337. The PCT shall remove the name of the Contractor from the list referred to in clause 336 where the Contractor's consent to dispense ceases to have effect pursuant to clause 317, or if the Contractor ceases to provide *dispensing services* to its patients for any other reason.

● Dispute resolution

Regulations

99. Local resolution of contract disputes

(1) Subject to sub-paragraph (3), in the case of any dispute arising out of or in connection with the contract, the contractor and the PCT must make every reasonable effort to communicate and co-operate with each other with a view to resolving the dispute, before referring the dispute for determination in accordance with the NHS dispute resolution procedure (or, where applicable, before commencing court proceedings).

(2) Either the contractor or the PCT may, if it wishes to do so, invite the LMC for the area of the PCT to participate in discussions which take place pursuant to sub-paragraph (1).

(3) In the case of a dispute which falls to be dealt with under the procedure specified in paragraph 36, sub-paragraph (1) does not apply where it is not practicable for the parties to attempt local resolution before the expiry of the period specified in paragraph 36(4).

100. Dispute resolution: non-NHS contracts

(1)   In the case of a contract which is not an NHS contract, any dispute arising out of or in connection with the contract, except matters dealt with under the complaints procedure pursuant to Part 6 of this Schedule, may be referred for consideration and determination to the Secretary of State, if –
(a) the PCT so wishes and the contractor has agreed in writing; or
(b) the contractor so wishes (even if the PCT does not agree).

(2)   In the case of a dispute referred to the Secretary of State under sub-paragraph (1) –
(a) the procedure to be followed is the NHS dispute resolution procedure; and
(b) the parties agree to be bound by any determination made by the adjudicator.

101. NHS dispute resolution procedure

(1)   Subject to sub-paragraph (2), the procedure specified in the following sub-paragraphs and paragraph 102 applies in the case of any dispute arising out of or in connection with the contract which is referred to the Secretary of State –
(a) in accordance with section 4(3) of the 1990 Act (where the contract is an NHS contract); or
(b) in accordance with paragraph 100(1) (where the contract is not an NHS contract).

(2)   The procedure specified in this paragraph and paragraph 102 does not apply where a contractor refers a matter for determination in accordance with paragraph 36(1) of this Schedule, and in such a case the procedure specified in that paragraph shall apply instead.

(3)   Any party wishing to refer a dispute as mentioned in sub-paragraph (1) shall send to the Secretary of State a written request for dispute resolution which shall include or be accompanied by –
(a) the names and addresses of the parties to the dispute;
(b) a copy of the contract; and
(c) a brief statement describing the nature and circumstances of the dispute.

(4)   Any party wishing to refer a dispute as mentioned in sub-paragraph (1) must send the request under sub-paragraph (3) within a period of 3 years beginning with the date on which the matter giving rise to the dispute happened or should reasonably have come to the attention of the party wishing to refer the dispute.

(5) Where the dispute relates to a contract which is not an NHS contract, the Secretary of State may determine the matter himself or, if he considers it appropriate, appoint a person or persons to consider and determine it.

(6) Before reaching a decision as to who should determine the dispute, either under sub-paragraph (5) or under section 4(5) of the 1990 Act, the Secretary of State shall, within the period of 7 days beginning with the date on which a matter was referred to him, send a written request to the parties to make in writing, within a specified period, any representations which they may wish to make about the matter.

(7) The Secretary of State shall give, with the notice given under sub-paragraph (6), to the party other than the one which referred the matter to dispute resolution a copy of any document by which the matter was referred to dispute resolution.

(8) The Secretary of State shall give a copy of any representations received from a party to the other party and shall in each case request (in writing) a party to whom a copy of the representations is given to make within a specified period any written observations which it wishes to make on those representations.

(9) Following receipt of any representations from the parties or, if earlier, at the end of the period for making such representations specified in the request sent under sub-paragraph (6) or (8), the Secretary of State shall, if he decides to appoint a person or persons to hear the dispute –
   (a) inform the parties in writing of the name of the person or persons whom he has appointed; and
   (b) pass to the person or persons so appointed any documents received from the parties under or pursuant to paragraph (3), (6) or (8).

(10) For the purpose of assisting him in his consideration of the matter, the adjudicator may –
   (a) invite representatives of the parties to appear before him to make oral representations either together or, with the agreement of the parties, separately, and may in advance provide the parties with a list of matters or questions to which he wishes them to give special consideration; or
   (b) consult other persons whose expertise he considers will assist him in his consideration of the matter.

(11) Where the adjudicator consults another person under sub-paragraph (10)(b), he shall notify the parties accordingly in writing and, where he considers that the interests of any party might be substantially affected by the result of the consultation, he shall give to the parties such

opportunity as he considers reasonable in the circumstances to make observations on those results.

(12) In considering the matter, the adjudicator shall consider –
   (a) any written representations made in response to a request under sub-paragraph (6), but only if they are made within the specified period;
   (b) any written observations made in response to a request under sub-paragraph (8), but only if they are made within the specified period;
   (c) any oral representations made in response to an invitation under sub-paragraph (10)(a);
   (d) the results of any consultation under sub-paragraph (10)(b); and
   (e) any observations made in accordance with an opportunity given under sub-paragraph (11).

(13) In this paragraph, "specified period" means such period as the Secretary of State shall specify in the request, being not less than 2, nor more than 4, weeks beginning with the date on which the notice referred to is given, but the Secretary of State may, if he considers that there is good reason for doing so, extend any such period (even after it has expired) and, where he does so, a reference in this paragraph to the specified period is to the period as so extended.

(14) Subject to the other provisions of this paragraph and paragraph 102 and to any agreement by the parties, the adjudicator shall have wide discretion in determining the procedure of the dispute resolution to ensure the just, expeditious, economical and final determination of the dispute.

102. Determination of dispute

(1) The adjudicator shall record his determination and the reasons for it, in writing and shall give notice of the determination (including the record of the reasons) to the parties.

(2) In the case of a contract referred for determination in accordance with paragraph 100(1), subsection (8) of section 4 of the 1990 Act shall apply as that subsection applies in the case of a contract referred for determination in accordance with subsection (3) of section 4 of that Act.

(3) In the case of a contract referred for determination in accordance with paragraph 100(1), subsection (5) of section 28W of the Act shall apply as that subsection applies in the case of a contract referred for determination in accordance with subsection (3) of section 4 of the 1990 Act.

103. Interpretation of Part 7

(1)   In this Part, "any dispute arising out of or in connection with the contract" includes any dispute arising out of or in connection with the termination of the contract.

(2)   Any term of the contract that makes provision in respect of the requirements in this Part shall survive even where the contract has terminated.

Standard Contract

Local resolution of contract disputes

517.   Subject to clause 519, in the case of any dispute arising out of or in connection with the Contract, the Contractor and the PCT must make every reasonable effort to communicate and co-operate with each other with a view to resolving the dispute, before referring the dispute for determination in accordance with the *NHS dispute resolution procedure* (or, where applicable, before commencing court proceedings).

518.   Either the Contractor or the PCT may, if it wishes to do so, invite the *Local Medical Committee* for the area of the PCT to participate in discussions which take place pursuant to clause 517.

519.   In the case of a dispute which falls to be dealt with under the procedure specified in paragraph 36 of Schedule 6 to *the Regulations*, clause 517 does not apply where it is not practicable for the parties to attempt local resolution before the expiry of the 7-day period specified in paragraph 36(4) of Schedule 6 to *the Regulations*.

Dispute resolution: non-NHS contracts[25]

520.   Any dispute arising out of or in connection with the Contract, except matters dealt with under the complaints procedure set out in clauses 499 to 515 of this Contract, may be referred for consideration and determination to *the Secretary of State*, if:
520.1 the PCT so wishes and the Contractor has agreed in writing; or
520.2 the Contractor so wishes (even if the PCT does not agree).

521.   In the case of a dispute referred to the Secretary of State under clause 520, the procedure to be followed is the *NHS dispute resolution procedure*,

---

25   These clauses are mandatory terms only if the contract is not an NHS contract. Otherwise, the clauses should be deleted from the Contract.

and the parties agree to be bound by a determination made by the
adjudicator.

NHS dispute resolution procedure

522. Subject to clause 523, the *NHS dispute resolution procedure* applies in the case of any dispute arising out of or in connection with the Contract which is referred to *the Secretary of State* in accordance with [section 4(3) of the *1990 Act* / clause 520 above],[26] and the PCT and the Contractor shall participate in the *NHS dispute resolution procedure* as set out in paragraphs 101 and 102 of Schedule 6 to *the Regulations*.

523. The *NHS dispute resolution procedure* does not apply where the Contractor refers a matter for determination in accordance with clause 262, and in such a case the procedure specified in paragraph 36 of Schedule 6 to *the Regulations* shall apply instead.

524. Any party wishing to refer a dispute shall send to *the Secretary of State* a written request for dispute resolution which shall include or be accompanied by –
    524.1 the names and addresses of the parties to the dispute;
    524.2 a copy of the Contract; and
    524.3 a brief statement describing the nature and circumstances of the dispute.

525. Any party wishing to refer a dispute as mentioned in clause 522 must send the request under clause 524 within a period of 3 years beginning with the date on which the matter giving rise to the dispute happened or should reasonably have come to the attention of the party wishing to refer the dispute.

526. In clauses 517 to 525 "any dispute arising out of or in connection with the contract" includes any dispute arising out of or in connection with the termination of the contract.

527. Part 24 shall survive the expiry or termination of the Contract.

Guidance

6.33 The new GMS contract contains comprehensive appeal processes, referred to as dispute resolution. These can cover issues ranging from

---

26 If the contract is an NHS contract, the parties must select the phrase "section 4(3) of the 1990 Act". If the contract is not an NHS contract, the parties must select the phrase "clause 520 above".

decisions about contractual sanctions and termination through to matters such as remuneration, list closure, practice area, patient assignment, and opt-outs. As a rule of thumb virtually all disputes will be capable of being referred for adjudication. Dispute resolution does not apply to complaints made under the NHS complaints system as set out in the GMS Contract Regulations.

6.34 It is expected that most contractual disputes can be resolved as part of the normal contractual relationship. Use of the formal dispute resolution procedures will usually represent a failure of that relationship and should be avoided where possible. PCTs and GMS contractors should make every reasonable effort to communicate and co-operate with each other in an attempt to resolve any disputes before considering referring the dispute for determination in accordance with the dispute resolution procedure, or to the Courts. This is a requirement under the contract. Reaching local solutions will make best use of the resources available for the local population, will help to develop a partnership approach between contractor and PCT, and will avoid additional bureaucracy and cost for both parties. Local resolution might involve, where necessary, board-level involvement in conciliation meetings and neither side should be afraid to use appropriately skilled and qualified advisers. In addition both the PCT and the GMS contractor may, if either so wishes, invite the LMC to participate in any discussions. If no solution can be found locally it will be open to either part to the dispute to refer a matter to dispute resolution.

Who appeals are determined by

6.35 Where a dispute arises out of or in connection with a NHS contract either party may refer to matter to the FHSAA (SHA) or, where appropriate, the SHA or FHSAA, for consideration and determination. The procedures are set out in paragraphs 36 and 100 to 101 of Schedule 6 to the GMS Regulations. Directions will provide for the FHSAA (SHA) to deal with most cases, but it will be able to appoint an adjudicator to act on its behalf. SHAs will deal with cases that involve the list closure or patient assignment procedures described in chapter 2.

6.36 Such disputes should therefore be addressed directly to either the FHSAA (SHA) or, where appropriate, the local SHA. The FHSAA (SHA) address is:

FHSAA(SHA)
30 Victoria Avenue
Harrogate HG1 5PR.

The Chief Executive of the FHSAA (SHA) is Mr Paul Burns.

6.37   The one exception to paragraphs 6.35 and 6.36 is a dispute concerning contract termination where the termination relates to a member of the contracting body (or the body itself) no longer meeting the conditions set out in paragraph 110 or 112 of Schedule 6 of the GMS Regulations. Appeals against a PCT decision that the relevant conditions have been broken go to the independent FHSAA. Its address is set out in paragraph 6.31.

6.38   Disputes where the contractor is not a NHS body can be referred to either the FHSAA (SHA) or a competent court. Where the contractor wishes to follow the NHS process it should express that choice in writing. Any such dispute should follow the procedure set out for NHS contracts. It is important to note that the resulting determination will be binding on both parties.

● Duty of co-operation

Regulations

12.   Duty of co-operation in relation to additional, enhanced and out-of-hours services

(1)   A contractor which does not provide to its registered patients or to persons whom it has accepted as temporary residents –
     (a) a particular additional service;
     (b) a particular enhanced service; or
     (c) out-of-hours services, either at all or in respect of some periods or some services,
shall comply with the requirements specified in sub-paragraph (2).

(2)   The requirements referred to in sub-paragraph (1) are that the contractor shall –
     (a) co-operate, insofar as is reasonable, with any person responsible for the provision of that service or those services;
     (b) comply in core hours with any reasonable request for information from such a person or from the PCT relating to the provision of that service or those services; and
     (c) in the case of out-of-hours services, take reasonable steps to ensure that any patient who contacts the practice premises during the out-of-hours period is provided with information about how to obtain services during that period.

(3)   Nothing in this paragraph shall require a contractor whose contract does not include the provision of out-of-hours services to make itself available during the out-of-hours period.

13.   Where a contractor is to cease to be required to provide to its patients –
(a) a particular additional service;
(b) a particular enhanced service; or
(c) out-of-hours services, either at all or in respect of some periods or some services,
it shall comply with any reasonable request for information relating to the provision of that service or those services made by the PCT or by any person with whom the Trust intends to enter into a contract for the provision of such services.

Standard Contract

Duty of co-operation in relation to *additional, enhanced* and *out-of-hours services*[27]

41.   If the Contractor is not, pursuant to the Contract, providing to its *registered patients* or to persons whom it has accepted as *temporary residents* –
41.1 a particular *additional service*;
41.2 a particular *enhanced service*; or
41.3 *out-of-hours services*, either at all or in respect of some periods or some services,
the Contractor shall comply with the requirements specified in clause 42.

42.   The requirements referred to in clause 41 are that the Contractor shall –
42.1 co-operate, insofar as is reasonable, with any person responsible for the provision of that service or those services;
42.2 comply in *core hours* with any reasonable request for information from such a person or from the PCT relating to the provision of that service or those services; and
42.3 in the case of *out-of-hours services*, take reasonable steps to ensure that any *patient* who contacts the *practice premises* during the *out-of-hours period* is provided with information about how to obtain services during that period.

---

27   Although not every aspect of clauses 41 to 44 will be relevant to every Contractor, these clauses should be left in every GMS Contract as, in many cases, a Contractor will not be providing each *additional service*, each *enhanced service* and *out-of-hours services*: these clauses have been drafted so that they can be left in the Contract even if that were to be the case. These clauses are required by paragraph 12 of Schedule 6 to *the Regulations*.

43.   Nothing in clauses 41 and 42 shall require the Contractor (if it is not providing *out-of-hours services* under the Contract) to make itself available during the *out-of-hours period*.

44.   If the Contractor is to cease to be required to provide to its *patients* –
44.1 a particular *additional service*;
44.2 a particular *enhanced service*; or
44.3 *out-of-hours services*, either at all or in respect of some periods or some services,
it shall comply with any reasonable request for information relating to the provision of that service or those services made by the PCT or by any person with whom the Trust intends to enter into a contract for the provision of such services.

Duty to secure primary medical services

Guidance

2.3   The Health and Social Care (Community Health and Standards) Act 2003 places PCTs under a new duty to provide or secure the provision of primary medical services. This will take effect from 1 April 2004. The Act says that a PCT must commission or provide primary medical services to the extent that it considers it necessary to meet all reasonable requirements. This duty underpins the Patient Services Guarantee set out in chapter 6 of *Investing in General Practice*. PCTs are advised that to fulfil the duty they must commission sufficient (i) essential services, (ii) additional services (or equivalent; the term only relates to GMS), and (iii) out-of-hours services, to meet the needs of their whole population. This means that where contractors opt out of additional services or out-of-hours care, PCTs must ensure effective alternative provision is in place at the time that opt-outs take effect.

Employment law

Guidance

4.16   GMS contractors are obliged to:
(i)   provide written terms and conditions of service in contracts

(ii)   not unfairly dismiss an employee

(iii)   allow for ante-natal care, maternity leave, paternity leave, adoption leave, and parental leave, if their employees satisfy the relevant entitlement conditions under employment legislation for those types of leave. Additionally, employees have common law rights to a reasonable amount of time off, where necessary, to care for dependants. Employees of contractors will, if they qualify, be entitled to statutory sick pay from the contractor for 28 weeks of absence on account of sickness in any 3 years

(iv)   not discriminate on the grounds of gender, marital status, race, colour, disability or Trade Union membership (additionally, as a matter of policy, we expect GMS providers not to discriminate on the grounds of age, religion, creed or sexual orientation)

(v)   not to make deductions from wages without agreement

(vi)   consult fully and make appropriate payments in a redundancy situation

(vii)   recognise the rights of staff transferred from another NHS employer, and

(viii)   comply with the Public Interest Disclosure Act 1998 which gives full protection of the law to all self-employed NHS professionals who act in the public interest. The Department of Health is working with Public Concern at Work to produce guidance on whistleblowing for use in primary medical services.

Enhanced services – definition and monitoring

Guidance

(i) Definition and monitoring arrangements

2.77   PCTs will be placed under a duty through directions to commission all six current Directed Enhanced Services (DES) to meet the needs of their population. In line with paragraph 2.13 of *Investing in General Practice*, the Contract Regulations define enhanced services as follows:

"medical services other than essential services, additional services or out-of-hours services; or

essential services, additional services or out-of-hours services or an element of such a service that a contractor agrees under the contract to provide in accordance with specifications set out in a plan, which requires of the contractor an enhanced level of service provision to that which it needs generally to provide in relation to that service or element of service".

The Contract Regulations allow the medical services to be of any type, in any setting, and to extend beyond the scope of primary medical services. There is no legal constraint as to what types of NHS medical services a PCT can commission through the four provider routes described in section A of this chapter. This will give PCTs a broad ability to develop more integrated services across the primary, secondary and acute sectors.

2.78 However, for the purposes of financial monitoring, the definition of enhanced services is drawn more tightly than the legal definition. PCTs will be notified of their enhanced services expenditure floor level in the January 2004 allocations, which they will be expected to meet but can exceed. PCTs will need to consider carefully what constitutes an enhanced service for the purpose of accurate financial monitoring. This will be undertaken at national level by the joint BMA/NHS Confederation/Health Departments Technical Steering Committee. Whilst a precise national definition would not be sufficiently sensitive to local issues, PCTs and contractors should bear in mind that, generally speaking, the following spend would count towards the floor:
   (i) commissioning, or direct PCT provision, of Directed, National or Locally Enhanced Services from any provider, not just GMS and PMS contractors
   (ii) Practitioners With a Special Interest (PWSIs) except in relation to essential or additional services
   (iii) the plus element of PMS Plus and the specialist element of specialist PMS arrangements
   (iv) local primary medical care incentive schemes commissioned from GMS or PMS providers
   (v) if the PCT proposed, for example, to re-commission a service that had previously been placed with a NHS trust it would count towards the floor, regardless of the outcome of the contest, but only providing that:
       (a) it was contestable for GMS and PMS contractors
       (b) it is a service that might reasonably be provided by GMS and PMS contractors, for example because looking across the UK there are other such contractors delivering similar services.

2.79 The following would not count:
   (i) spend on primary medical services that is funded through other routes described in chapter 5, such as primary care administered funding (e.g. spend on appraisal), spend on essential services (including greenfield and brownfield sites), and spend on any

additional or out-of-hours services (except where spend is for the purpose of delivering services to a higher standard than that normally required)

(ii) baseline spend on services provided through Trusts or other providers, for example an accident and emergency-based minor injuries service commissioned from an acute trust, or existing services delivered by GPs in community hospitals or as clinical assistants. These baseline services cannot be included for as long as the existing contracts are simply rolled forward.

2.80   PCTs are expected to draw up initial plans for commissioning of enhanced services to meet, or exceed, their local floor during February 2004. These should include proposals for commissioning the six DESs. These should then be signed off by their Professional Executive Committee. The LMC should be consulted about the proposed level of spend, and the PCT should seek to obtain LMC agreement that the proposed services count within the above definition for financial monitoring purposes. Where there is a dispute over what counts towards the floor, the LMC and PCT should seek to resolve this locally in the first instance. Disputes over what counts towards the floor should not delay the commissioning of the service. Where a dispute remains unresolved, the PCT would need to indicate in its financial returns to the Department that the level of spend is disputed. The TSC would then in turn note that some of the funding within its assessment of spend is disputed. It is important that PCTs keep copies of correspondence with LMCs; they may need to send these to the Department to inform the TSC's monitoring of the Gross Investment Guarantee, which is described in chapter 5.

PCT commissioning of

2.82   PCTs will be under a legal obligation to commission services for violent patients (from 1 February 2004), influenza immunisations, and minor surgery (both from 1 April 2004). These can be commissioned from any provider, or the PCT can provide the service itself. However, it is likely that PCTs will in most instances want to commission these services from the patients' own GMS and PMS contractors, to ensure continuity of care.

2.83   The main purpose of enhanced services is to expand the range of local services to meet local need, improve convenience and choice and ensure value for money. Before making commissioning decisions PCTs are advised to bear in mind what contractors are legally obliged to provide under the definitions of essential and additional services set out in sections B and D of this chapter.

2.84   The PCT commissions enhanced services as primary medical services; they only become GMS services when they are provided as part of a GMS contract. The PCT has discretion to draw up specifications on the basis of local need and it can also decide when it wants to commission most enhanced services. For example, a PCT could choose to commission minor surgery from a PMS or commercial contractor using a different specification and at a different price from the GMS NES specification. Nonetheless, PCTs may wish to be guided by the twelve GMS Nationally Enhanced Specifications in the *Supplementary Documents*. GMS contractors may expect, and may only be willing, to offer enhanced services on the basis of the GMS NES specifications and prices. Commissioning decisions are entirely a matter of local negotiation (and the contract dispute resolution procedure described in chapter 6 does not apply); PCTs will want to make commissioning decisions on the basis of quality, accessibility, choice, and value for money. PCTs will also want to consider the duration of such contracts.

Entire agreement

Standard Contract

601.   Subject to Part 10 (opt-outs of *additional* and *out-of-hours services*), clauses 376, 385 and 406 and any variations made in accordance with Part 25, this Contract constitutes the entire agreement between the parties with respect to its subject matter.

602.   The Contract supersedes any prior agreements, negotiations, promises, conditions or representations, whether written or oral, and the parties confirm that they did not enter into the Contract on the basis of any representations that are not expressly incorporated into the Contract. However, nothing in this Contract purports to exclude liability on the part of either party for fraudulent misrepresentation.

Equity and probity – ensuring of

Guidance

3.66   All contractors have a legitimate expectation that the QOF will be applied in a fair manner within and across PCTs. This will be ensured through:

(i) application of the national rules set out in this chapter, and mechanisms to ensure that they are not being misapplied (including through dispute resolution procedures described in chapter 6), or deliberately flouted

(ii) QMAS providing consistency of calculations

(iii) consistency of approach for PCT visits and training of assessors.

3.67 PCTs should note that the QOF is built on the principle of high trust. The systems described thus far in this chapter have been designed to minimise bureaucracy and intrusion for the vast majority of contractors that will submit accurate QOF data. In order for the high trust system to operate, it is necessary to have robust mechanisms in place to deal with the extremely small minority of contractors that may seek to submit incorrect claims and obtain falsely inflated levels of rewards. PCTs have a duty both to financial auditors in respect of the proper use of public funds, and to ensure fairness for the honest majority.

3.68 The PCT is required to confirm all achievement payments before they are made. For most contractors this will be automatic. In the following exceptional cases, the achievement payment may not automatically be paid by April:

(i) where monthly reports and/or annual visits throw up issues around data accuracy, and these have not been remedied in sufficient time to the satisfaction of the PCT. This could for example include –

(a) inexplicably low or high numbers of patients on disease registers given the PCT average prevalence, e.g. as a result of not coding or miscoding patient records, or

(b) unusually high levels of exception-reporting.

These should normally be assessed during the practice visit. In the event of data accuracy being questioned during a visit, the contractor and PCT will draw up a remedial plan, which the contractor will normally implement within a month of the visit, and the PCT will seek to confirm it has been implemented within a further 2 weeks. Given the last visits would take place by the end of January, this would then enable achievement payments to be made by the end of April. In the event of remedial action not having taken place to the satisfaction of the PCT, the PCT could re-score the achievement points, following consultation with the LMC. This is in line with paragraph 3.31 of *Investing in General Practice*. Contractors would be able to challenge such decisions under the dispute resolution procedure

(ii) if a PCT has evidence which shows that a contractor has been systematically and inappropriately referring patients to secondary care in order to maximise quality achievement points, the PCT could re-score the achievement points calculation. Again, this would follow consultation with the LMC, and be subject to appeal. The QOF is intended to reward contractors for the work that they are doing, rather than for work that is carried out on their patients in secondary care and funded by the PCT

(iii) where there is a substantial unexplained variation between aspiration and achievement. The assessment of likely achievement arising from the PCT visit should normally significantly reduce the likelihood of this occurrence. If such variations do occur, the PCT would be under a financial obligation to make further inquiries to satisfy itself of the validity of the claim before making payment

(iv) in the event of suspected fraud or other illegality.

3.69   If the PCT has concerns in relation to 3.68 (i)–(iii), it should discuss these in the first instance with the contractor. The PCT can ask the practice for more information to support its achievement claim. The PCT may also wish to check the practice's records in more detail, or ask to see certain documents.

3.70   Where the PCT has good reason to suspect fraud, it should involve the NHS Counter Fraud and Security Management Services (CFSMS) at the earliest opportunity. Any fraud or attempt to defraud relating to QOF payments will be treated as seriously as other forms of NHS fraud, and could lead to criminal prosecution. It could also lead to visits without notice or the contractor's consent.

3.71   A random 5% sample of contractors will also be checked thoroughly as part of counter-fraud measures. Wherever possible, this will draw on the pre-existing written material provided for the annual review, to minimise bureaucracy. Where checks require a visit, this would normally occur as part of the following year's annual visit, to minimise disruption to contractors and their patients.

● Essential services

Standard Contract

45.   The Contractor must provide the services described in clauses 46 to 51 (*essential services*) at such times, within *core hours*, as are appropriate to meet the reasonable needs of its patients, and to have in place arrangements for its patients to access such services throughout the *core hours* in case of emergency.[28]

---

28   This clause is also required by regulation 20 of *the Regulations*.

46.   The Contractor must provide –

46.1   services required for the management of the Contractor's *registered patients* and *temporary residents* who are, or believe themselves to be –

46.1.1 ill with conditions from which recovery is generally expected;

46.1.2 terminally ill; or

46.1.3 suffering from chronic disease

delivered in the manner determined by the *practice* in discussion with the patient;

46.2   appropriate ongoing treatment and care to all *registered patients* and *temporary residents* taking account of their specific needs including –

46.2.1 the provision of advice in connection with the patient's health, including relevant health promotion advice; and

46.2.2 the referral of the patient for other services under *the Act*; and

46.2.3 primary medical services required in *core hours* for the immediately necessary treatment of any person to whom the Contractor has been requested to provide treatment owing to an accident or emergency at any place in its *practice area.*

47.   For the purposes of clause 46.1, "management" includes –

47.1   offering a consultation and, where appropriate, physical examination for the purpose of identifying the need, if any, for treatment or further investigation; and

47.2   the making available of such treatment or further investigation as is necessary and appropriate, including the referral of the patient for other services under *the Act* and liaison with other *health care professionals* involved in the patient's treatment and care.

48.   For the purposes of clause 46.3, "emergency" includes any medical emergency whether or not related to services provided under the Contract.

49.   The Contractor must provide primary medical services required in *core hours* for the immediately necessary treatment of any person falling within clause 50 who requests such treatment, for the period specified in clause 51.

50.   A person falls within this clause if he is a person –

50.1   whose application for inclusion in the Contractor's list of patients has been refused in accordance with clauses 180 to 183 and who is not registered with another provider of *essential services* (or their equivalent) in the area of the PCT;

50.2 whose application for acceptance as a *temporary resident* has been rejected under clauses 180 to183; or

50.3 who is present in the Contractor's *practice area* for less than 24 hours.

51. The period referred to in clause 49 is –

51.1 in the case of clause 50.1, 14 days beginning with the date on which that person's application was refused or until that person has been registered elsewhere for the provision of *essential services* (or their equivalent), whichever occurs first;

51.2 in the case of clause 50.2, 14 days beginning with the date on which that person's application was rejected or until that person has been subsequently accepted elsewhere as a *temporary resident*, whichever occurs first; and

51.3 in the case of clause 50.3, 24 hours or such shorter period as the person is present in the Contractor's *practice area.*

Guidance

2.18 Chapter 2 of *Investing in General Practice* defined essential services. The Department of Health, the NHS Confederation and the GPC have agreed that this definition is best translated into regulation 15 of the Contract Regulations as follows:

"(3) The services described in this paragraph are services required for the management of its registered patients and temporary residents who are –

(a) ill, or believe themselves to be ill, with conditions from which recovery is generally expected;

(b) terminally ill; or

(c) suffering from chronic disease,

delivered in the manner determined by the practice in discussion with the patient.

(4) For the purposes of paragraph (3) –

"disease" means a disease included in the list of three-character categories contained in the tenth revision of the International Statistical Classification of Diseases and Related Health Problems;[29] and

"management" includes –

(a) offers of consultation to and, where appropriate, physical examination for the purpose of identifying the need, if any, for treatment or further investigation; and

29 World Health Organisation, 1992, ISBN 92 4 1544 19 8 (v. I). NLM Classification: WB 15.

(b) the making available of such treatment or further investigation as is necessary and appropriate, including the referral of the patient for other services under the Act and liaison with other health care professionals involved in the patient's treatment and care.

(5) The other services described in this paragraph are the provision of appropriate ongoing treatment and care to all registered patients and temporary residents taking account of their specific needs including –

(a) the provision of advice in connection with the patient's health, including relevant health promotion advice; and

(b) the referral of the patient for other services under the Act."

2.19 PCTs and contractors are invited to note the following points:

(i) chronic disease is as defined in the International Statistical Classification of Diseases and Related Health Problems. This includes, for example, patients with disabilities, patients suffering from long-term conditions including for example hypertension or infertility but who are otherwise healthy, and patients suffering from mild to moderate psychopathic disorders. The contractor must provide services to the extent that the condition can be dealt with appropriately in a primary care setting

(ii) paragraph (5) of Regulation 15 reflects paragraph 2.10 of *Investing in General Practice*, which refers to "continuous holistic treatment and care". To reflect this paragraph (5) provides an obligation for all contractors to provide "appropriate ongoing treatment and care for all registered patients and temporary residents taking account of their specific needs". Paragraph (5) includes an obligation on the contractor to provide advice in connection with the patient's health, including relevant health promotion advice.

Additional services are not essential services and so if a contractor has opted out of providing these, it clearly does not have to provide them under essential services.

(iii) the specifications for enhanced services in *Supplementary Documents* make clear that "no part of the specification by commission, omission or implication defines or redefines essential or additional services". PCTs should note that, with certain exceptions, GMS contractors are funded through the global sum and MPIG to provide the equivalent services for which they were previously funded under existing GMS. Exceptions are set out in the mapping diagram in *Supplementary Documents*:

(a) influenza immunisation is now commissioned as a DES, and the childhood vaccinations and immunisation target payments are also a DES

(b) part of the funding for cervical cytology is in the Quality and Outcomes Framework

(c) the funding for intra partum care is also in enhanced services

(d) part of the funding for minor surgery is in enhanced services. In addition, following the new definition of the contraceptive additional service, intrauterine contraceptive devices and contraceptive implants are not funded through the global sum and MPIG, but through enhanced services.

Essential services – definition of

Regulations

15. Essential services

(1) For the purposes of section 28R(1) of the Act (requirement to provide certain primary medical services), the services which must be provided under a general medical services contract ("essential services") are the services described in paragraphs (3), (5), (6) and (8).

(2) Subject to regulation 20, a contractor must provide the services described in paragraphs (3) and (5) throughout the core hours.

(3) The services described in this paragraph are services required for the management of its registered patients and temporary residents who are, or believe themselves to be –

(a) ill, with conditions from which recovery is generally expected;

(b) terminally ill; or

(c) suffering from chronic disease,

delivered in the manner determined by the practice in discussion with the patient.

(4) For the purposes of paragraph (3) –

"disease" means a disease included in the list of three-character categories contained in the tenth revision of the International Statistical Classification of Diseases and Related Health Problems; and

"management" includes –

(a) offering consultation and, where appropriate, physical examination for the purpose of identifying the need, if any, for treatment or further investigation; and

    (b) the making available of such treatment or further investigation as is necessary and appropriate, including the referral of the patient for other services under the Act and liaison with other health care professionals involved in the patient's treatment and care.

(5)   The services described in this paragraph are the provision of appropriate ongoing treatment and care to all registered patients and temporary residents taking account of their specific needs including –
    (a) the provision of advice in connection with the patient's health, including relevant health promotion advice; and
    (b) the referral of the patient for other services under the Act.

(6)   A contractor must provide primary medical services required in core hours for the immediately necessary treatment of any person to whom the contractor has been requested to provide treatment owing to an accident or emergency at any place in its practice area.

(7)   In paragraph (6), "emergency" includes any medical emergency whether or not related to services provided under the contract.

(8)   A contractor must provide primary medical services required in core hours for the immediately necessary treatment of any person falling within paragraph (9) who requests such treatment, for the period specified in paragraph (10).

(9)   A person falls within paragraph (8) if he is a person –
    (a) whose application for inclusion in the contractor's list of patients has been refused in accordance with paragraph 17 of Schedule 6 and who is not registered with another provider of essential services (or their equivalent) in the area of the PCT;
    (b) whose application for acceptance as a temporary resident has been rejected under paragraph 17 of Schedule 6; or
    (c) who is present in the contractor's practice area for less than 24 hours.

(10)   The period referred to in paragraph (8) is –
    (a) in the case of paragraph (9)(a), 14 days beginning with the date on which that person's application was refused or until that person has been subsequently registered elsewhere for the provision of essential services (or their equivalent), whichever occurs first;
    (b) in the case of paragraph (9)(b), 14 days beginning with the date on which that person's application was rejected or until that person has been subsequently accepted elsewhere as a temporary resident, whichever occurs first; and
    (c) in the case of paragraph (9)(c), 24 hours or such shorter period as the person is present in the contractor's practice area.

Flexible Career Scheme

Statement of Financial Entitlement.

16. FLEXIBLE CAREERS SCHEME

16.1 This is an established Scheme for certain part-time doctors. It is managed locally by Postgraduate Deaneries and is for employed doctors only. Contractors are eligible for contractor payments under this Scheme, but will also receive payments to be forwarded to doctors.

Flexible Careers Scheme Contractor Payments

16.2 A PCT must pay to a contractor under its GMS contract a Flexible Career Scheme (FCS) Contractor Payment if –
(a) it employs a part-time doctor who is a member of the FCS; and
(b) that FCS doctor performs primary medical services under its GMS contract, as a medical practitioner, with a working commitment that generates a Time Commitment Fraction of at least one-fifth but not more than five-ninths, except that the doctor may also work –
　(i) an additional 28 hours, during the membership year, of funded education time for personal and professional development, and
　(ii) a limited amount of additional time in the NHS, with the approval of his local Director of Postgraduate GP Education.

16.3 For the purposes of the calculation of time commitment in paragraph 16.2(b), the following periods of leave are discounted –
(a) annual leave up to a maximum of 6 weeks pro rata (compared to full-time);
(b) maternity, paternity, parental or adoption leave endorsed by the PCT;
(c) sickness leave endorsed by the PCT;
(d) special leave in an emergency, which is granted in accordance with employment law and guidance issued by the Department of Trade and Industry; and
(e) other special leave for pressing personal or family reasons, endorsed by the PCT.

Amount of FCS Contractor Payments

16.4 PCTs will need to obtain from the contractor at the end of each quarter a return of the actual cost to the contractor, rounded to the nearest pound, of it employing the FCS doctor while he is a member of the scheme. This is –

(a) to include salary, national insurance contributions and NHS pension scheme contributions;

(b) not to include costs relating to any additional work the FCS doctor is permitted, with the approval of his local Director of Postgraduate GP Education, to undertake outside the FCS.

16.5 A percentage of that amount is then payable as the contractor's FCS Contractor Payment, as calculated (subject to the following provisions of this Section) in accordance with the following table.

In respect of doctors whose applications to join the FCS have been received by their local Director of Postgraduate GP Education before 1 January 2004 and who join the scheme before 1 April 2004	
Year 1	50%
Year 2	50%
Year 3	25%
Year 4	10%
In respect of other FCS doctors	
Year 1	50%
Year 2	25%
Year 3	10%

16.6 For these purposes –

(a) the qualifying date for the first payment, and so the start of the doctor's first year in the Scheme, is the date the doctor joins the Scheme;

(b) if, in relation to any period of leave referred to in paragraph 16.3 the local Director of Postgraduate GP Education reasonably determines that, for exceptional reasons, the year of membership of the FCS in which the period of leave started should be extended, that year of membership shall not be taken to have elapsed until a full year has elapsed from the start of that year of membership, discounting the period of leave, and his qualifying date for payments must be adjusted accordingly; and

(c) if the quarterly return relates to costs incurred in respect of different years of membership of the FCS, the contractor must specify which costs relate to which year of membership of the scheme.

Amount of FCS Doctor Payments

16.7   Subject to the following provisions of this Section, if a contractor is eligible for a FCS contractor payment, the PCT must also pay to the contractor under its GMS contract, in respect of the doctor who is a member of the FCS, an annual FCS Doctor Payment of £1050.

Payments in respect of part years

16.8   If –
(a) an FCS doctor's membership of the FCS ceases during a year of membership; or
(b) an FCS doctor moves to a new employer during a year of membership of the FCS but remains a member of the scheme,
the amount of the FCS Doctor Payment payable to the contractor is to be adjusted by multiplying the amount of the payment otherwise payable by the following fraction: the number of days for which the FCS doctor is contracted to work for the contractor during the membership year, divided by 365.

Payments in respect of educational sessions

16.9   In respect of each of up to eight educational sessions attended in a year of membership of the FCS by an FCS doctor, and on the basis of a return from the contractor at the end of each quarter, the PCT must reimburse the contractor who employs the FCS doctor under its GMS contract for–
(a) the actual cost of employing the FCS doctor during those sessions (to be determined in accordance with paragraph 16.5 above); and
(b) any expenses claimed by and paid to the FCS doctor by the contractor to cover the cost of his actual travel and subsistence in attending those sessions, if these costs are reasonable in the opinion of the PCT.

Payment arrangements

16.10   FCS Doctor Payments to the contractor are to fall due on the last day of the month during which his qualifying date falls, taking account of any adjustment of his qualifying date in accordance with paragraph 16.6.

16.11   The other payments under this Section are to fall due on the last day of the month following the quarter in respect of the quarterly return is made.

Conditions attached to Flexible Career Scheme payments and overpayments

16.12 FCS Contractor Payments and payments under paragraph 16.9(a), or any part thereof, are only payable if the contractor satisfies the following conditions –

(a) the contractor must make available to the PCT any information which the PCT does not have but needs, and the contractor either has or could reasonably be expected to obtain, in order to calculate the payment. In particular, the contractor must, on request, provide the PCT with written records demonstrating the actual costs it is seeking to recover; and

(b) all information supplied pursuant to or in accordance with this paragraph must be accurate.

16.13 FCS Doctor Payments, or any part thereof, are only payable if the following conditions are satisfied –

(a) a contractor that receives an FCS Doctor Payment in respect of a doctor must give that payment to that doctor –

  (i) within one calendar month of it receiving that payment, and

  (ii) as an element of the personal income of that doctor, subject to any lawful deduction of income tax, national insurance and superannuation contributions,

  once it has secured from the doctor an enforceable undertaking that he will repay to the contractor any amount repayable by the contractor to the PCT under this Section in respect of him;

(b) the contractor must inform the PCT if the doctor in respect of whom the payment is made ceases to be a member of the FCS.

16.14 Payments in respect of expenses under paragraph 16.9(b) are only payable if the following conditions are satisfied –

(a) the contractor must make available to the PCT any information which the PCT does not have but needs (including receipts), and the contractor either has or could reasonably be expected to obtain in order to calculate the payment; and

(b) all information provided pursuant to or in accordance with sub-paragraph (a) must be accurate.

16.15 If a contractor breaches the conditions set out in paragraph 16.12 or 16.14, the PCT may in appropriate circumstances withhold payment of any or any part of a payment to which the conditions relate that is otherwise payable.

16.16 If a contractor breaches the conditions in paragraph 16.13, the PCT may require repayment of any payment paid to which the condition relates, or may withhold payment of any other sum payable to the contractor under this SFE, to the value of the payment paid.

16.17 If as a result of the doctor leaving the FCS, the PCT has paid a larger amount to the contractor in respect of a FCS Doctor Payment than the amount to which the contractor is entitled, the PCT may require repayment of the excess paid, or may withhold payment of any other sum payable to the contractor under this SFE, to the value of the excess paid.

16.18 Where, pursuant to paragraph 16.16 or 16.17, a contractor is required to repay any or any part of a RS Doctor Payment, the arrangements by which the contractor may seek to enforce the undertaking referred to in paragraph 16.13(a) as a consequence of that repayment are a matter for the contractor.

Force majeure[30]

Standard Contract

607. Neither party shall be responsible to the other for any failure or delay in performance of its obligations and duties under this Contract which is caused by circumstances or events beyond the reasonable control of a party. However, the affected party must promptly on the occurrence of such circumstances or events:

607.1 inform the other party in writing of such circumstances or events and of what obligation or duty they have delayed or prevented being performed; and

607.2 take all action within its power to comply with the terms of this Contract as fully and promptly as possible.

608. Unless the affected party takes such steps, clause 607 shall not have the effect of absolving it from its obligations under this Contract. For the avoidance of doubt, any actions or omissions of either party's personnel or any failures of either party's systems, procedures, premises or equipment shall not be deemed to be circumstances or events beyond the reasonable control of the relevant party for the purposes of this clause, unless the cause of failure was beyond reasonable control.

609. If the affected party is delayed or prevented from performing its obligations and duties under the Contract for a continuous period of 3 months, then either party may terminate this Contract by notice in

---

30 This clause is not required by the Regulations, but is recommended.

writing within such period as is reasonable in the circumstances (which shall be no shorter than 28 days).

610. The termination shall not take effect at the end of the notice period if the affected party is able to resume performance of its obligations and duties under the Contract within the period of notice specified in accordance with clause 609 above, or if the other party otherwise consents.

Gifts

Regulations

124. Gifts

(1) The contractor shall keep a register of gifts which –
  (a) are given to any of the persons specified in sub-paragraph (2) by or on behalf of –
    (i) a patient,
    (ii) a relative of a patient, or
    (iii) any person who provides or wishes to provide services to the contractor or its patients in connection with the contract; and
  (b) have, in its reasonable opinion, an individual value of more than £100.00.

(2) The persons referred to in sub-paragraph (1) are –
  (a) the contractor;
  (b) where the contract is with two or more individuals practising in partnership, any partner;
  (c) where the contract is with a company –
    (i) any person legally and beneficially holding a share in the company, or
    (ii) a director or secretary of the company;
  (d) any person employed by the contractor for the purposes of the contract;
  (e) any general medical practitioner engaged by the contractor for the purposes of the contract;
  (f) any spouse of a contractor (where the contractor is an individual medical practitioner) or of a person specified in paragraphs (b) to (e); or
  (g) any person (whether or not of the opposite sex) whose relationship with a contractor (where the contractor is an individual medical practitioner) or with a person specified in paragraphs (b) to (e) has the characteristics of the relationship between husband and wife.

(3)   Sub-paragraph (1) does not only apply where –
        (a) there are reasonable grounds for believing that the gift is
            unconnected with services provided or to be provided by the
            contractor;
        (b) the contractor is not aware of the gift; or
        (c) the contractor is not aware that the donor wishes to provide services
            to the contractor.

(4)   The contractor shall take reasonable steps to ensure that it is informed of
        gifts which fall within sub-paragraph (1) and which are given to the
        persons specified in sub-paragraph (2)(b) to (g).

(5)   The register referred to in sub-paragraph (1) shall include the following
        information –
        (a) the name of the donor;
        (b) in a case where the donor is a patient, the patient's NHS number or,
            if the number is not known, his address;
        (c) in any other case, the address of the donor;
        (d) the nature of the gift;
        (e) the estimated value of the gift; and
        (f) the name of the person or persons who received the gift.

(6)   The contractor shall make the register available to the PCT on request.

Standard Contract

492.   The Contractor shall keep a register of gifts which –
        492.1 are given to any of the persons specified in clause 493 by, or on
              behalf of, a patient, a relative of a patient or any person who
              provides or wishes to provide services to the Contractor or its
              patients in connection with the Contract; and
        492.2 have, in its reasonable opinion, a value of more than £100.00.

493.   The persons referred to in clause 492 are –
        493.1 the Contractor;
        493.2 if the Contractor is a partnership, any partner;
        493.3 if the Contractor is a company, any person legally and beneficially
              holding a share in the company, or a director or secretary of the
              company;
        493.4 any person employed by the Contractor for the purposes of the
              Contract;
        493. 5 any *general medical practitioner* engaged by the Contractor for the
              purposes of the Contract;

493.6 any spouse of the Contractor (if the Contractor is an individual medical practitioner) or of a person specified in clauses 493.2 to 493.5; or

493.7 any person (whether or not of the opposite sex) whose relationship with the Contractor (where the Contractor is an individual medical practitioner) or with a person specified in clauses 493.2 to 493.5 has the characteristics of the relationship between husband and wife.

494. Clause 492 does not apply where –

494.1 there are reasonable grounds for believing that the gift is unconnected with services provided or to be provided by the Contractor;

494.2 the Contractor is not aware of the gift; or

494.3 the Contractor is not aware that the donor wishes to provide services to the Contractor.

495. The Contractor shall take reasonable steps to ensure that it is informed of gifts which fall within clause 492 and which are given to the persons specified in clauses 493.2 to 493.7.

496. The register referred to in clause 492 shall include the following information –

496.1 the name of the donor;

496.2 in a case where the donor is a patient, the patient's NHS number or, if the number is not known, his address;

496.3 in any other case, the address of the donor;

496.4 the nature of the gift;

496.5 the estimated value of the gift; and

496.6 the name of the person or persons who received the gift.

497. The Contractor shall make the register available to the PCT on request.

● Global sum

Statement of Financial Entitlement

GLOBAL SUM PAYMENTS

2.1. Global Sum Payments are a contribution towards the contractor's costs in delivering essential and additional services, including its staff costs. Although the Global Sum Payment is notionally an annual amount, it is to be revised quarterly and a proportion paid monthly.

Calculation of a contractor's first Initial Global Sum Monthly Payment

2.2   PCTs must calculate for each contractor the first value of its Initial Global Sum Monthly Payment ("Initial GSMP"). This calculation is to be made by first establishing the contractor's Contractor Registered Population (CRP) –

(a) if the contract takes effect on 1 April 2004 – or is treated as taking effect for payment purposes on 1 April 2004, which will be the case for GMS contracts replacing default contracts – on that date; or

(b) if the contract takes effect (for payment purposes) after 1 April 2004, on the date the contract takes effect.

2.3   Once the contractor's CRP has been established, this number is to be adjusted by the Global Sum Allocation Formula, a summary of which is included in annex B of this SFE. The resulting figure, which is the contractor's Contractor Weighted Population for the quarter, is then to be multiplied by £54. If the PCT is within the area of a London SHA, a London Adjustment is thereafter to be added, which is the contractor's CRP multiplied by £2.18.

2.4   Then, the PCT will need to add to the total produced by paragraph 2.3 (with or without the London Adjustment, as appropriate) these further amounts –

(a) the annual amount of the contractor's Temporary Patients Adjustment. The method of calculating contractors' Temporary Patients Adjustments is set out in annex C;

(b) a Superannuation Premium, which is the contractor's Contractor Weighted Population for the Quarter multiplied by £0;[31] and

(c) from 1 July 2004, an Appraisal Premium, which is the contractor's Contractor Weighted Population for the Quarter multiplied by £0.[32] (The purpose of the appraisal premium is to contribute to the contractor's costs in respect of the appraisal of medical practitioners performing primary medical services under the GMS contract, including the costs of employing locums and the costs of preparing portfolios.)

The resulting amount is then to be divided by 12, and the resulting amount from that calculation is the contractor's first Initial GSMP.

---

31   It is expected that the amount for the financial year 2004/05 will be agreed and inserted in April 2004.

32   It is expected that the amount for the financial year 2004/05 will be agreed and inserted in April 2004.

Calculation of Adjusted Global Sum Monthly Payments

2.5   If the GMS contract stipulates from the outset that the contractor is not to provide one or more of the Additional or Out-of-Hours Services listed in column 1 of the table in this paragraph, the PCT is to calculate an Adjusted GSMP for that contractor as follows. If the contractor is not going to provide –

(a)   one of the Additional or Out-of-Hours Services listed in column 1 of the table, the contractor's Adjusted GSMP will be its Initial GSMP reduced by the percentage listed opposite the service it is not going to provide in column 2 of the table;

(b)   more than one of the Additional or Out-of-Hours Services listed in column 1 of the Table, an amount is to be deducted in respect of each service it is not going to provide. The value of the deduction for each service is to be calculated by reducing the contractor's Initial GSMP by the percentage listed opposite that service in column 2 of the Table, without any other deductions from the Initial GSMP first being taken into account. The total of all the deductions in respect of each service is then deducted from the Initial GSMP to produce the Adjusted GSMP.

Column 1 Additional or out-of-hours services	Column 2 Percentage of initial GSMP
Cervical screening services	1.1
Child health surveillance	0.7
Minor surgery	0.6
Maternity medical services	2.1
Contraceptive services	2.4
Childhood immunisations and pre-school boosters	1.0
Vaccinations and immunisations	2.0
Out-of-hours services	6.0

First Payable Global Sum Monthly Payment

2.6   Once the first value of a contractor's Initial GSMP, and where appropriate Adjusted GSMP have been calculated, the PCT must determine the gross amount of the contractor's Payable GSMP. This is its Initial GSMP or, if it has one, its Adjusted GSMP. The net amount of a contractor's Payable GSMP, i.e. the amount actually to be paid each month, is the gross amount of its Payable GSMP minus any monthly deductions in respect of superannuation determined in accordance with Section 22 (see paragraph 22.6).

2.7 The PCT must pay the contractor its Payable GSMP, thus calculated, monthly (until it is next revised). The Payable GSMP is to fall due on the last day of each month. However, if the contract took effect on a day other than the first day of a month, the contractor's Payable GSMP in respect of the first part-month of its contract is to be adjusted by the fraction produced by dividing –
(a) the number of days during the month in which the contractor was under an obligation under its GMS contract to provide the Essential Services by
(b) the total number of days in that month.

Revision of Payable Global Sum Monthly Payment

2.8 The amount of the contractor's Payable GSMP is thereafter to be reviewed –
(a) at the start of each quarter (when the contractor may have a new Contractor Weighted Population for the quarter);
(b) if there are to be new Additional or Out-of-Hours Services opt-outs (whether temporary or permanent); or
(c) if the contractor is to start or resume providing specific Additional Services that it has not been providing.

2.9 Whenever the Payable GSMP needs to be revised, the PCT will first need to calculate a new Initial GSMP for the contractor (unless this cannot have changed). This is to be calculated in the same way as the contractor's first Initial GSMP (as outlined in paragraphs 2.3 and 2.4 above) but –
(a) using the most recently established CRP of the contractor (the number is to be established quarterly); and
(b) from 1 July 2004, adding in the Appraisal Premium.

2.10 Any deductions for Additional or Out-of-Hours Services opt-outs are then to be calculated in the manner described in paragraph 2.5. If the contractor starts or resumes providing specific Additional Services under its GMS contract to patients it is required to provide essential services to, then any deduction that had been made in respect of those services will need to be reversed. The resulting amount (if there are to be any deductions in respect of Additional or Out-of-Hours Services) is the contractor's new (or possibly first) Adjusted GSMP.

2.11 Once any new values of the contractor's Initial GSMP and Adjusted GSMP have been calculated, the PCT must determine the gross amount of the contractor's new Payable GSMP. This is its (new) Initial GSMP or, if it has one, its (new or possibly first) Adjusted GSMP. The net amount of a contractor's Payable GSMP, i.e. the amount actually to be paid each month, is the gross amount of its Payable GSMP minus any monthly deductions in respect of superannuation determined in accordance with Section 22 (see paragraph 22.6).

2.12   Payment of the new Payable GSMP must (until it is next revised) be made monthly, and it is to fall due on the last day of each month. However, if a change is made to the Additional or Out-of-Hours Services that a contractor is under an obligation to provide and that change takes effect on any day other than the first day of the month, the contractor's Payable GSMP for that month is to be adjusted accordingly. Its amount for that month is to be the total of –

(a)   the appropriate proportion of its previous Payable GSMP. This is to be calculated by multiplying its previous Payable GSMP by the fraction produced by dividing –

   (i)   the number of days in the month during which it was providing the level of services based upon which its previous Payable GSMP was calculated, by

   (ii)   the total number of days in the month; and

(b)   the appropriate proportion of its new Payable GSMP. This is to be calculated by multiplying its new Payable GSMP by the fraction produced by dividing –

   (i)   the number of days left in the month after the change to which the new Payable GSMP relates takes effect, by

   (ii)   the total number of days in the month.

2.13   Any overpayment of Payable GSMP in that month as a result of the PCT paying the previous Payable GSMP before the new Payable GSMP has been calculated is to be deducted from the first payment in respect of a complete month of the new Payable GSMP. If there is an underpayment for the same reason, the shortfall is to be added to the first payment in respect of a complete month of the new Payable GSMP.

Conditions attached to Payable Global Sum Monthly Payments

2.14   Payable GSMPs, or any part thereof, are only payable if the contractor satisfies the following conditions –

(a)   the contractor must make available to the PCT any information which the PCT does not have but needs, and the contractor either has or could reasonably be expected to obtain, in order to calculate the contractor's Payable GSMP;

(b) the contractor must make any returns required of it (whether computerised or otherwise) to the Exeter Registration System, and do so promptly and fully;

(c) the contractor must immediately notify the PCT if for any reason it is not providing (albeit temporarily) any of the services it is under an obligation to provide under its GMS contract; and

(d) all information supplied to the PCT pursuant to or in accordance with this paragraph must be accurate.

2.15 If the contractor breaches any of these conditions, the PCT may, in appropriate circumstances, withhold payment of any or any part of a Payable GSMP that is otherwise payable.

2.16 It is also a condition of every contractor's Payable GSMPs that it achieves in respect of the financial year 2004/05 an Achievement Points Total of at least 100. If it breaches this condition, the PCT must withhold from the contractor £7500 multiplied by its Contractor Population Index (i.e. for the last quarter) in respect of its Payable GSMPs for the financial year 2004/05 (the contractor will, however, receive an Achievement Payment in respect of the points it does score pursuant to paragraph 5.39).

2.17 However, if the contractor's GMS contract either takes effect after 1 April 2004 or is terminated before 31 March 2005, the amount to be withheld pursuant to paragraph 2.16 is to be adjusted by the fraction produced by dividing the number of days during which the financial year 2004/05 for which its GMS contract had effect by 365."

● Golden Hello Scheme

Statement of Financial Entitlement

14. GOLDEN HELLO SCHEME

14.1 Under the Golden Hello Scheme, a lump sum "golden hello" payment is made to doctors who are starting out as GP performers in their first eligible post. All eligible doctors receive a standard payment and those starting work in specified PCT areas also receive an additional payment.

Standard payments under the Golden Hello Scheme

14.2 A doctor will be eligible for a standard payment under the Golden Hello Scheme if, after 1 April 2004, he takes up a post as a GP performer and –

(a) the post is as a GP performer employed or engaged by a contractor (including a member of the Flexible Careers Scheme);
(b) the post, if part-time –
  (i) involves a working commitment that generates a Time Commitment Fraction of at least one-fifth, or
  (ii) with any other post held by the doctor that also entails performing primary medical services together involve working commitment that generates a Time Commitment Fraction of at least one-fifth;
(c) if the doctor is an employee of the contractor, he is on a contract –
  (i) for an indefinite period (but not a fixed number of sessions), or
  (ii) for a fixed term of more than 2 years,
  unless he is a member of the Flexible Careers Scheme and he has given the PCT a written undertaking that he will remain in general practice at the end of his membership of the Flexible Careers Scheme;
(d) subject to paragraph 14.3, prior to starting work in that post, he has not –
  (i) been included in the medical performers list, services list or medical list of any Health Authority or PCT (unless this was because of temporary arrangements made by a PCT for the provision of general medical services or the performance of primary medical services following the suspension of a doctor),
  (ii) been employed or engaged (except as a locum) by a GP principal to assist, as a medical practitioner, in the provision of general medical services, or worked (except as a locum) as a GP performer –
    (aa) either full-time, or part-time with a working commitment generating a Time Commitment Fraction of at least one-quarter, if he took up post before 29 November 2002, or at least one-fifth if he took up post on or after 29 November 2002, and
    (bb) under a contract for an indefinite period (but not for a fixed number of sessions) or for a fixed term of more than 2 years, or
  (iii) been engaged (except as a locum) as a pilot scheme provider or an employee of a pilot scheme provider, or worked (except as a locum) as a medical practitioner performing primary medical services under a PMS contract –
    (aa) either full-time, or part-time with a working commitment generating a Time Commitment Fraction of at least one-quarter, if he took up the post before 29 November 2002 or at least one-fifth, if he took up the post on or after 29 November 2002, and

> (bb) under a contract for an indefinite period (but not for a fixed number of sessions) or for a fixed term of more than 2 years,
>
> unless he only comes within heads (i) to (iii) because of his participation in the GP Retainer Scheme and the claim pursuant to this Section relates to his first post after leaving the GP retainer scheme; and
>
> (e) subject to the provisions in this Section for making further payments because of new commitments, he has not previously received a standard payment under–
>
> (i) this Section,
>
> (ii) paragraph 38 of the Red Book,
>
> (iii) the Golden Hello Scheme under a PMS contract,
>
> (iv) Schedule 1 to the New Entrant, Delayed Retirement and Flexible Careers Schemes (Personal Medical Services) (England) Directions 2003, or
>
> (v) Part 2 of the Personal Medical Services Contracts (Payments for Specific Purposes) Directions 2004.

14.3 Paragraph 14.2(d) shall not apply to a GP performer who did not perform general medical services or personal medical services between 24 June 2002 and 24 September 2002 (except as a locum).

Additional payments under the Golden Hello Scheme

14.4 If –

(a) a doctor is eligible for a standard payment under paragraph 14.2; and

(b) the post to which his claim pursuant to this Section relates was with a contractor whose sole or main surgery is, when he takes up the post, within the area of a PCT included in annex H,

the doctor is potentially eligible for an additional payment under the Golden Hello Scheme. To be eligible for such a payment, the doctor's working commitment to the post to which the claim for an additional payment relates must generate a Time Commitment Fraction of at least one-fifth.

Calculation of standard and additional payments under the Golden Hello Scheme

14.5 Subject to the following provisions of this Section, PCTs must pay to contractors, in respect of doctors –

(a) who are eligible for standard or additional payments under the Golden Hello Scheme, and

(b) whose eligibility arises because of a work commitment that relates to the primary medical services that the contractor has undertaken to provide under its GMS contract,

any standard or additional payment for which that doctor is eligible, and at the following rates –

Standard payment	
Full-time, or part-time with a Time Commitment Fraction of at least ½	£5000
Part-time with a Time Commitment Fraction of less than ½	£3000
Additional payment	
Full-time, or part-time with a Time Commitment Fraction of at least ½	£7000
Part-time with a Time Commitment Fraction of less than ½	£4200

Further payments for new commitments

14.6 If, under the Golden Hello Scheme (whether under this Section or the other provisions listed in paragraph 14.2(e)), the lower level of the standard payment has been paid to or in respect of a doctor, or a standard payment was made to or in respect of the doctor but either no additional payment or the lower level of the additional payment was paid, the contractor may be entitled to a further payment from the PCT under his GMS contract if, after 1 April 2004, the doctor's work commitment changes, and –

(a) this is within 2 years of the doctor taking up the post that made him eligible for a standard payment under the Golden Hello Scheme ("the eligible post"); or

(b) the doctor took up the post that made him eligible for the standard payment while he was a member of the Flexible Careers Scheme, and the change to his work commitment is within 2 years of leaving that Scheme.

14.7 In these circumstances, if –

(a) the doctor increases his time commitment to the contractor, whether in the eligible post or by moving to a new post or by taking on an additional post; or

(b) with or without an increased time commitment, the doctor moves from a post that did not attract an additional payment to a post that would (for a new entrant) attract an additional payment,

he will be eligible for the further payments set out in paragraphs 14.8 and 14.9.

14.8 In a case where the doctor increases his time commitment –
  (a) if work relating to the new time commitment starts –
    (i) within 6 months of the doctor taking up the eligible post, or
    (ii) as regards a doctor who is in or has left the Flexible Careers Scheme, within 2 years of him leaving that Scheme,
    the further payment for which he is eligible is the difference between the standard (and where applicable additional) payment the doctor would have received if the new time commitment had been the doctor's time commitment when he first took up the eligible post and the standard (and where applicable additional) payment already awarded to him under the Golden Hello Scheme; or
  (b) if –
    (i) work relating to the new time commitment starts within 2 years of the doctor taking up the eligible post, but more than 6 months after he took up the post, and
    (ii) the doctor is not and has not been in the Flexible Careers Scheme,
    the further payment for which he is eligible is half the difference between the standard (and where applicable additional) payment the doctor would have received if the new time commitment had been the doctor's time commitment when he first took up the eligible post and the standard (and where applicable additional) payment already awarded to him under the Golden Hello Scheme.

14.9 In a case where the doctor –
  (a) moves from a post that did not attract an additional payment to a post that would (for a new entrant) attract an additional payment; or
  (b) takes on an extra post that would (for a new entrant) attract an additional payment,
  the further payment is to be the additional payment that the doctor would have received if the new work commitment (also taking into account any additional time commitment) had been the doctor's work commitment when he first took up the eligible post.

14.10 Subject to the following provisions of this Section, PCTs must pay to contractors, in respect of doctors –
  (a) who are eligible for further payments under the Golden Hello Scheme, pursuant to paragraphs 14.6 to 14.9, and

(b) whose eligibility arises because of a work commitment that relates to the primary medical services that the contractor has undertaken to perform under its GMS contract,

any further payment for which that doctor is eligible.

Conditions attached to payments under the Golden Hello Scheme

14.11 Payments under this Section, or any part thereof, are only payable if the following conditions are satisfied –

(a) applications for standard, additional and further payments under the Golden Hello Scheme must be made –

   (i) in the case of standard or additional payments, within 12 months of the date on which the doctor took up the eligible post,

   (ii) in the case of an additional payment, within 12 months of the date on which the new work commitment starts;

(b) a contractor who receives a payment under the Golden Hello Scheme in respect of a doctor must give that payment to that doctor –

   (i) within one calendar month of it receiving that payment, and

   (ii) as an element of the personal income of that doctor, subject to any lawful deduction of income tax, national insurance and superannuation contributions,

once it has secured from the doctor an enforceable undertaking that he will repay to the contractor any amount repayable by the contractor to the PCT under this Section in respect of him;

(c) if, within 2 years of starting in an eligible post giving rise to a standard payment (and any related additional payment) under this Section, the doctor in respect of whom the payment was made ceases to practise as a medical practitioner anywhere in the United Kingdom, the contractor that received the standard payment (and any related additional payment) must repay to the PCT –

   (i) the whole of the standard payment (and any related additional payment) paid to the contractor, if the doctor ceases to practise within 6 months of him starting in the eligible post, or

   (ii) half the standard payment (taken together with any related additional payment) paid to the contractor, if the doctor ceases to practise within 2 years of him starting in the eligible post but more than 6 months after him starting in that post;

(d) if within 2 years of starting in an eligible post giving rise to an additional payment (or a further payment in place of an additional payment) under this Section, the doctor in respect of whom the payment is made ceases to practise as a medical practitioner anywhere in the United Kingdom or moves to a post which would not, for a new entrant, attract an additional payment, the contractor that received the additional payment (or further payment in place of an additional payment) must repay to the PCT –

(i)   the whole of the additional payment (or further payment) paid to the contractor, if the move takes place or the doctor ceases to practise within 6 months of the doctor starting in the post that gave rise to the payment, or

(ii) half of the additional payment (or further payment), if the move takes place or the doctor ceases to practise within 2 years of him starting in the post that gave rise to the payment but more than 6 months after him starting in that post.

14.12   For the purposes of calculating the time periods referred to in paragraph 14.11(c) and (d), the following periods are discounted –

(a)   periods of maternity, paternity, adoption or parental leave, if the doctor –

(i)   in the case of –

(aa) ordinary or additional maternity, paternity or adoption leave, gives an undertaking that he will return to general practice after not more than 2 years' absence, or

(bb) extended maternity, paternity or adoption leave, or parental leave, agrees the leave with the PCT and undertakes to return to general practice at the end of the agreed period of leave, and

(ii) honours that undertaking;

(b)   periods of absence due to exceptional personal circumstances known to and endorsed by the PCT.

14.13   If the condition in paragraph 14.11(a) is breached, the payment to which the application relates is not payable.

14.14   If the condition in paragraph 14.11(b) is breached, the PCT may require repayment of the payment paid to the contractor, or may withhold payment of any other payment payable to the contractor under this SFE, to the value of the payment paid.

14.15   If the conditions in paragraph 14.11(c) and (d) are breached because the doctor ceases to practise because of –

(a)   death; or

(b)   forced early retirement because of illness or injury,

then no amount is repayable, but otherwise, the PCT may require repayment of the payment paid, or the excess amount paid, or may withhold payment of any other payment payable to the contractor under this SFE, to the value of the payment or excess amount paid.

14.16   Where, pursuant to paragraph 14.14, a contractor is required to repay any or any part of a standard, additional or further payment under this

Section, the arrangements by which the contractor may seek to enforce the undertaking referred to in paragraph 14.11(b) as a consequence of that repayment are a matter for the contractor.

Governing law and jurisdiction[33]

Standard Contract

603. This Contract shall be governed by and construed in accordance with English law.

604. Without prejudice to the dispute resolution procedures contained in this Contract, in relation to any legal action or proceedings to enforce this Contract or arising out of or in connection with this Contract, each party agrees to submit to the exclusive jurisdiction of the courts of England and Wales.

605. Clauses 603 and 604 shall continue to apply notwithstanding the termination of the Contract.

Greenfield sites

See also: Premises

Guidance

2.14 Paragraph 7.20 of *Investing in General Practice* explained that when looking to commission for greenfield sites (i.e. new surgeries that cover essential services as a result of significant increases in population), the PCT "could advertise and seek applications through a two-stage process". It also made clear that the PCT's ability to provide such services itself would not be circumscribed by this process; if a PCT was not free to establish its own provision, its ability to reduce patient assignments to GMS and PMS providers with closed lists would be constrained.

2.15 In the first stage, PCTs would draw up a specification of what they want by way of the range of and access to services and the quality of care. They

---

33 This clause is not required by *the Regulations*, but is recommended.

could then invite bids for existing GMS and PMS contractors. The PCT would not be expected to go to stage two (inviting bids from alternative providers) unless there was no interest, or if those contractors did not in the PCT's view satisfy the criteria set out in the specification. In most circumstances it is likely to make best sense to contract with existing GMS or PMS practices. This could be through a variation to their main contract, or a separate contract, which could be time-limited, should both parties agree. In some areas where there is a shortage of primary care professionals alternative providers may offer much needed additional local capacity.

Gross Investment Guarantee

Guidance

5.3 UK spend on primary medical services will rise by 33% between 2002/03 and 2005/06, from £6.1 billion in 2002/03 to £8 billion. This will be delivered through the Gross Investment Guarantee (GIG) mechanism. The UK GIG total is the aggregate of the national GIGs in England, Scotland, Wales and Northern Ireland. In England resources are expected to rise from £5 billion in 2002/03 to £6.8 billion in 2005/06. This includes funds for PMS.

5.4 Part 7 of *Supplementary Documents* set out a notional distribution of resources within the England GIG. The England GIG is being revised and key changes include:
(i)   reflecting the Minimum Practice Income Guarantee (MPIG) deal
(ii) revising the 2002/03 spend on fees and allowances. Provisional data show that expenditure relating to the GMS non-cash-limited (GMSNCL) baseline was higher than estimated
(iii) revising the assumption about growth in GMS cash-limited (GMSCL) monies
(iv) reflecting higher than expected projected spend on dispensing, mainly as a result of higher drugs costs
(v)   increasing the provision for superannuation contributions from the existing 7% GP and practice staff employer superannuation contributions already contained in the global sum and MPIG. The increase will take account of the rise in contributions to 14% from 1 April 2004, and additionally reflect an expected increase in net contractor income which itself requires 14% contributions
(vi) making adjustments either upwards or downwards for projected under or over-spends in 2003/04.

In the light of these changes, and further consideration by the Technical Steering Committee (TSC), the England Gross Investment Guarantee figures for 2004/05 and 2005/06 will be amended and published in January 2004.

5.5 As is currently the case, in-year financial pressures will need to be effectively managed by PCTs from within their overall resource envelope. In-year financial pressures will not lead to in-year changes to contractor entitlements. Paragraph 5.7 of *Investing in General Practice* also made clear that "to ensure delivery of the GIG the pricing of the contract could be adjusted". Were the need to arise for such adjustments to be made, the Department of Health or its agents would be required to consult the General Practitioners Committee before making changes to the Statement of Financial Entitlements for subsequent years.

5.6 Future increases in resources beyond 2005/06 would lead to increases in both the GIG and the SFE entitlements. These will be considered as part of future negotiations between the four Health Departments or their agents and the GPC.

● Health service body status

See also: Contract – NHS or private

Regulations

10. Health service body status

(1) Where a proposed contractor elects in a written notice served on the PCT at any time prior to the contract being entered into to be regarded as a health service body for the purposes of section 4 of the 1990 Act, it shall be so regarded from the date on which the contract is entered into.

(2) If, pursuant to paragraph (1) or (5), a contractor is to be regarded as a health service body, that fact shall not affect the nature of, or any rights or liabilities arising under, any other contract with a health service body entered into by a contractor before the date on which the contractor is to be so regarded.

(3) Where a contract is made with an individual medical practitioner or two or more persons practising in partnership, and that individual, or that partnership is to be regarded as a health service body in accordance with paragraph (1) or (5), the contractor shall, subject to paragraph (4), continue to be regarded as a health service body for the purposes of

section 4 of the 1990 Act for as long as that contract continues irrespective of any change in –

(a) the partners comprising the partnership;

(b) the status of the contractor from that of an individual medical practitioner to that of a partnership; or

(c) the status of the contractor from that of a partnership to that of an individual medical practitioner.

(4) A contractor may at any time request in writing a variation of the contract to include provision in or remove provision from the contract that the contract is an NHS contract, and if it does so –

(a) the PCT shall agree to the variation; and

(b) the procedure in paragraph 104(1) of Schedule 6 shall apply.

(5) If, pursuant to paragraph (4), the PCT agrees to the variation to the contract, the contractor shall –

(a) be regarded; or

(b) subject to paragraph (7), cease to be regarded,

as a health service body for the purposes of section 4 of the 1990 Act from the date that variation is to take effect pursuant to paragraph 104(1) of Schedule 6.

(6) Subject to paragraph (7), a contractor shall cease to be a health service body for the purposes of section 4 of the 1990 Act if the contract terminates.

(7) Where a contractor ceases to be a health service body pursuant to –

(a) paragraph (5) or (6), it shall continue to be regarded as a health service body for the purposes of being a party to any other NHS contract entered into after it became a health service body but before the date on which the contractor ceased to be a health service body (for which purpose it ceases to be such a body on the termination of that NHS contract);

(b) paragraph (5), it shall, if it or the PCT has referred any matter to the NHS dispute resolution procedure before it ceases to be a health service body, be bound by the determination of the adjudicator as if the dispute had been referred pursuant to paragraph 100 of Schedule 6;

(c) paragraph (6), it shall continue to be regarded as a health service body for the purposes of the NHS dispute resolution procedure where that procedure has been commenced –

(i) before the termination of the contract, or

(ii) after the termination of the contract, whether in connection with or arising out of the termination of the contract or otherwise,

for which purposes it ceases to be such a body on the conclusion of that procedure.

Guidance

6.12 The Health and Social Care (Community Health and Standards) Act 2003 provides that a GMS contract may be treated as a NHS contract. An NHS contract is an arrangement between one Health Service Body and another for the provision of goods and services. Examples of Health Service Bodies include SHAs, PCTs, NHS trusts, Special Health Authorities and most PMS providers. Where the contract is an NHS contract disputes about the terms of a contract are dealt with through the NHS disputes resolution procedures rather than through the courts, thus potentially reducing bureaucracy and cost for both sides. It should also be noted that contractors with private law contracts would be able to choose to use the NHS dispute procedure instead of the Courts should they so wish to do so.

6.13 For a GMS contract to become a NHS contract the provider will need to elect to become a Health Service Body. Potential GMS providers will therefore need to give written notice to the PCT to this effect. It would be helpful if this could be done by 13 February 2004. Health Service Body status would then commence from the date that the contract is entered into.

6.14 The choice of being or not being a Health Service Body is entirely a matter for the GMS contractor. The PCT should not attempt to force such status onto, or deny such status to, a GMS contractor. Key points to note about Health Service Body status are:
   (i) if a GMS provider becomes a Health Service Body, it may enter into other NHS contracts with another Health Service Body
   (ii) becoming a Health Service Body does not affect other contracts the provider may have entered into before Health Service Body status takes effect. If for any reason the GMS contract is terminated, the contractor stops being a Health Service Body, unless it already holds a separate NHS contract in which case it can continue to be a Health Service Body for the purpose of that contract
   (iii) partnership changes do not affect Health Service Body status
   (iv) contractors can at any time seek to vary their contract to remove or include provision that it is to be considered a Health Service Body.

● Home visiting

Guidance

2.23 (i) home-visiting. Under the new contract, the contractor must attend a patient outside practice premises if the patient's medical condition is such that, in the reasonable opinion of the contractor, it is necessary to do so. This does not stop the PCT from investing in a home-visiting service if it so wishes, as set out in paragraph 2.26 of *Investing in General Practice*.

Infection control

Regulations

9.   Infection control

The contractor shall ensure that it has appropriate arrangements for infection control and decontamination.

Standard Contract

40.   The Contractor shall ensure that it has appropriate arrangements for infection control and decontamination.

Information management and technology – clinical coding

Guidance

4.35   Detailed specifications to enable suppliers to develop solutions to support the Quality and Outcome Framework have now been released. Contractors and PCTs should not, therefore, develop local queries to support the Quality and Outcomes Framework with respect to quality points generation. Contractors should not develop local Read Codes as these will result in a loss of earnings for contractors and poor quality data for PCTs. An interim release of Read Codes was made on 1 October 2003 containing the new exception codes for the Quality and Outcomes Framework. This, together with the logical query specification and associated business rules, contains the complete set of Read Codes products. As the Quality and Outcome Framework requires an up-to-date set of Read Codes to be present in clinical systems for payment purposes, contractors will need to ensure that they are working with the correct versions at all times. Further information on Read Codes is available from the NHS IA (tel. 0121 3330333) or at http://www.nhsia.nhs.uk/terms/pages/default.asp.

Service Level Agreements

4.36   Chapter 4 of *Investing in General Practice* states that "a national template SLA will be developed to support the development of future primary care IT systems providing practices with assurances on training, maintenance and support. The national template will allow local enhancements and additions in line with national programmes". Work is continuing to develop a template SLA for England which needs to take into account the current relationships between practices, PCTs and system suppliers as well as the emergence of national and local service providers.

National Information Management and Payment Systems

4.37   The GMS Payments Project will shortly be defining the functionality that will be required in GP clinical and PCT systems to support Quality and Outcomes Framework Payments. These specifications will also cover the proposed new national QOF Management System (QMAS) and the National Payments System. GP clinical system suppliers have been fully informed of these developments and are currently working to develop the required enhancements to their systems.

4.38   A national testing and certification programme is being developed with the support of the profession and the NHS Confederation to ensure that the outputs from GP clinical systems for QOF payments are produced in compliance with national standards.

Training and support

4.39   The project will ensure that contractors and PCTs are supported with training products and services so that they are able to use the systems and utilities described above. This should be complementary to the longer term IT training initiatives that PCTs should already have in place to help practice staff to develop the skills that they need to make best use of clinical systems and information. The training programme will be delivered in stages to ensure that all agencies have the necessary training to ensure that the payments are made in accordance with the GMS contract.

Preparing for the GMS new contract

4.40 There are a number of actions that PCTs and contractors can be taking before 1 April 2004 to prepare for the contract:

(i) PCTs should carry out a baseline survey of practice clinical systems and ensure that contractors have RFA 99 compliant clinical systems

(ii) contractors may wish to review system management and information governance in the light of the "Good Practice Guidance" recently published by the Department of Health, BMA and Royal College of General Practitioners and available at http//www.doh.gov.uk/pricare/computing/index.htm

(iii) contractors will want to set up and maintain disease registers in accordance with good practice guidance published at http://www.nelh.nhs.uk/nsf/chd/sig/secondary/appendix1.htm

(iv) contractors must ensure that the correct clinical codes associated with the Quality and Outcomes Framework are being used. Detailed further information on the codes is at http://www.doh.gov.uk/gmscontract/implementation.htm

(v) contractors may want to review existing templates and protocols with system suppliers to ensure that they meet the requirements of the new contract

(vi) contractors may want to undertake training needs assessment as part of ongoing contractor development programmes.

New NPfIT Service Delivery Arrangements

4.41 Five Local Service Providers (LSPs) will be appointed to manage the implementation of national applications including NHS care record systems in five regional 'clusters' of SHAs. All LSP contracts will be signed by December 2003. National Application Service Providers (NASPs) have been appointed to build and run the central applications for e-bookings, e-prescriptions and the data spine. PCTs can get further information via SHA Chief Information.

● Information management and technology – data flows

Guidance

3.72 IM&T support for the QOF will be provided through three mechanisms:

(i) the Interim Aspiration Utility (an aspiration spreadsheet), described in paragraphs 3.18 and 3.19, for assessing quality aspiration levels in 2004/05

(ii) all contractors having clinical systems that are compliant with national system specifications for GMS contract functionality. PCTs should provide funding to upgrade the clinical systems of those relatively few contractors that will not have compliant systems, as set out in John Hutton's letter to Dr John Chisholm of 14 October 2003 (available at http://www.doh.gov.uk/gmscontract/ITfunding.PDF). In addition, all practices are expected to have RFA99 compliant clinical systems

(iii) the introduction of the Quality and Outcomes Framework Management and Analysis System (QMAS). This system will ensure consistency in how quality achievement and prevalence are calculated, and will be linked to the Exeter payment systems. Data from clinical systems will be extracted through automated links to the QMAS, while non-clinical information (the yes/no organisational, patient experience and additional services indicators) will be added to the QMAS by the practice using a web-based interface. Clinical systems will be subject to a process of certification by the National Programme for IT (NPfIT) to ensure that they are compliant with the QMAS. It is expected that this process will be complete, and the QMAS introduced, by August 2004. This will be accompanied by guidance and training provided by NPfIT. Figure 13 illustrates how the QMAS will work.

Data flows

3.73 QMAS will enable contractors to:
(i) assess their current quality achievement points, estimated relative prevalence and current achievement payment whenever they wish
(ii) compare their current position with the average achievement in the PCT, the SHA and nationally. Such comparisons would not involve disclosure of information that identifies other contractors. This facility will be available later after the main system has gone live
(iii) check that the data they are providing are correct and complete.

3.74 PCTs will also have links to the QMAS. When planning cashflow, PCTs should note that QOF achievement could rise disproportionately during the last few months of 2005/06 as practices strive to maximise their QOF achievement payments. The QMAS will provide information for each PCT on:
(i) current individual practice points achievement, prevalence, and payments. This information is essential for financial planning and risk management purposes. This functionality will go live later than the basic payments system. PCTs must ensure that monthly practice identifiable information is not submitted to the PEC or main board

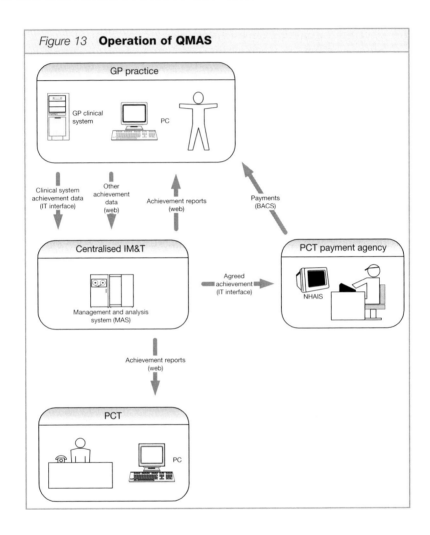

Figure 13 **Operation of QMAS**

(ii) overall PCT achievement against the QOF, compared with other PCTs in the SHA and nationally. This would not include information that identifies individual contractors. This functionality will also go live later than the basic payments system.

3.75 The QMAS will also provide:

(i) monthly information to SHAs on likely PCT points achievement, prevalence and spend. This is also necessary for financial management purposes. Such reports would not include information that identifies individual contractors

(ii) information to inform national policy development, e.g. the reviews of the QOF and the global sum allocation formula, or approved research. Where this includes data on individual contractors it would be anonymised

(iii) information to statutory authorities including NHS Counter Fraud Management and Security Services, auditors and CHAI. Access to identifiable contractor level information would normally be at the request of the PCT and with the permission of the contractor. In exceptional circumstances, e.g. serious fraud the PCT may need to access data without the contractor's permission.

These functions will be available later than the basic payments system.

3.76   PCTs should not use this information for performance management purposes as the QOF is voluntary. PCTs could, however, use the information as a way of offering support to the contractor.

3.77   Access to data (including, where appropriate, patient identifiable data by PCT assessors and staff from other organisations) will be subject to a code of practice. This will be published in spring 2004.

3.78   *Investing in General Practice* made clear that PCT-wide achievement against the QOF would be independently inspected by CHAI. CHAI is still in the early stages of developing its plans. The Department with CHAI will also be reviewing how PCT star ratings might best capture achievement against the QOF, again from 2005.

● Information management and technology – funding

Statement of Financial Entitlement

20.1   With effect from 1 April 2003, PCTs, rather than contractors, have become responsible for the purchase, maintenance, future upgrades and running costs of integrated IM&T systems for providers of services under GMS contracts, as well as for telecommunications links within the NHS.

20.2   Pending the transfer of these responsibilities, PCTs must in respect of the financial year 2004/05 pay to contractors under their GMS contracts amounts representing the reasonable costs of contractors in respect of IT maintenance and minor upgrades (i.e. where these costs are not met directly by the PCT). For these purposes –

(a) "maintenance" means routine support that is normally provided under annual contracts by GP clinical system suppliers or third parties. For the purposes of determining whether maintenance costs are reasonable, PCTs should review and consolidate existing maintenance contracts to ensure that they represent value for money and provide the required levels of support; and

(b) "minor upgrades" means upgrades required to ensure that existing clinical systems continue to perform efficiently (e.g. memory or hard disk upgrades, and replacement of broken or defective items such as printers, screens and back-up devices).

20.3 Payments under this Section are not to cover the cost of system replacements or significant upgrades (such as the purchase of new hardware, other than new hardware covered by paragraph 20.2(b)). Payment in respect of these items of expenditure is not covered in this SFE.

Guidance

4.29 The GMS Payments Project, which is part of the National Programme for IT (NPfIT), is developing and implementing the information systems that are required to support the new contract. This will coincide and be backed up by the new Local Service Providers (LSPs) delivering high quality primary care IM&T services throughout the NHS in England. Changes to the payment systems will be supported by a centrally funded training programme to smooth the transition. Further detailed information on the IM&T work programme will be made available on: http://www.doh.gov.uk/gmscontract/infotech.htm and http://www.natpact.nhs.uk.

Funding for maintenance and upgrades

4.30 In the period before the full implementation of the NPfIT programme GMS contractors are entitled through the SFEs to full funding of the costs of maintenance and minor upgrades for existing systems.

4.31 Maintenance is defined as the routine support that is normally provided under annual contracts by GP clinical system suppliers or third parties. PCTs are being encouraged to review and consolidate existing maintenance contracts to ensure that they represent value for money and provide the required levels of support.

4.32 Minor upgrades are defined as those required to ensure that existing clinical systems continue to perform efficiently: for example, memory or hard disk upgrades, replacement of broken or defective items such as printers, screens or back-up devices. This also includes the installation of cut-sheet feeder-printers to support new prescription requirements and replacement of critical items, e.g. servers, where these are no longer fit for purpose.

4.33 Any other upgrades, including system replacement, should be subject to local business case processes and the local availability of funding. It is not expected that systems which have been accredited to RFA 99 standards should be replaced at this time. In most cases RFA 99 systems will provide the platform on which new integrated systems will be built with new functionality being provided as national rollout of the NPfIT progresses.

4.34 Contractors currently using systems which are not RFA 99 accredited should replace those systems by April 2004 in order to ensure compliance with national GMS payments systems and the availability of key national initiatives, for example pathology results and security, confidentiality and prescribing requirements. The cost of pre-RFA 99 system replacement should be met in full by the PCT, which should apply appropriate procurement processes to ensure value for money. Regulations currently state that contractors must use RFA 99 compliant systems if they are to gain PCT consent to reliance on electronic patient records. Contractors that do not have any computer systems currently should be encouraged and supported to implement RFA 99 v1.1 (or greater) accredited systems and the purchase and maintenance of those systems should be fully funded by the PCT by April 2004.

Insurance

Regulations

122. Insurance

(1) The contractor shall at all times hold adequate insurance against liability arising from negligent performance of clinical services under the contract.

(2) The contractor shall not sub-contract its obligations to provide clinical services under the contract unless it has satisfied itself that the sub-contractor holds adequate insurance against liability arising from negligent performance of such services.

(3) In this paragraph –
(a) "insurance" means a contract of insurance or other arrangement made for the purpose of indemnifying the contractor; and

(b) a contractor shall be regarded as holding insurance if it is held by an employee of its in connection with clinical services which that employee provides under the contract or, as the case may be, sub-contract.

123. The contractor shall at all times hold adequate public liability insurance in relation to liabilities to third parties arising under or in connection with the contract which are not covered by the insurance referred to in paragraph 122(1).

Standard Contract

488. The Contractor shall at all times hold adequate insurance against liability arising from negligent performance of clinical services under the Contract.

489. The Contractor shall not sub-contract its obligations to provide clinical services under the Contract unless it is satisfied that the sub-contractor holds adequate insurance against liability arising from negligent performance of such services.

490. For the purposes of clauses 488 to 490.2 –
490.1 "insurance" means a contract of insurance or other arrangement made for the purpose of indemnifying the Contractor; and
490.2 the Contractor shall be regarded as holding insurance if it is held by an employee of its in connection with clinical services which that employee provides under the contract or, as the case may be, sub-contract.

491. The Contractor shall at all times hold adequate public liability insurance in relation to liabilities to third parties arising under or in connection with the Contract which are not covered by the insurance referred to in clause 488.

Level of skill

Regulations

67. Level of skill

The contractor shall carry out its obligations under the contract with reasonable care and skill.

Standard Contract

Level of skill

24. The Contractor shall carry out its obligations under the Contract in a timely manner and with reasonable care and skill.

List removals

See also: Administrative removals

Regulations

19. Removals from the list at the request of the patient

(1) The contractor shall notify the PCT in writing of any request for removal from its list of patients received from a registered patient.

(2) Where the PCT –
(a) receives notification from the contractor under sub-paragraph (1); or
(b) receives a request from the patient to be removed from the contractor's list of patients,
it shall remove that person from the contractor's list of patients.

(3) A removal in accordance with sub-paragraph (2) shall take effect –
(a) on the date on which the PCT receives notification of the registration of the person with another provider of essential services (or their equivalent); or
(b) 14 days after the date on which the notification or request made under sub-paragraph (1) or (2) respectively is received by the PCT, whichever is the sooner.

(4) The PCT shall, as soon as practicable, notify in writing –
(a) the patient; and
(b) the contractor,
that the patient's name will be or has been removed from the contractor's list of patients on the date referred to in sub-paragraph (3).

(5) In this paragraph and in paragraphs 20(1)(b) and (10), 21(6) and (7), 23 and 26, a reference to a request received from or advice, information or notification required to be given to a patient shall include a request received from or advice, information or notification required to be given to –

(a) in the case of a patient who is a child, a parent or other person referred to in paragraph 15(4)(a); or

(b) in the case of an adult patient who is incapable of making the relevant request or receiving the relevant advice, information or notification, a relative or the primary carer of the patient.

20. Removals from the list at the request of the contractor

(1) Subject to paragraph 21, a contractor which has reasonable grounds for wishing a patient to be removed from its list of patients, which do not relate to the applicant's race, gender, social class, age, religion, sexual orientation, appearance, disability or medical condition shall –

(a) notify the PCT in writing that it wishes to have the patient removed; and

(b) subject to sub-paragraph (2), notify the patient of its specific reasons for requesting removal.

(2) Where, in the reasonable opinion of the contractor –

(a) the circumstances of the removal are such that it is not appropriate for a more specific reason to be given; and

(b) there has been an irrevocable breakdown in the relationship between the patient and the contractor,

the reason given under sub-paragraph (1) may consist of a statement that there has been such a breakdown.

(3) Except in the circumstances specified in sub-paragraph (4), a contractor may only request a removal under sub-paragraph (1), if, within the period of 12 months prior to the date of its request to the PCT, it has warned the patient that he is at risk of removal and explained to him the reasons for this.

(4) The circumstances referred to in sub-paragraph (3) are that –

(a) the reason for removal relates to a change of address;

(b) the contractor has reasonable grounds for believing that the issue of such a warning would –

(i) be harmful to the physical or mental health of the patient, or

(ii) put at risk the safety of one or more of the persons specified in sub-paragraph (5); or

(c) it is, in the opinion of the contractor, not otherwise reasonable or practical for a warning to be given.

(5) The persons referred to in sub-paragraph (4) are –

(a) the contractor, where it is an individual medical practitioner;

(b) in the case of a contract with two or more individuals practising in partnership, a partner in that partnership;

    (c) in the case of a contract with a company, a legal and beneficial owner of shares in that company;

    (d) a member of the contractor's staff;

    (e) a person engaged by the contractor to perform or assist in the performance of services under the contract; or

    (f) any other person present –

        (i) on the practice premises, or

        (ii) in the place where services are being provided to the patient under the contract.

(6) The contractor shall record in writing –

    (a) the date of any warning given in accordance with sub-paragraph (3) and the reasons for giving such a warning as explained to the patient; or

    (b) the reason why no such warning was given.

(7) The contractor shall keep a written record of removals under this paragraph which shall include –

    (a) the reason for removal given to the patient;

    (b) the circumstances of the removal; and

    (c) in cases where sub-paragraph (2) applies, the grounds for a more specific reason not being appropriate,

and shall make this record available to the PCT on request.

(8) A removal requested in accordance with sub-paragraph (1) shall, subject to sub-paragraph (9), take effect from –

    (a) the date on which the PCT receives notification of the registration of the person with another provider of essential services (or their equivalent); or

    (b) the eighth day after the PCT receives the notice referred to in sub-paragraph (1)(a),

whichever is the sooner.

(9) Where, on the date on which the removal would take effect under sub-paragraph (8), the contractor is treating the patient at intervals of less than 7 days, the contractor shall notify the PCT in writing of the fact and the removal shall take effect –

    (a) on the eighth day after the Trust receives notification from the contractor that the person no longer needs such treatment; or

    (b) on the date on which the PCT receives notification of the registration of the person with another provider of essential services (or their equivalent),

whichever is the sooner.

(10) The PCT shall notify in writing –

    (a) the patient; and

    (b) the contractor,

that the patient's name has been or will be removed from the contractor's list of patients on the date referred to in sub-paragraph (8) or (9).

21. Removals from the list of patients who are violent

(1) A contractor which wishes a patient to be removed from its list of patients with immediate effect on the grounds that –
   (a) the patient has committed an act of violence against any of the persons specified in sub-paragraph (2) or behaved in such a way that any such person has feared for his safety; and
   (b) it has reported the incident to the police,
   shall notify the PCT in accordance with sub-paragraph (3).

(2) The persons referred to in sub-paragraph (1) are –
   (a) the contractor where it is an individual medical practitioner;
   (b) in the case of a contract with two or more individuals practising in partnership, a partner in that partnership;
   (c) in the case of a contract with a company, a legal and beneficial owner of shares in that company;
   (d) a member of the contractor's staff;
   (e) a person engaged by the contractor to perform or assist in the performance of services under the contract; or
   (f) any other person present –
      (i) on the practice premises, or
      (ii) in the place where services were provided to the patient under the contract.

(3) Notification under sub-paragraph (1) may be given by any means including telephone or fax but if not given in writing shall subsequently be confirmed in writing within 7 days (and for this purpose a faxed notification is not a written one).

(4) The PCT shall acknowledge in writing receipt of a request from the contractor under sub-paragraph (1).

(5) A removal requested in accordance with sub-paragraph (1) shall take effect at the time that the contractor –
   (a) makes the telephone call to the PCT; or
   (b) sends or delivers the notification to the PCT.

(6) Where, pursuant to this paragraph, the contractor has notified the PCT that it wishes to have a patient removed from its list of patients, it shall inform the patient concerned unless –
   (a) it is not reasonably practicable for it to do so; or
   (b) it has reasonable grounds for believing that to do so would –
      (i) be harmful to the physical or mental health of the patient, or

        (ii) put at risk the safety of one or more of the persons specified in sub-paragraph (2).

(7)   Where the PCT has removed a patient from the contractor's list of patients in accordance with sub-paragraph (5) it shall give written notice of the removal to that patient.

(8)   Where a patient is removed from the contractor's list of patients in accordance with this paragraph, the contractor shall record in the patient's medical records that the patient has been removed under this paragraph and the circumstances leading to his removal.

22.   Removals from the list of patients registered elsewhere

(1)   The PCT shall remove a patient from the contractor's list of patients if –
    (a) he has subsequently been registered with another provider of essential services (or their equivalent) in the area of the PCT; or
    (b) it has received notice from another PCT, a Local Health Board, a Health Board or a Health and Social Services Board that he has subsequently been registered with a provider of essential services (or their equivalent) outside the area of the PCT.

(2)   A removal in accordance with sub-paragraph (1) shall take effect –
    (a) on the date on which the PCT receives notification of the registration of the person with the new provider; or
    (b) with the consent of the PCT, on such other date as has been agreed between the contractor and the new provider.

(3)   The PCT shall notify the contractor in writing of persons removed from its list of patients under sub-paragraph (1).

23.   Removals from the list of patients who have moved

(1)   Subject to sub-paragraph (2), where the PCT is satisfied that a person on the contractor's list of patients has moved and no longer resides in that contractor's practice area, the PCT shall –
    (a) inform that patient and the contractor that the contractor is no longer obliged to visit and treat the person;
    (b) advise the patient in writing either to obtain the contractor's agreement to the continued inclusion of the person on its list of patients or to apply for registration with another provider of essential services (or their equivalent); and
    (c) inform the patient that if, after the expiration of 30 days from the date of the advice mentioned in paragraph (b), he has not acted in accordance with the advice and informed it accordingly, the PCT will remove him from the contractor's list of patients.

(2)   If, at the expiration of the period of 30 days referred to in sub-paragraph (1)(c), the PCT has not been notified of the action taken, it shall remove the patient from the contractor's list of patients and inform him and the contractor accordingly.

24.   Where the address of a patient who is on the contractor's list of patients is no longer known to the PCT, the PCT shall –

(a) give to the contractor notice in writing that it intends, at the end of the period of 6 months commencing with the date of the notice, to remove the patient from the contractor's list of patients; and

(b) at the end of that period, remove the patient from the contractor's list of patients unless, within that period, the contractor satisfies the PCT that it is still responsible for providing essential services to that patient.

25.   Removals from the list of patients absent from the United Kingdom etc.

(1)   The PCT shall remove a patient from the contractor's list of patients where it receives notification that that patient –

(a) intends to be away from the United Kingdom for a period of at least 3 months;

(b) is in Her Majesty's Forces;

(c) is serving a prison sentence of more than 2 years or sentences totalling in the aggregate more than that period;

(d) has been absent from the United Kingdom for a period of more than 3 months; or (e) has died.

(2)   A removal in accordance with sub-paragraph (1) shall take effect –

(a) in the cases referred to in sub-paragraph (1)(a) to (c) from the date of the departure, enlistment or imprisonment or the date on which the PCT first receives notification of the departure, enlistment or imprisonment whichever is the later; or

(b) in the cases referred to in sub-paragraph (1)(d) and (e) from the date on which the PCT first receives notification of the absence or death.

(3)   The PCT shall notify the contractor in writing of patients removed from its list of patients under sub-paragraph (1).

26.   Removals from the list of patients accepted elsewhere as temporary residents

(1)   The PCT shall remove from the contractor's list of patients a patient who has been accepted as a temporary resident by another contractor or other provider of essential services (or their equivalent) where it is satisfied, after due inquiry –

(a) that the patient's stay in the place of temporary residence has exceeded 3 months; and

(b) that he has not returned to his normal place of residence or any other place within the contractor's practice area.

(2) The PCT shall notify in writing of a removal under sub-paragraph (1) –

(a) the contractor; and

(b) where practicable, the patient.

(3) A notification to the patient under sub-paragraph (2)(b) shall inform him of –

(a) his entitlement to make arrangements for the provision to him of essential services (or their equivalent), including by the contractor by which he has been treated as a temporary resident; and

(b) the name and address of the PCT in whose area he is resident.

27. Removals from the list of pupils etc. of a school

(1) Where the contractor provides essential services under the contract to persons on the grounds that they are pupils at or staff or residents of a school, the PCT shall remove from the contractor's list of patients any such persons who do not appear on particulars of persons who are pupils at or staff or residents of that school provided by that school.

(2) Where the PCT has made a request to a school to provide the particulars mentioned in sub-paragraph (1) and has not received them, it shall consult the contractor as to whether it should remove from its list of patients any persons appearing on that list as pupils at, or staff or residents of, that school.

(3) The PCT shall notify the contractor in writing of patients removed from its list of patients under sub-paragraph (1).

Standard Contract

Removals from the list at the request of the patient

186. The Contractor shall notify the PCT in writing of any request for removal from its list of patients received from a *registered patient*.

187. Where the PCT receives notification from the Contractor under clause 186, or receives a request from the patient to be removed from the Contractor's list of patients, it shall remove that person from the Contractor's list of patients.

188. A removal under clause 187 shall take effect –

188.1 on the date on which the PCT receives notification of the registration of the person with another provider of *essential services* (or their equivalent); or

188.2 14 days after the date on which the notification or request made under clause 186 or 187 respectively is received by the PCT, whichever is the sooner.

189. The PCT shall, as soon as practicable, notify in writing –

189.1 the patient; and

189.2 the Contractor,

that the patient's name will be or has been removed from the Contractor's list of patients on the date referred to in clause 188.

190. In clauses 189, 191, 200.1, 206, 207, 212, 213 and 219 a reference to a request received from, or advice, information or notification required to be given to, a patient shall include a request received from or advice, information or notification required to be given to –

190.1 in the case of a patient who is a *child*, a *parent* or other person referred to in clause 173.1; or

190.2 in the case of an adult patient who is incapable of making the relevant request or receiving the relevant advice, information or notification, a relative or the *primary carer* of the patient.

Removals from the list at the request of the Contractor

191. Subject to clauses 201 to 207, where the Contractor has reasonable grounds for wishing a patient to be removed from its list of patients which do not relate to the applicant's race, gender, social class, age, religion, sexual orientation, appearance, disability or medical condition, the Contractor shall –

191.1 notify the PCT in writing that it wishes to have the patient removed; and

191.2 subject to clause 192, notify the patient in writing of its specific reasons for requesting removal.

192. Where, in the reasonable opinion of the Contractor, the circumstances of the removal are such that it is not appropriate for a more specific reason to be given, and there has been an irrevocable breakdown in the relationship between the patient and the Contractor, the reason given under clause 191 may consist of a statement that there has been such a breakdown.

193. Except in the circumstances specified in clause194, the Contractor may only request a removal under clause 191, if, within the period of 12 months prior to the date of its request to the PCT, it has warned the patient that he is at risk of removal and explained to him the reasons for this.

194. The circumstances referred to in clause 193 are that –
    194.1 the reason for removal relates to a change of address;
    194.2 the Contractor has reasonable grounds for believing that the issue of such a warning would be harmful to the physical or mental health of the patient or would put at risk the safety of one or more of the persons specified in clause 195; or
    194.3 it is, in the opinion of the Contractor, not otherwise reasonable or practical for a warning to be given.

195. The persons referred to in clause 194 are –
    195.1 if the Contractor is an individual medical practitioner, the Contractor;
    195.2 if the Contractor is a partnership, a partner in the partnership;
    195.3 if the Contractor is a company, a legal and beneficial owner of shares in that company;
    195.4 a member of the Contractor's staff;
    195.5 a person engaged by the Contractor to perform or assist in the performance of services under the Contract; or
    195.6 any other person present on the *practice premises* or in the place where services are being provided to the patient under the Contract.

196. The Contractor shall record in writing the date of any warning given in accordance with clause 193 and the reasons for giving such a warning as explained to the patient, or the reason why no such warning was given.

197. The Contractor shall keep a written record of removals under clause 191 which shall include the reason for removal given to the patient, the circumstances of the removal and in cases where clause 192 applies, the grounds for a more specific reason not being appropriate, and the Contractor shall make this record available to the PCT on request.

198. A removal requested in accordance with clause 191 shall, subject to clause 199, take effect from the date on which the person is registered with another provider of *essential services*, or the eighth day after the Trust receives the notice, whichever is the sooner.

199. Where, on the date on which the removal would take effect under clause 198, the Contractor is treating the patient at intervals of less than 7 days, the Contractor shall inform the PCT in writing of that fact and the removal shall take effect on the eighth day after the Trust receives notification from the Contractor that the person no longer needs such treatment, or on the date on which the person is registered with another provider of *essential services*, whichever is the sooner.

200. The PCT shall notify in writing –
    200.1 the patient; and

200.2 the Contractor

that the patient's name has been or will be removed from the Contractor's list of patients on the date referred to in clause 198 or 199.

Removals from the list of patients who are violent

201. Where the Contractor wishes a patient to be removed from its list of patients with immediate effect on the grounds that –

201.1 the patient has committed an act of violence against any of the persons specified in clause 202 or behaved in such a way that any such person has feared for his safety; and

201.2 it has reported the incident to the police,

the Contractor shall notify the PCT in accordance with clause 203.

202. The persons referred to in clause 201 are –

202.1 if the Contract is with an individual medical practitioner, that individual;

202.2 if the Contract is with a partnership, a partner in that partnership;

202.3 if the Contract is with a company, a legal and beneficial owner of shares in that company;

202.4 a member of the Contractor's staff;

202.5 a person employed or engaged by the Contractor to perform or assist in the performance of services under the Contract; or

202.6 any other person present on the *practice premises* or in the place where services were provided to the patient under the Contract.

203. Notification under clause 201 may be given by any means including telephone or fax but if not given in writing shall subsequently be confirmed in writing within 7 days (and for this purpose a faxed notification is not a written one).

204. The PCT shall acknowledge in writing receipt of a request from the Contractor under clause 201.

205. A removal requested in accordance with clause 201 shall take effect at the time the Contractor makes the telephone call to the PCT, or sends or delivers the notification to the PCT.

206. Where, pursuant to clauses 201 to205, the Contractor has notified the PCT that it wishes to have a patient removed from its list of patients, it shall inform the patient concerned unless –

206.1 it is not reasonably practicable for it to do so; or

206.2 it has reasonable grounds for believing that to do so would be harmful to the physical or mental health of the patient or would put at risk the safety of one or more of the persons specified in clause 202.

207. Where the PCT has removed a patient from the Contractor's list of patients in accordance with clause 205 it shall give written notice of the removal to that patient.

208. Where a patient is removed from the Contractor's list of patients in accordance with clauses 201 to 207, the Contractor shall record in the patient's medical records that the patient has been removed under this paragraph and the circumstances leading to his removal.

Removals from the list of patients registered elsewhere

209. The PCT shall remove a patient from the Contractor's list of patients if he has subsequently been registered with another provider of essential services (or their equivalent) in the area of the PCT or it has received notice from another PCT, a *Health Board*, a Local Health Board or a *Health and Social Services Board* that the patient has subsequently been registered with a provider of *essential services* (or their equivalent) outside the area of the PCT.

210. A removal in accordance with clause 209 shall take effect on the date on which notification of acceptance by the new provider was received or with the consent of the PCT, on such other date as has been agreed between the Contractor and the new provider.

211. The PCT shall notify the Contractor in writing of persons removed from its list of patients under clause 209.

Removals from the list of patients who have moved

212. Subject to clause 213, where the PCT is satisfied that a person on the Contractor's list of patients no longer resides in that Contractor's *practice area*, the PCT shall –
    212.1 inform that patient and the Contractor that the Contractor is no longer obliged to visit and treat the patient;
    212.2 advise the patient in writing either to obtain the Contractor's agreement to the continued inclusion of the patient on its list of patients or to apply for registration with another provider of *essential services* (or their equivalent); and
    212.3 inform the patient that if, after the expiration of 30 days from the date of the advice referred to in clause 212.2, he has not acted in accordance with the advice and informed it accordingly, the PCT will remove him from the Contractor's list of patients.

213. If, at the expiration of the period of 30 days referred to in clause 212.3, the PCT has not been notified of the action taken, it shall remove the patient from the Contractor's list of patients and inform him and the Contractor accordingly.

214. Where the address of a patient who is on the Contractor's list is no longer known to the PCT, the PCT shall –
    214.1 give to the Contractor notice in writing that it intends, at the end of the period of 6 months commencing with the date of the notice, to remove the patient from the Contractor's list of patients; and
    214.2 at the end of that period, remove the patient from the Contractor's list of patients unless, within that period, the Contractor satisfies the PCT that it is still responsible for providing *essential services* to that patient.

Removals from the list of patients absent from the United Kingdom etc.

215. The PCT shall remove a patient from the Contractor's list of patients where it receives notification that that patient –
    215.1 intends to be away from the United Kingdom for a period of at least 3 months;
    215.2 is in Her Majesty's Forces;
    215.3 is serving a prison sentence of more than 2 years or sentences totalling in the aggregate more than that period;
    215.4 has been absent from the United Kingdom for a period of more than 3 months; or
    215.5 has died.

216. A removal in accordance with clause 215 shall take effect –
    216.1 in the cases referred to in clauses 215.1 to 215.3 from the date of the departure, enlistment or imprisonment or the date on which the PCT first receives notification of the departure, enlistment or imprisonment whichever is the later;
    216.2 in the cases referred to in clauses 215.4 and 215.5 from the date on which the PCT first receives notification of the absence or death.

217. The PCT shall notify the Contractor in writing of patients removed from its list of patients under clause 215.

Removals from the list of patients accepted elsewhere as *temporary residents*

218. The PCT shall remove from the Contractor's list of patients a patient who has been accepted as a *temporary resident* by another contractor or other provider of *essential services* (or their equivalent) where it is satisfied, after due inquiry –
    218.1 that the patient's stay in the place of temporary residence has exceeded 3 months; and

218.2 that the patient has not returned to his normal place of residence or any other place within the Contractor's *practice area*.

219. The PCT shall notify the Contractor and, where practicable, the patient, of a removal under clause 218.

220. A notification to the patient under clause 219 shall inform him of –
     220.1 his entitlement to make arrangements for the provision to him of *essential services* (or their equivalent), including by the Contractor by whom he has been treated as a *temporary resident*; and
     220.2 the name and address of the PCT in whose area he is resident.

Removals from the list of pupils etc. of a school

221. Where the Contractor provides *essential services* under the Contract to persons on the grounds that they are pupils at or staff or residents of a school, the PCT shall remove from the Contractor's list of patients any such persons who do not appear on particulars of persons who are pupils at or staff or residents of that school provided by that school.

222. Where the PCT has made a request to a school to provide the particulars mentioned in clause 221 and has not received them, it shall consult the Contractor as to whether it should remove from its list of patients any persons appearing on that list as pupils at, or staff or residents of, that school.

223. The PCT shall notify the Contractor in writing of patients removed from its list of patients under clause 221.

Guidance

Reasons for removing patients

2.43 When patients register or stop being registered with the contractor, the contractor must supply the necessary information as soon as practicable to the PCT through the registration system. Where either the PCT or contractors remove patients from lists they must notify the patients and inform them of their right to receive primary medical services from another contractor. Patients may be removed from contractors' lists for a variety of reasons. A simple summary is provided in Table 4 (again, the Contract Regulations provide the definitive statement of law).

Table 4 **Reasons for removing patients**	
Reason	**Point of removal**
1. Patient chooses to register elsewhere	14 days after PCT is notified by the contractor or patient or date when PCT receives notification that patient is registered with another provider, whichever is the sooner
2. Teacher or pupil was receiving primary medical services through a school but has left	When PCT receives list from the school which does not include the patient
3. Patient moves outside the practice area	Date PCT is notified by the contractor or patient or 30 days after writing to patient
4. Patient's address is no longer known	PCT notifies the contractor that the patient's name will be removed from the list after 6 months
5. Patient joins the armed forces	Enlistment date, or date PCT is notified by the contractor or patient, whichever is sooner
6. Patient sentenced to a prison sentence for more than 2 years	Start of sentence, or date PCT is notified by the contractor or patient, whichever is sooner
7. Patient leaves the country for more than 3 months	Date patient leaves UK, or date PCT receives notification from the contractor or patient of intention to leave or that patient has left, whichever is sooner
8. Patient death	Date the PCT is notified by the contractor of the patient's death. Contractors must notify the PCT by the end of the first working day following the death where death occurs on the practice's premises – otherwise as soon as is practicable

Table 4 – continued	
Reason	**Point of removal**
9. Contractor requests that an individual patient is removed	1. Immediate for violent patients
2. When the patient is accepted by/ assigned to another practice, or 8 days after the date of the request by the contractor to the PCT for removal, whichever is sooner
3. If at the date of removal, a patient is receiving treatment at intervals of 7 days or less, the practice will be required to inform the PCT of this and removal will take place on the eighth day after the PCT has received notification from the practice that the person no longer needs such treatment, or on the date that the person is accepted/assigned to another practice. Doctors are also under an obligation under *GMC Good Medical Practice* guidance to take steps to ensure the continuing care of patients
10. Contractor requests administrative removal of groups of patients	Removal date

Removals proposed by contractors

2.44 Where contractors remove patients from their lists they must always inform the PCT in writing. For individual cases contractors must have reasonable grounds for wishing a patient to be removed. Those reasons cannot be due to the person's disability or medical condition, appearance, age, race, gender, social class, age, religion, or sexual orientation. Legitimate grounds for removal may include for example –

(i) violence, or threatening behaviour. This could involve, for example in relation to home visits, the patient, a relative, a household member or pets such as unchained dogs

(ii) crime and deception, for example fraudulently obtaining drugs for non-medical reasons, stealing from the premises or causing criminal damage

(iii) where the relationship between the contractor/practitioner and patient has been broken to the extent that it is necessary to end the professional relationship with the patient. Contractors should note they should not remove patients simply because they are exacting or highly dependent, exhibit high levels of anxiety or demand about perceived serious symptoms, or because they have made a complaint against a practitioner or the contractor.

Warnings and giving reasons for removal

2.45 Contractors should warn the patients before steps are taken for their removal. They may do so by any means they feel appropriate in the circumstances. It may not always be practically possible for a warning to be given to the patient, for example where a warning could result in physical or mental harm to the patient, or put at risk the safety of other people. Warnings should be recorded in writing. This record should note the date that the warning was given. Where a removal does take place and no warning was given, the contractor should also record why. A warning is not required where a patient is removed from a list because that patient moves out of the practice area.

2.46 Contractors will be required to explain in writing to patients their specific reasons for taking action for removing them from their list. In certain cases it may be sufficient to say that there has been a breakdown of the doctor–patient relationship. The Contract Regulations also require the contractor to keep a written record of the reasons and the circumstances for removing a patient, and these records should be shown to the PCT if it so requests.

● Local Discipline Committees and the NHS

Guidance

4.9 Outstanding proceedings involving GP Principals, that are taking place under the NHS (Service Committees & Tribunal) Regulations, will need to be concluded consistently and in a timely and orderly fashion when the new GMS contract comes into force. Since terms of service for individual GPs disappear under new GMS there will be no further need for local disciplinary committees constituted under these regulations to investigate alleged breaches of terms of service. The Service Committees

& Tribunal Regulations will be revoked for GMS (but not for general dental services, general ophthalmic services or pharmaceutical services). Transitional and consequential provisions will provide a way in which unresolved local disciplinary investigations involving GPs' terms of service should be concluded on or after the date the new GMS contract comes into force. Advice will be available on the Department's website in March 2004.

4.10 Under new GMS, questions arising from the operation of contracts with providers will be dealt with using the contract disputes mechanisms described in chapter 6. Questions relating to the suitability, efficiency or probity of individual doctors who are performing primary medical services will be dealt with by using regulations made under section 28X of the 1977 NHS Act (the NHS (Performers Lists) Regulations 2004).

Local Medical Committees – functions of

Regulations

27. (1) The functions of a Local Medical Committee which are prescribed for the purposes of section 45A(9) (Local Medical Committees) of the Act [55] are –

(a) the consideration of any complaint made to it by any medical practitioner against a medical practitioner specified in paragraph (2) providing services under a contract in the relevant area involving any question of the efficiency of those services;

(b) the reporting of the outcome of the consideration of any such complaint to the PCT with whom the contract is held in cases where that consideration gives rise to any concerns relating to the efficiency of services provided under a contract;

(c) the making of arrangements for the medical examination of a medical practitioner specified in paragraph (2), where the contractor or the PCT is concerned that the medical practitioner is incapable of adequately providing services under the contract and it so requests with the agreement of the medical practitioner concerned; and

(d) the consideration of the report of any medical examination arranged in accordance with sub-paragraph (c) and the making of a written report as to the capability of the medical practitioner of adequately providing services under the contract to the medical practitioner concerned, the contractor and the PCT with whom the contractor holds a contract.

(2) The medical practitioner referred to in paragraph (1)(a) and (c)[e] is a medical practitioner who is –
  (a) a contractor;
  (b) one of two or more individuals practising in partnership who hold a contract; or
  (c) a legal and beneficial shareholder in a company which holds a contract.

(3) In this regulation, "the relevant area" means the area for which the Local Medical Committee is formed.

Locums – payments for covering maternity, paternity and adoption leave

Statement of Financial Entitlement

9.1 Employees of contractors will have rights to time off for ante-natal care, maternity leave, paternity leave, adoption leave and parental leave, if they satisfy the relevant entitlement conditions under employment legislation for those types of leave. The rights of partners in partnerships to these types of leave is a matter for their partnership agreement.

9.2 If an employee or partner who takes any such leave is a performer under a GMS contract, the contractor may need to employ a locum to maintain the level of services that it normally provides. Even if the PCT is not directed in this SFE to pay for such cover, it may do so as a matter of discretion. However, if –
  (a) the performer is a GP performer; and
  (b) the leave is ordinary maternity, paternity leave or ordinary adoption leave,
the contractor may be entitled to payment of, or a contribution towards, the costs of locum cover under this SFE.

Entitlement to payments for covering ordinary maternity, paternity and ordinary adoption leave

9.3 In any case where a contractor actually and necessarily engages a locum (or more than one such person) to cover for the absence of a GP performer on ordinary maternity leave, paternity leave or ordinary adoption leave, and –
  (a) the leave of absence is for more than 1 week (the maximum periods are: 26 weeks for ordinary maternity leave and for ordinary adoption

leave for the parent who is the main care provider; and 2 weeks for paternity leave and for adoption leave for the parent who is not the main care provider);

(b) the performer on leave is entitled to that leave either under –
  (i) statute,
  (ii) a partnership agreement or other agreement between the partners of a partnership, or
  (iii) a contract of employment, provided that the performer on leave is entitled under their contract of employment to be paid their full salary by the contractor during their leave of absence;

(c) the locum is not a partner or shareholder in the contractor, or already an employee of the contractor, unless the performer on leave is a job-sharer; and

(d) the contractor is not also claiming another payment for locum cover in respect of the performer on leave pursuant to this Part,

then subject to the following provisions of this Section, the PCT must provide financial assistance to the contractor under its GMS contract in respect of the cost of engaging that locum (which may or may not be the maximum amount payable, as set out in paragraph 9.5).

9.4 It is for the PCT to determine whether or not it is or was in fact necessary to engage the locum, or to continue to engage the locum, but it is to have regard to the following principles –

(a) it should not normally be considered necessary to employ a locum if the PCT has offered to provide the locum cover itself and the contractor has refused that offer without good reason;

(b) it should not normally be considered necessary to employ a locum if the performer on leave had a right to return but that right has been extinguished; and

(c) it should not normally be considered necessary to employ a locum if the contractor has engaged a new employee or partner to perform the duties of the performer on leave and it is not carrying a vacancy in respect of another position which the performer on leave will fill on his return.

Ceilings on the amounts payable

9.5 The maximum amount payable under this Section by the PCT in respect of locum cover for a GP performer is £948.33 per week.

Payment arrangements

9.6 The contractor is to submit claims for costs actually incurred after they have been incurred, at a frequency to be agreed between the PCT and the contractor, or if agreement cannot be reached, within 14 days of the end of month during which the costs were incurred. Any amount payable falls due 14 days after the claim is submitted.

Conditions attached to the amounts payable

9.7 Payments under this Section, or any part thereof, are only payable if the contractor satisfies the following conditions –

(a) if the leave of absence is maternity leave, the contractor must supply the PCT with a certificate of expected confinement as used for the purposes of obtaining statutory maternity pay, or a private certificate providing comparable information;

(b) if the leave of absence is for paternity leave, the contractor must supply the PCT with a letter written by the GP performer confirming prospective fatherhood and giving the date of expected confinement;

(c) if the leave of absence is for adoption leave, the contractor must supply the PCT with a letter written by the GP performer confirming the date of the adoption and the name of the main care provider, countersigned by the appropriate adoption agency;

(d) the contractor must, on request, provide the PCT with written records demonstrating the actual cost to it of the locum cover; and

(e) once the locum arrangements are in place, the contractor must inform the PCT –

(i) if there is to be any change to the locum arrangements, or

(ii) if, for any other reason, there is to be a change to the contractor's arrangements for performing the duties of the performer on leave,

at which point the PCT is to determine whether it still considers the locum cover necessary.

9.8 If the contractor breaches any of these conditions, the PCT may, in appropriate circumstances, withhold payment of any sum otherwise payable under this Section.

● Movement between GMS and PMS

Guidance

6.20 Under the terms of the National Health Service (Primary Care) Act 1997 any GP who entered into a PMS pilot arrangement has a preferential right (if so determined by the Secretary of State) to return to GMS. The new primary care performers' list described in chapter 4, taken together with the new GMS contracts and the "permanent" PMS provisions under section 28C, means that the right of individual PMS GPs to return to GMS will end. Instead a new right for the whole PMS contract to transfer to a GMS contract will be introduced. GMS contractors will also be able to continue to seek to enter into a local PMS contract should they so wish.

6.21 Where a PMS provider seeks to transfer to a GMS contract, the PCT will be required to offer that provider a GMS contract, so long as it meets all the provider conditions laid down in the GMS Contract Regulations. PMS providers that return to GMS would be entitled to the GMS payments set out in the SFE. They can also apply to the PCT to receive an MPIG and the way in which this should be calculated will be set out in the Department of Health's forthcoming guidance on PMS.

Minimum Practice Income Guarantee (MPIG)

Statement of Financial Entitlement

3.1 The Minimum Practice Income Guarantee (MPIG) is based on the historic revenue of a contractor's GPs from the list in Annex D essentially of Red Book fees and allowances, and is essentially designed to protect those income levels. A 1 year aggregate of these protected income amounts is the contractor's Initial Global Sum Equivalent (GSE), which is then adjusted to produce first its Adjusted GSE and then its Final GSE.

CALCULATION OF GLOBAL SUM EQUIVALENT

3.2 In order to calculate a contractor's GSE, a calculation will first need to be made of its Initial and Adjusted GSE. This is to be done by the PCT –
(a) on the basis of information obtained by it from the contractor about payments to the contractor (or the GPs comprising the contractor) under the Red Book, and in particular in the year preceding 1 July 2003; and
(b) in accordance with the Department of Health guidance reproduced in Annex D. Paragraphs 1–7 cover the calculation of the Initial GSE, and adjustments to take account, for example, of practice mergers and splits are covered in paragraphs 8–19.

3.3 Whether or not any adjustments are in fact necessary to the Initial GSE, the final total produced as a result of the calculation in accordance with

Annex D is known as the contractor's Adjusted GSE. That amount is then subject to three further adjustments –

(a) the amount is increased by 2.85% to bring prices in respect of the year ending 30 June 2003 up to 31 March 2004 levels (i.e. re-basing for the financial year 2003/04); then

(b) the sub-paragraph (a) amount is increased by 1.47% to take account of projected price increases in respect of the financial year 2004/05 (i.e. re-basing for the financial year 2004/05); then

(c) the sub-paragraph (b) amount is added to the contractor's GSE Superannuation Adjustment. This is an adjustment to take account of the additional 7% employer's superannuation contributions in respect of practice staff as a result of the Treasury transfer. The contractor's GSE Superannuation Adjustment is its Contractor Weighted Population for the Quarter multiplied by £1.46.

The resulting amount is the contractor's Final GSE.

CALCULATION OF CORRECTION FACTOR MONTHLY PAYMENTS

3.4 The contractor's Final GSE is then to be compared to the paragraph 2.3 total in respect of the contractor taking away from that paragraph 2.3 total any Historic Opt-Outs Adjustment to which it is entitled.

3.5 A contractor is entitled to the Historic Opt-Outs Adjustment if –

(a) since 1 July 2002 the GPs comprising the contractor have not been providing, within GMS services, services which as far as possible are equivalent to one or more of the Additional or Out-of-Hours Services listed in the Table in paragraph 2.5; and

(b) the contractor will not be providing those services in the financial year 2004/05.

3.6 The amount of the contractor's Historic Opt-Outs Adjustment is calculated as follows. If the contractor is claiming an Historic Opt-Outs Adjustment in respect of –

(a) one of the Additional or Out-of-Hours Services listed in column 1 of the Table in paragraph 2.5, the value of the contractor's Historic Opt-Outs Adjustment is the amount by which its paragraph 2.3 total is reduced if it is reduced by the percentage listed opposite that service in column 2 of the Table;

(b) more than one of the Additional or Out-of-Hours Services listed in column 1 of the Table in paragraph 2.5, the value of the contractor's Historic Opt-Outs Adjustment is to include an amount in respect of each service. The value of the amount for each service is the amount by which the contractor's paragraph 2.3 total is reduced if it is reduced by the percentage listed opposite that service in column 2 of the Table, without any other deductions from the paragraph 2.3 total first being taken into account. The total of all the amounts in respect of each service is then aggregated to produce the final amount of the contractor's Historic Opt-Outs Adjustment.

3.7 Accordingly, a contractor's paragraph 2.3 total minus any Historic Opt-Outs Adjustment to which it is entitled, is its Global Sum Comparator.

3.8 If the contractor's Final GSE is less than its Global Sum Comparator, a Correction Factor is not payable in respect of that contractor. However, if its Final GSE is greater than its Global Sum Comparator, Correction Factor Monthly Payments (CFMPs) must be paid by the PCT to the contractor under its GMS contract. The amount of the CFMPs payable is the difference between the contractor's Final GSE and its Global Sum Comparator, divided by 12. CFMPs are to fall due on the last day of each month.

3.9 Unless the contractor is subject to a partnership merger or split, the amount of the contractor's CFMPs is to remain unchanged throughout the financial year 2004/05, even if the amount of the contractor's Payable GSMP changes.

Practice mergers or splits

3.10 The MPIG calculation is a one-off calculation, which will remain unchanged. It is only to be made in respect of GMS contracts that take effect, or are treated as taking effect, on 1 April 2004. Except as provided for in paragraphs 3.11 to 3.14, a contractor with a GMS contract which takes effect, or is treated as taking effect, after 1 April 2004 will not be entitled to an MPIG (or therefore to CFMPs).

3.11 If the new contractor comes into existence as the result of a merger between one or more other contractors, and that merger led to the termination of GMS contracts and the agreement of a new GMS contract, the new contractor is to be entitled to a CFMP that is the total of any CFMPs payable under the previous GMS contracts.

3.12 If –
   (a) a new contractor comes into existence as the result of the split of a previous contractor;
   (b) at least some of the members of the new contractor were members of the previous contractor; and
   (c) the split led to the termination of the previous contractor's GMS contract,
   the new contractor will be entitled to a proportion of any CFMP payable under the terminated contract. The proportions are to be worked out on a *pro rata* basis, based upon the number of patients registered with the

previous contractor (i.e. immediately before its contract is terminated) who will be registered with the new contractor when its new contract takes effect.

3.13 If a new GMS contract is agreed by a contractor which has split from a previously established contractor, but the split did not lead to the termination of the previously established contractor's GMS contract, the new contractor will not be entitled to any of the previously established contractor's CFMP unless, as a result of the split, an agreed number, or a number ascertainable by the PCT(s) for the contractors, of patients have transferred to the new contractor at or before the end of the first full quarter after the new GMS contract takes effect.

3.14 If such a transfer has taken place, the previously established contractor and the new contractor are each to be entitled to a proportion of the CFMP that has been payable under the previously established contractor's GMS contract. The proportions are to be worked out on a *pro rata* basis. The new contractor's fraction of the CFMP will be –
    (a) the number of patients transferred to it from the previously established contractor; divided by
    (b) the number of patients registered with the previously established contractor immediately before the split that gave rise to the transfer
    and the old contractor's CFMP is to be reduced accordingly.

Conditions attached to payment of Correction Factor Monthly Payments

3.15 CFMPs, or any part thereof, are only payable if the contractor satisfies the following conditions –
    (a) the contractor must make available any information which the PCT does not have but needs, and the contractor either has or could reasonably be expected to obtain, in order to calculate the contractor's CFMP; and
    (b) all information supplied pursuant to or in accordance with this paragraph must be accurate.

3.16 If the contractor breaches any of these conditions, the PCT may, in appropriate circumstances, withhold payment of any or any part of a CFMP that is otherwise payable.

Future years

3.17 In future years, Correction Factor Payments will be uprated by the same percentage as Global Sum Payments.

Newly Registered Patients

Regulations

Newly registered patients

4.   (1) Where a patient has been –
        (a) accepted on a contractor's list of patients under paragraph 15; or
        (b) assigned to that list by the PCT,
        the contractor shall, in addition and without prejudice to its other obligations in respect of that patient under the contract, invite the patient to participate in a consultation either at its practice premises or, if the medical condition of the patient so warrants, at one of the places referred to in paragraph 3(2).
    (2) An invitation under sub-paragraph (1) shall be issued within 6 months of the date of the acceptance of the patient on, or their assignment to, the contractor's list.
    (3) Where a patient (or, where appropriate, in the case of a patient who is a child, his parent) agrees to participate in a consultation mentioned in sub-paragraph (1) the contractor shall, in the course of that consultation make such inquiries and undertake such examinations as appear to it to be appropriate in all the circumstances.

Standard Contract

Newly registered patients

32.   Where a patient has been accepted on the Contractor's list of patients under clauses 170 to 175 or assigned to that list by the PCT, the Contractor shall, in addition and without prejudice to its other obligations in respect of that patient under the Contract, invite the patient to participate in a consultation either at its practice premises or, if the medical condition of the patient so warrants, at one of the places referred to in clause 30. Such an invitation shall be issued within 6 months of the date of the acceptance of the patient on, or their assignment to, the Contractor's list of patients.

33.   Where a patient (or, where appropriate, in the case of a patient who is a *child*, his *parent*) agrees to participate in a consultation referred to in clause 32 above, the Contractor shall, in the course of that consultation,

make such inquiries and undertake such examinations as appear to it to be appropriate in all the circumstances.

Guidance

2.23 (ii) newly registered patients. The contractor is obliged to invite all newly registered patients for a consultation within 6 months. The extra workload involved is reflected in the list-turnover adjustment within the global sum

Notices/notification to PCTs

Regulations

85. Notice provisions specific to a contract with a company limited by shares

(1) A contractor which is a company limited by shares shall give notice in writing to the PCT forthwith when –
  (a) any share in the contractor is transmitted or transferred (whether legally or beneficially) to another person on a date after the contract has been entered into;
  (b) it passes a resolution or a court of competent jurisdiction makes an order that the contractor be wound up;
  (c) circumstances arise which might entitle a creditor or a court to appoint a receiver, administrator or administrative receiver for the contractor;
  (d) circumstances arise which would enable the court to make a winding up order in respect of the contractor; or
  (e) the contractor is unable to pay its debts within the meaning of section 123 of the Insolvency Act 1986 (definition of inability to pay debts).

(2) A notice under sub-paragraph (1)(a) shall confirm that the new shareholder, or, as the case may be, the personal representative of a deceased shareholder –
  (a) is a medical practitioner, or that he satisfies the conditions specified in section 28S(2)(b)(i) to (iv) of the Act (persons eligible to enter into GMS contracts); and
  (b) meets the further conditions imposed on shareholders by virtue of regulations 4 and 5.

86. Notice provisions specific to a contract with two or more individuals practising in partnership

(1) A contractor which is a partnership shall give notice in writing to the PCT forthwith when –
   (a) a partner leaves or informs his partners that he intends to leave the partnership, and the date upon which he left or will leave the partnership;
   (b) a new partner joins the partnership.

(2) A notice under sub-paragraph (1)(b) shall –
   (a) state the date that the new partner joined the partnership;
   (b) confirm that the new partner is a medical practitioner, or that he satisfies the conditions specified in section 28S(2)(b)(i) to (iv) of the Act;
   (c) confirm that the new partner meets the conditions imposed by regulations 4 and 5; and
   (d) state whether the new partner is a general or a limited partner.

87. Notification of deaths

(1) The contractor shall report in writing to the PCT the death on its practice premises of any patient no later than the end of the first working day after the date on which the death occurred.

(2) The report shall include –
   (a) the patient's full name;
   (b) the patient's NHS number where known;
   (c) the date and place of death;
   (d) a brief description of the circumstances, as known, surrounding the death;
   (e) the name of any medical practitioner or other person treating the patient whilst on the practice premises; and
   (f) the name, where known, of any other person who was present at the time of the death.

(3) The contractor shall send a copy of the report referred to in sub-paragraph (1) to any other PCT in whose area the deceased was resident at the time of his death.

88. Notifications to patients following variation of the Contract

Where the Contract is varied in accordance with Part 8 of this Schedule and, as a result of that variation –

(a) there is to be a change in the range of services provided to the contractor's registered patients; or

(b) patients who are on the contractor's list of patients are to be removed from that list,

the PCT shall notify those patients in writing of the variation and its effect and inform them of the steps they can take to obtain elsewhere the services in question or, as the case may be, register elsewhere for the provision of essential services (or their equivalent).

Standard Contract

Notice provision specific to a Contractor that is a company limited by shares[34]

457.   The Contractor shall give notice in writing to the PCT forthwith when –

457.1 any share in the Contractor is transmitted or transferred (whether legally or beneficially) to another person on a date after the Contract has been entered into;

457.2 it passes a resolution or a court of competent jurisdiction makes an order that the Contractor be wound up;

457.3 circumstances arise which might entitle a creditor or a court to appoint a receiver, administrator or administrative receiver for the Contractor;

457.4 circumstances arise which would enable the court to make a winding up order in respect of the Contractor; or

457.5 the Contractor is unable to pay its debts within the meaning of section 123 of the Insolvency Act 1986.

458.   A notice under clause 457.1 shall confirm that the new shareholder, or, as the case may be, the personal representative of a deceased shareholder –

458.1 is a medical practitioner, or that he satisfies the conditions specified in section 28S(2)(b)(i) to (iv) of *the Act*; and

458.2 meets the further conditions imposed on shareholders by virtue of regulations 4 and 5 of *the Regulations*.

Notice provision specific to a Contractor that is a partnership[35]

459.   The Contractor shall give notice in writing to the PCT forthwith when –

459.1 a partner leaves or informs his partners that he intends to leave the partnership, and the date upon which he left or will leave the partnership; and

459.2 a new partner joins the partnership.

460. A notice under clause 459.2 shall –
    460.1 state the date that the new partner joined the partnership;
    460.2 confirm that the new partner is a medical practitioner, or that he satisfies the condition specified in section 28S(2)(b)(i) to (iv) of *the Act*;
    460.3 confirm that the new partner meets the conditions imposed by regulations 4 and 5; and
    460.4 state whether the new partner is a general or limited partner.

Notification of deaths

461. The Contractor shall report in writing to the PCT the death on its *practice premises* of any patient no later than the end of the first working day after the date on which the death occurred.

462. The report shall include –
    462.1 the patient's full name;
    462.2 the patient's NHS number where known;
    462.3 the date and place of death;
    462.4 a brief description of the circumstances, as known, surrounding the death;
    462.5 the name of any doctor or other person treating the patient whilst on the *practice premises*; and
    462.6 the name, where known, of any other person who was present at the time of the death.

463. The Contractor shall send a copy of the report referred to in clause 461 to any other PCT in whose area the deceased was resident at the time of his death.

Notifications to patients following a variation of the Contract

464. Where the Contract is varied in accordance with Part 25 of this Contract and, as a result of that variation –
    464.1 there is to be a change in the range of services provided to the Contractor's patients; or
    464.2 patients who are on the Contractor's list of patients are to be removed from that list,

---

34 Clauses 457 and 458 only need to be included in the Contract if the Contractor is a company limited by shares. If the Contractor is not a company limited by shares, these clauses can be deleted.

35 Clauses 459 and 460 only need to be included in the Contract if the Contractor is a partnership. If the Contractor is not a partnership, these clauses can be deleted.

the PCT shall notify those patients in writing of the variation and its effect and inform them of the steps they can take to obtain elsewhere the services in question or, as the case may be, register elsewhere for the provision of *essential services* (or their equivalent).

Out-of-hours services

See also: Out-of-hours opt-outs · Out-of-hours services

Regulations

Criteria for out-of-hours services

10. A contractor whose contract includes the provision of out-of-hours services shall only be required to provide such services if, in the reasonable opinion of the contractor in the light of the patient's medical condition, it would not be reasonable in all the circumstances for the patient to wait for the services required until the next time at which he could obtain such services during core hours.

Standards for out-of-hours services

11. From 1 January 2005, a contractor which provides out-of-hours services must, in the provision of such services, meet the quality standards set out in the document entitled "Quality Standards in the Delivery of GP Out-of-Hours Services" published on 20 June 2002.

Out-of-hours services – before 1 January 2005

Regulations

30.

(1) Subject to paragraph 10 of Schedule 6, a contract under which services are to be provided before 1 January 2005 (whether or not such services will be provided after that date) must provide for the services specified in paragraph (2) to be provided throughout the out-of-hours period unless –

(a) the PCT has accepted in writing, prior to the signing of the contract, a written request from the contractor that the contract should not require the contractor to make such provision;

(b) the contract is, at the date on which it is signed, with –

    (i) a medical practitioner who is, or was on 31 March 2004, relieved of responsibility for providing services to his patients under paragraph 18(2) of Schedule 2 to the National Health Service (General Medical Services) Regulations 1992,

    (ii) a partnership in which all of the partners who are general medical practitioners are, or were on 31 March 2004, relieved of responsibility for providing services to their patients under that paragraph, or

    (iii) a company in which all of the general medical practitioners who own shares in that company are, or were on 31 March 2004, relieved of responsibility for providing services to their patients under that paragraph;

(c) the contractor has opted out in accordance with paragraph 4 or 5 of Schedule 3; or

(d) the contract has been otherwise varied to exclude a requirement to make such provision.

(2)   The services referred to in paragraph (1) are –

(a) the services which must be provided in core hours under regulation 15; and

(b) such additional services as are included in the contract pursuant to regulation 29.

31.

(1)   Where the contract is with –

(a) an individual medical practitioner who is, or was on 31 March 2004, responsible for providing services during all or part of the out-of-hours period to the patients of a medical practitioner who meets the requirements in paragraph (2);

(b) two or more individuals practising in partnership at least one of whom is, or was on 31 March 2004, a medical practitioner responsible for providing such services; or

(c) a company in which one or more of the shareholders is, or was on 31 March 2004, a medical practitioner responsible for providing such services,

the contract with that contractor must require the contractor to continue to provide such services to the patients of the exempt contractor until the happening of one of the events in paragraph (3).

(2)   The requirements referred to in paragraph (1)(a) are that –

(a) the medical practitioner was relieved of responsibility for providing services to his patients under paragraph 18(2) of Schedule 2 to the

National Health Service (General Medical Services) Regulations 1992; and (b) he –

    (i) has entered or intends to enter into a contract which does not include out-of-hours services pursuant to regulation 30(1)(b)(i),

    (ii) is one of two or more individuals practising in partnership who have entered or intends to enter into a contract which does not include out-of-hours services pursuant to regulation 30(1)(b)(ii), or

    (iii) is the owner of shares in a company which has entered or intends to enter into a contract which does not include out-of-hours services pursuant to regulation 30(1)(b)(iii).

(3)   The events referred to in paragraph (1) are –

    (a) the contractor has opted out of the provision of out-of-hours services in accordance with paragraph 4 or 5 of Schedule 3; or

    (b) the PCT (and, if it is different, the PCT with whom the exempt contractor holds its contract) has or have agreed in writing that the contractor need no longer provide some or all of those services to some or all of those patients.

(4)   In this regulation "exempt contractor" means a contractor who is exempt from providing out-of-hours services pursuant to regulation 30(1)(b).

32.   A contract which includes the provision of out-of-hours services pursuant to regulation 30 or 31 must contain terms which have the same effect as those set out in Schedule 7.

Standard Contract

Out-of-hours services[36]

82.   [Subject to clause 83, the Contractor shall provide-

    82.1 the services which must be provided in *core hours* pursuant to clauses 45 to 51; and

    82.2 such additional services (if any) as are included in the Contract pursuant to clause 55

    during the *out-of-hours period*[37]].

83.   The Contractor shall only be required to provide the services specified in clause 82 during the *out-of-hours period* to a patient if, in the reasonable opinion of the Contractor in the light of the patient's medical condition, it would not be reasonable in all the circumstances for the patient to wait for the services required until the next time at which he could obtain such services during *core hours*.[38]

36   A contractor is required to provide *out-of-hours* services under the Contract if it falls within the categories specified in regulations 30 to 31 of *the Regulations*: otherwise it is a matter for negotiation between the parties. This means that the Contractor must provide *out-of-hours services* under the Contract in the following circumstances –

1. (regulation 30) if, under the Contract, the Contractor will be providing any services before 1 January 2005 (whether or not services will be provided after that date), the Contract must provide for *out-of-hours services* to be provided to patients by the Contractor unless –

    (a) the PCT has accepted in writing, prior to the signing of the Contract, a written request from the Contractor that the Contract should not require the Contractor to make such provision; or

    (b) the Contract is, at the date on which it is signed, with –
    - a medical practitioner who is or was, on 31 March 2004 relieved of responsibility for providing services to his patients under paragraph 18(2) of Schedule 2 to the National Health Service (General Medical Services) Regulations 1992;
    - a partnership in which all of the partners who are *general medical practitioners* are, or were on 31 March 2004 relieved of responsibility for providing services to their patients under that paragraph on that date;
    - a company in which all of the *general medical practitioners* who own shares in that company are, or were on 31 March 2004 relieved of responsibility for providing services to their patients under that paragraph on that date

    (c) the Contractor opts out of the provision of *out-of-hours services* pursuant to the Contract (which will not affect the need to include the provision of *out-of-hours services* in the Contract at the point the Contract is entered into); or

    (d) the Contract has been otherwise varied to exclude a requirement to make such provision (this will not be relevant at the point where the Contract is being entered into because there will not be any such variation until there is a contract to vary); AND

2. (regulation 31) if the Contract is with any of the persons specified in (a) to (c) below, the Contract must require the Contractor to continue providing *out-of-hours services* to patients of an exempt contractor where the Contractor is –

    (a) an individual medical practitioner who is, or was on 31 March 2004, responsible for providing services during all or part of the out-of-hours period to the patients of a medical practitioner who meets the requirements set out in paragraph 3 below ("exempt contractor");

    (b) two or more individuals practising in partnership at least one of whom is, or was on 31 March 2004, a medical practitioner responsible for providing such services; or

    (c) a company in which one or more of the shareholders is, or was, on 31 March 2004, a medical practitioner responsible for providing such services

    and the Contractor must continue to provide such services until it has opted out of the provision of *out-of-hours services* in accordance with Part 10 of the Contract, or the PCT (or if it is different, the PCT with whom the exempt contractor holds its contract)) has or have agreed in writing that the Contractor need no longer provide some or all of those services to some or all of those patients.

3. the requirements referred to in 2(a) are that –

    (a) the medical practitioner was relieved of responsibility for providing services to his patients under paragraph 18(2) of Schedule 2 to the National Health Service (General Medical Services) Regulations 1992; and

    (b) he –
    - has entered or intends to enter into a contract which does not include *out-of-hours services* pursuant to paragraph 1(b) above,
    - is one of two or more individuals practising in partnership who have entered or intend to enter into a contract which does not includes *out-of-hours services* pursuant to paragraph 1(b) above;
    - is the owner of shares in a company which has entered or intends to enter into a contract which does not include *out-of-hours services* pursuant to paragraph 1(b) above.

84.   From 1 January 2005, the Contractor must, in the provision of *out-of-hours services*, meet the quality standards set out in the document entitled "Quality Standards in the Delivery of GP Out-of-Hours Services" published on 20 June 2002 (the document is published by the Department of Health on its website at http://www.doh.gov.uk/pricare/qualitystandards.htm or a copy may be obtained by writing to Primary Care, Room 7E28, Department of Health, Quarry House, Quarry Hill, Leeds LS2 7UE or by e-mailing OOHAccreditation@doh.gov.uk).[39]

85.   If the Contractor is required to provide *out-of-hours services* under the Contract pursuant to regulation 31 of *the Regulations* to the patients of an exempt contractor it shall provide such services, and continue to provide such services until –

  85.1 it has opted out of the provision of *out-of-hours services* in accordance with Part 10 of this Contract;

  85.2 the PCT and, where applicable, the PCT that holds a contract with the contractor for whom *out-of-hours services* are being provided by the Contractor under the Contract, has or have agreed in writing that the Contractor need no longer provide some or all of those services to some or all of those patients.[40]

86.   [If the Contractor is required to provide *out-of-hours services* under the Contract, pursuant to article 20 of the *Transitional Order*, to the patients of a party to a *default contract* who is an exempt contractor (within the meaning of that article) it shall provide such services to those patients, and continue to provide such services until –

  86.1 the exempt contractor's *default contract* referred to in article 20(3)(a) of the *Transitional Order* has come to an end and not been succeeded by a *general medical services contract* which does not include *out-of-hours services* pursuant to regulation 30(1)(b) of *the Regulations*;

---

37   This clause is mandatory only if *out-of-hours services* are being provided pursuant to regulation 30 or 31 of *the Regulations*: if *out-of-hours services* are included in the Contract other than by virtue of regulation 30 or 31, details of what services are to be provided by the Contractor during the *out-of-hours period* should be included here instead, and the provision can be re-drafted depending on what is agreed between the parties.

38   This clause is required whenever *out-of-hours services* will be provided, whether pursuant to regulation 30 or 31 of *the Regulations* or not.

39   This clause is required whenever *out-of-hours services* will be provided, whether pursuant to regulation 30 or 31 of *the Regulations* or not.

40   This clause is only required if the Contractor is providing *out-of-hours services* pursuant to regulation 31 of *the Regulations*. Otherwise this clause should be deleted.

86.2 the Contractor has opted out of the provision of *out-of-hours services* in accordance with Part 10 of the Contract; or

86.3 the PCT and, if it is different, the PCT that holds a contract with the contractor for whom *out-of-hours services* are being provided by the Contractor under the Contract, has or have agreed in writing that the Contractor need no longer provide some or all of those services to some or all of those patients.][41]

Out-of-hours services – application for approval for out-of-hours arrangement

Regulations

2.

(1) An application to the PCT for approval of an out-of-hours arrangement shall be made in writing and shall state –

(a) the name and address of the accredited service provider or the proposed transferee doctor;

(b) the periods during which the contractor's obligations under the contract are to be transferred;

(c) how the accredited service provider or proposed transferee doctor intends to meet the contractor's obligations during the periods specified under paragraph (b);

(d) the arrangements for the transfer of the contractor's obligations under the contract to and from the accredited service provider or transferee doctor at the beginning and end of the periods specified under paragraph (b);

(e) whether the proposed arrangement includes the contractor's obligations in respect of maternity medical services; and

(f) how long the proposed arrangements are intended to last and the circumstances in which the contractor's obligations under the contract during the periods specified under paragraph (b) would revert to it.

---

41   Clause 86 only needs to be included if, pursuant to article 20 of the *Transitional Order*, the Contractor will be responsible for providing *out-of-hours services* to the patients of a party to a *default contract*. If it is not relevant to the Contractor, the clause can be deleted.

(2) The PCT shall determine the application before the end of the period of 28 days beginning with the day on which the PCT received it.

(3) The PCT shall grant approval to a proposed out-of-hours arrangement if it is satisfied –
   (a) having regard to the overall provision of primary medical services provided in the out-of-hours period in its area, that the arrangement is reasonable and will contribute to the efficient provision of such services in the area;
   (b) having regard, in particular, to the interests of the contractor's patients, that the arrangement is reasonable;
   (c) having regard, in particular, to all reasonably foreseeable circumstances, that the arrangement is practicable and will work satisfactorily;
   (d) that any arrangement with a person referred to in paragraph 1(5)(b) will be of an equivalent standard to an arrangement with a person referred to in paragraph 1(5)(a);
   (e) that in the case of an arrangement with a person referred to in paragraph 1(5)(a), the practice premises are within the geographical area in respect of which approval is given under regulation 5 of the Out-of-Hours Regulations;
   (f) that it will be clear to the contractor's patients how to seek primary medical services during the out-of-hours period;
   (g) where maternity medical services are to be provided under the out-of-hours arrangement, that they will be performed by a medical practitioner who has such medical experience and training as are necessary to enable him properly to perform such services; and
   (h) that if the arrangement comes to an end, the contractor has in place proper arrangements for the immediate resumption of its responsibilities,
   and shall not refuse to grant approval without first consulting the Local Medical Committee (if any) for its area.

(4) The PCT shall give notice to the contractor of its determination and, where it refuses an application, it shall send the contractor a statement in writing of the reasons for its determination.

(5) A contractor which wishes to refer the matter in accordance with the NHS dispute resolution procedure must do so before the end of the period of 30 days beginning with the day on which the PCT's notification under sub-paragraph (4) was sent.

3. Effect of approval of an arrangement with a transferee doctor

Where the PCT has approved an out-of-hours arrangement with a transferee doctor the PCT and the transferee doctor shall be deemed to have agreed a variation of their contract which has the effect of including in it, from the date on which the out-of-hours arrangement commences and for so long as that arrangement is not suspended or terminated, the services covered by that arrangement and paragraph 104(1) of Schedule 6 shall not apply.

4. Review of approval

(1) Where it appears to the PCT that it may no longer be satisfied of any of the matters referred to in paragraphs (a) to (h) of paragraph 2(3), it may give notice to the contractor that it proposes to review its approval of the out-of-hours arrangement.

(2) On any review under sub-paragraph (1), the PCT shall allow the contractor a period of 30 days, beginning with the day on which it sent the notice, within which to make representations in writing to the PCT.

(3) After considering any representations made in accordance with sub-paragraph (2), the PCT may determine to –
(a) continue its approval;
(b) withdraw its approval following a period of notice; or
(c) if it appears to it that it is necessary in the interests of the contractor's patients, withdraw its approval immediately.

(4) Except in the case of an immediate withdrawal of approval, the PCT shall not withdraw its approval without first consulting the Local Medical Committee (if any) for its area.

(5) Where the PCT determines to withdraw its approval immediately, it shall notify the Local Medical Committee (if any) for its area.

(6) The PCT shall give notice to the contractor of its determination under sub-paragraph (3).

(7) Where the PCT withdraws its approval, whether immediately or on notice, it shall include with the notice a statement in writing of the reasons for its determination.

(8) A contractor which wishes to refer the matter in accordance with the NHS dispute resolution procedure must do so before the end of the period of 30 days beginning with the day on which the PCT's notification under sub-paragraph (6) was sent.

(9) Where the PCT determines to withdraw its approval following a period of notice, the withdrawal shall take effect at the end of the period of 2 months beginning with –
(a) the date on which the notice referred to in sub-paragraph (6) was sent; or

(b) where there has been a dispute which has been referred under the NHS dispute resolution procedure and the dispute is determined in favour of withdrawal, the date on which the contractor receives notice of the determination.

(10)   Where the PCT determines to withdraw its approval immediately, the withdrawal shall take effect on the day on which the notice referred to in sub-paragraph (6) is received by the contractor.

5.   Suspension of approval

(1)   Where the PCT suspends its approval of an accredited service provider under regulation 9 of the Out-of-Hours Regulations or receives notice of suspension of such approval under regulation 11 of those Regulations, it shall forthwith suspend its approval of any out-of-hours arrangement made by the contractor with that accredited service provider.

(2)   A suspension of approval under sub-paragraph (1) shall take effect on the day on which the contractor receives notice of suspension of approval of the accredited service provider under regulation 11 of the Out-of-Hours Regulations.

6.   Immediate withdrawal of approval other than following review

(1)   The PCT shall withdraw its approval of an out-of-hours arrangement immediately –

    (a) in the case of an arrangement with a person referred to in paragraph 1(5)(a), if it withdraws its approval of the accredited service provider under regulation 8 of the Out-of-Hours Regulations or receives notice of withdrawal of such approval under regulation 11 of those Regulations;

    (b) in the case of an arrangement with a person referred to in paragraph 1(5)(b), if the person with whom it is made ceases to hold a general medical services contract with the PCT which includes the provision of out-of-hours services; or

    (c) where, without any review having taken place under paragraph 4, it appears to the PCT that it is necessary in the interests of the contractor's patients to withdraw its approval immediately.

(2)   The PCT shall give notice to the contractor of a withdrawal of approval under sub-paragraph (1)(b) or (c) and shall include with the notice a statement in writing of the reasons for its determination.

(3)   An immediate withdrawal of approval under sub-paragraph (1) shall take effect –

(a) in the case of a withdrawal under sub-paragraph (1)(a), on the day on which the contractor receives notice of withdrawal of approval of the accredited service provider under Regulation 11 of the Out-of-Hours regulations; or

(b) in the case of a withdrawal under sub-paragraph (1)(b) or (c), on the day on which the notice referred to in sub-paragraph (2) is received by the contractor.

(4)   The PCT shall notify the Local Medical Committee (if any) for its area of a withdrawal of approval under sub-paragraph (1)(c).

(5)   A contractor which wishes to refer a withdrawal of approval under sub-paragraph (1)(c) in accordance with the NHS dispute resolution procedure must do so before the end of the period of 30 days beginning with the day on which the PCT's notification under sub-paragraph (2) was sent.

7.   Suspension or termination of an out-of-hours arrangement

(1)   The contractor shall suspend an arrangement made with an accredited service provider under paragraph 1(2) on receipt of the notice of suspension of approval of that provider under regulation 11 of the Out-of-Hours Regulations.

(2)   The contractor shall terminate an out-of-hours arrangement made under paragraph 1(2) with effect from the date of the taking effect of the withdrawal of the PCT's approval of that arrangement under paragraph 4 or 6.

● Out-of-hours services – opt-out

Guidance

(ii) Opt-outs

2.63   The opt-out process for out-of-hours is set out in the Contract Regulations and is largely the same as for permanent opt-out from additional services. The opt-out tariff is 6% of the global sum. Key points in relation to out-of-hours opt-outs are –

(i)   PCTs are encouraged to find out contractors' intentions as early as possible, and confirm these before the end of February 2004

Out-of-hours services – opt-out

Guidance

(ii) where PCTs have firm plans for implementing alternative out-of-hours provision, the easiest approach is for the PCT and contractor to agree an opt-out date when they are discussing the content of contracts in February 2004. This avoids the need to go through the formal procedure

(iii) PCTs and contractors can give opt-out notices after signing their contracts. Unlike additional service opt-outs, there is no preliminary notice process

(iv) opt-out from out-of-hours services is permanent; there is no temporary opt-out

(v) opt-out is all or nothing. The contractor cannot for example, opt out only at weekends, or only in respect of certain groups of patients; though once the opt-out has happened, it could be commissioned by the PCT to provide such services

(vi) unlike additional services, the contractor does not have to give reasons for opting out. It has to specify the date it wants the opt-out to come into effect. This must be either three or 6 months from the notice date

(vii) when responding to the notice (within no more than 28 days), the PCT cannot refuse the opt-out request. For notices given before 1 October 2004, it can however set a different target date for the opt-out to take effect. This can be any day from the date specified by the contractor up to 1 January 2005. For notices given after 1 October 2004, the PCT must specify the date given by the contractor in its opt-out notice (that is, 3 or 6 months from the date of the notice)

(viii) the PCT must do its best to put in place the necessary arrangements for the contractor to opt out by that target date. Where this is not possible the PCT can, if necessary, extend the period to 9 months or until 1 January 2005, whichever is the later by following the procedure in the Contract Regulations. This means that all contractors who wish to opt out by 1 January 2005 should do so immediately after they have signed their GMS contracts, in writing by 1 April 2004. The 9 month rule means that, for example, a contractor that gives notice on 1 May 2004 may not be able to opt out until 1 February 2005, if the PCT is unable to secure alternative provision before then

(ix) the PCT can only refuse or further delay opt-out in exceptional circumstances, for example if the contractor's location is so remote or isolated that there is no realistic alternative to the contractor continuing to provide its own out-of-hours services. In England, exceptional circumstances are expected to be extremely rare and the PCT would require the SHA's permission. SHAs will also be performance managing PCT progress towards effective re-provision, to ensure that there is no slippage

(x) nothing in the opt-out procedures prevents PCTs and contractors at
any time agreeing a different date for the opt-out to take effect.

(iii) Sub-contracting, transfer of responsibility and accreditation

2.64 Sub-contracting of out-of-hours services is subject to specific rules –
(i) contractors who provide out-of-hours services will normally have to
obtain permission from PCTs before they sub-contract those services
to other out-of-hours providers. PCTs will be able to withhold (or
subsequently withdraw) this permission if they are not satisfied that
the terms of the contract (including, from 1 January 2005, the
national quality standards) will be met
(ii) contractors who want to sub-contract will need formally to apply in
writing for permission, giving details of the provider and the
proposed arrangements. This does not apply to occasional, short-
term arrangements, nor to sub-contracts to locum doctors, informal
rotas or to other GMS or PMS practices that provide out-of-hours
services. PCTs will be expected to respond as soon as possible to a
contractor's request to sub-contract, and normally within 28 days
(iii) where the contractor plans to sub-contract to a provider with which
the PCT is familiar (e.g. an out-of-hours provider with which it has a
contract itself) then this is likely to be largely a formality, unless
there are concerns about the provider's ability to cope with the
additional workload
(iv) where the provider is unfamiliar – or is one about which the PCT has
other concerns – the PCT will want to assure itself that the proposed
provider will be able to deliver an appropriate service. The PCT may,
if necessary, request further information before making a decision,
and it may also attach conditions to its approval.

2.65 The requirement to gain permission for sub-contracting applies from the
date of the new contract, and therefore applies to contractors that are
waiting to opt out. However, until 31 December 2004 contractors will
continue to be able to transfer responsibility for out-of-hours services, so
they will generally not need to sub-contract. During the transitional
period the current arrangements for transfers will continue more or less
as per the old GMS regulations. Contractors will be able to continue to
transfer responsibility for out-of-hours services to another provider in
accordance with any arrangements approved by a PCT and in force at 31
March 2004 in relation to any of the GPs who make up the contractor.
Contractors will also be able to apply for approval to make new transfer
arrangements. The information they need to supply will be largely the
same as under the old system, and the detail is set out in Schedule 7 to
the Contract Regulations.

2.66   The effect of a transfer is that, whilst the service will still be provided
        under the contractor's GMS contract, the contractor will not be liable for
        any breaches of the terms of the contract by the other provider. Transfer
        is only available in respect of out-of-hours services automatically
        included in the GMS contract, not for any other out-of-hours services it
        may have voluntarily agreed to provide. As now, PCTs that are not
        satisfied that transfer arrangements are (or continue to be) satisfactory
        will be able to refuse or withdraw permission as necessary. If contractors
        disagree with these decisions, they will be able use the contract dispute
        resolution procedure to challenge them (rather than appealing to the
        Secretary of State as at present). Where PCT decisions under the old
        Terms of Service are already the subject of an appeal at 31 March 2004,
        the appeals process will continue unless the parties agree otherwise, and
        the decision will be treated as if it had been made under the dispute
        resolution procedure.

2.67   Until 31 December 2004, if transfer arrangements end for whatever
        reason, the contractor will continue to be responsible for making
        alternative arrangements. However, PCTs should also have contingency
        arrangements in place for considering what support, if any, they should
        provide to contractors in this situation. As now, transfer arrangements
        with accredited providers will end automatically if accreditation is
        withdrawn or suspended

2.68   All transfer arrangements will end automatically on 31 December 2004.
        Contractors which still have transfer arrangements in place on 31
        December 2004 will automatically be treated as having permission to
        convert the arrangement into a sub-contract. The continuation of the
        transfer arrangements until December 2004 means that PCTs will need to
        continue to operate the accreditation system until then, unless it has
        become redundant because all the contractors in the PCT's area have
        already opted out. PCTs will also have to deal with new applications for
        accreditation during that period. Many of these applications will be from
        existing accredited providers which have merged or reorganised. In some
        cases, the PCT may already be familiar with the organisation(s)
        concerned. The procedure will therefore be amended to allow PCTs to
        accredit the applicant without first referring it to another PCT for
        assessment. However, the PCT may refer the applicant for assessment by
        another PCT if it wishes. Guidance on the accreditation system is
        available from http://www.out-of-hours/info.

(iv) Commissioning alternative out-of-hours services

2.69   By 1 January 2005 it is expected that all PCTs will be fully responsible for
        securing out-of-hours services for their local populations, whether

through APMS contracts, specialist PMS contracts, contracts with GMS or PMS contractors, or by providing services themselves. The Department issued guidance to PCTs on setting up new out-of-hours arrangements in October 2003. This is available at http://www.out-of-hours.info, as are details of allocations for the Out-of-Hours Development Fund, which will be one of the sources of funding available to PCTs to commission out-of-hours services and (as appropriate) to support those contractors which continue to provide their own out-of-hours services. The funding arrangements are further described in chapter 5. By the end of February 2004 PCTs are expected to have developed robust plans for re-provision.

2.70   The new commissioning responsibility is a major opportunity to shape and deliver better quality more integrated services; it is not just an operational challenge. In planning provision, PCTs will wish to take a strategic view looking across the delivery of primary, acute and emergency services. They will wish to work with other PCTs in their area. All the services they commission will need to meet the National Quality Standards.

2.71   GMS contractors, including those who have opted out of out-of-hours, can at any time approach the PCT with a view to providing out-of-hours services to their own patients or those of other contractors. PCTs should consider such requests within the context of their overall strategy for out-of-hours services. When agreeing that the contractor will provide such services, the contractor and the PCT will also need to agree the terms on which the arrangement can be ended (which can, but need not, be the same as the opt-out procedures).

2.72   Contractors that opt out still have an interest in the out-of-hours services that are provided to their patients, as well as a responsibility to help ensure that their patients receive seamless care. PCTs will want to keep contractors informed of the out-of-hours services available to their patients, including any proposed changes.

2.73   All GMS contracts will include a term requiring contractors to co-operate with other people who provide out-of-hours services to their patients. Co-operation might include providing and receiving information about patients, although members of the contractor cannot be required to make themselves available during the out-of-hours period. There will need, for example, to be a system in place for the transmission of information to providers about patients with special needs (including violent and vulnerable patients, and those who are terminally ill) and for contractors in turn to receive timely details of the out-of-hours care provided to their patients. Contractors which opt out, or otherwise stop providing services, will also be required to provide any information reasonably requested by the PCT or the alternative provider which is to take over the service.

2.74   It is vital that patients are fully informed of how to access out-of-hours services. PCTs will want to have developed plans for effective public engagement well in advance of opt-outs taking effect. They may wish to develop these as part of the wider process of planning, by January 2004, community engagement on the new contract generally. Patients will benefit from more integrated services, all of which, for the first time, will have to meet the OOH national standards from 1 January 2005. GPs will benefit from a better work/life balance. The change will help improve recruitment and retention of GPs and enable primary care capacity to be expanded. The change will also enable GPs to focus on delivering better quality services in hours.

2.75   All GMS contacts will include a term requiring contractors to include information about how to access out-of-hours services in their practice leaflets. Contractors which do not provide out-of-hours services must also take reasonable steps to ensure that patients who contact the practice by telephone during the out-of-hours period get accurate information about how to obtain out-of-hours services. Contractors with clear telephone messages, or whose calls are transferred automatically to out-of-hours providers, will also be able to gain points in the organisational domain of the quality and outcomes framework.

● Out-of-hours services – temporary arrangements

Regulations

1.   Temporary arrangements for transfer of obligations and liabilities in relation to certain out-of-hours services

(1)   In this Schedule –

"accredited service provider" has the meaning given to it by regulation 2 of the Out-of-Hours Regulations;

"Out-of-Hours Regulations" means the National Health Service (Out-of-Hours Medical Services) and National Health Service (General Medical Services) Amendment Regulations 2002;

"out-of-hours arrangement" means an arrangement under sub-paragraph (2); and "transferee doctor" means a person referred to in sub-paragraph (5)(b) who has undertaken to carry out the obligations of a contractor during all or part of the out-of-hours period in accordance with an out-of-hours arrangement referred to in sub-paragraph (2).

(2) Subject to the provisions of this Schedule, where a contractor is required to provide out-of-hours services pursuant to regulation 30 or 31, it may, with the approval of the PCT, make an arrangement with one of the persons specified in sub-paragraph (5) as if regulations 1 to 11 of the Out-of-Hours Regulations, subject to the modifications specified in sub-paragraph (6), were still in force.

(3) Any arrangement made pursuant to sub-paragraph (2) shall cease to have effect on 1 January 2005.

(4) An arrangement made in accordance with sub-paragraph (2) shall, for so long as it continues, or is not suspended under paragraph 7(1), relieve the contractor of –
(a) its obligations to provide out-of-hours services pursuant to regulation 30 or 31; and
(b) all liabilities under the contract in respect of those services.

(5) The persons referred to in sub-paragraph (2) are –
(a) an accredited service provider; or
(b) a person who holds a general medical services contract with the PCT which includes the provision of out-of-hours services.

(6) The modifications referred to in sub-paragraph (2) are –
(a) as if out-of-hours period had the meaning given in regulation 2 of these Regulations;
(b) as if the requirements relating to an assessing authority in regulation 4(5) to (8) did not apply in cases where, in the opinion of the accrediting authority, it was appropriate and safe to dispense with them;
(c) as if the reference to a medical practitioner in regulation 11(2)(c) was a reference to a contractor;
(d) as if the reference to section 44 in regulation 11(2)(d) was to section 45A of the Act; and
(e) as if the reference to a medical list or supplementary list in paragraph 7 of the Schedule was to a medical performers list and the words "or he is named in an agreement under section 2 of the 1997 Act as a performer of personal medical services" were omitted.

(7) A contractor may make more than one out-of-hours arrangement and may do so (for example) with different transferee doctors or accredited service providers and in respect of different patients, different times and different parts of its practice area.

(8)   A contractor may retain responsibility for, or make separate out-of-hours arrangements in respect of, the provision to any patients of maternity medical services during the out-of-hours period which the contractor is required to provide pursuant to regulation 30 or 31 and any separate out-of-hours arrangements it makes may encompass all or any part of the maternity medical services it provides.

(9)   Nothing in this paragraph prevents a contractor from retaining or resuming its obligations in relation to named patients.

Guidance

2.58   This section explains the arrangements for out-of-hours services in the new contract. It considers:
(i)   out-of-hours services in GMS contracts
(ii) opt-out arrangements
(iii) sub-contracting, transfer and accreditation
(iv) commissioning alternative out-of-hours services.
Each is described in turn.

(i) Out-of-hours services in GMS contracts

2.59   The out-of-hours period is the converse of core hours; that is before 8 a.m. and after 6.30 p.m. on Mondays to Fridays, and all day Saturdays, Sundays and Bank Holidays, Good Friday and Christmas Day. Key features of the new arrangements for out-of-hours services in GMS contracts are:
(i)   contractors that wish to retain their existing responsibilities will have the right to do so, provided they can meet national quality standards from 1 January 2005
(ii) where the PCT agrees, contractors will be able to opt out of their current out-of-hours responsibilities between 1 April and 31 December 2004. From 1 January 2005, contractors will have a right to opt out in all but exceptional circumstances.

2.60   All GMS contracts that come into effect before 1 January 2005 must include out-of-hours services unless the PCT has agreed to the opt-out, or the contractor is exempt. After 1 January 2005, new GMS contracts will only include out-of-hours services where both parties agree. Where out-of-hours services are required to be included in a contract, the contractor must provide throughout the out-of-hours period both essential services and any additional services that are part of the core hours contract. However, this does not mean the contractor must provide the same level of service that it provides during core hours. The contractor must meet the urgent needs of patients that cannot safely be deferred. In deciding what service to provide, the contractor is allowed to consider whether the patient could reasonably be expected to wait until core hours to obtain the service.

2.61 Contractors that do not opt out can continue providing those services indefinitely, subject to termination rules set out in chapter 6. From 1 January 2005, all out-of-hours services included in GMS contracts must meet the National Quality Standards for Out-of-Hours Services. These quality standards, available at http://www.doh.gov.uk/pricare/oohquality.pdf, are currently being reviewed, and will be re-published in spring 2004.

2.62 Some GPs have preserved rights under old GMS paragraph 18(2) to be exempt from out-of-hours services. Where all the GPs in a contractor are exempt in this way, then (unless or until the relevant PCT agrees otherwise) the duty to provide out-of-hours services to that contractor's patients will fall instead to any contractor that includes a GP who was responsible for providing out-of-hours services to those patients on 31 March 2004 under the old GMS terms.

Over 75 year checks

Regulations

6.   Patients aged 75 years and over

(1) Where a registered patient who –
(a) has attained the age of 75 years; and
(b) has not participated in a consultation under this paragraph within the period of 12 months prior to the date of his request,
requests a consultation, the contractor shall, in addition and without prejudice to its other obligations in respect of that patient under the contract, provide such a consultation in the course of which it shall make such inquiries and undertake such examinations as appear to it to be appropriate in all the circumstances.

(2) A consultation under sub-paragraph (1) shall take place in the home of the patient where, in the reasonable opinion of the contractor, it would be inappropriate, as a result of the patient's medical condition, for him to attend at the practice premises.

Guidance

2.23 (iv) patients of 75 years or over. The contractor is obliged to provide a consultation to patients aged 75 or over who request it if the patient has not had a consultation within the last 12 months. The workload associated with these checks is reflected in the age/sex cost curve in the global sum formula. The new GMS arrangements represent a change from the existing GMS rules, where the GP has to write offering the consultation. This reflects the objective of promoting self-responsibility for health, and will reduce bureaucracy for contractors. The ongoing need for these consultations to be retained will be reviewed in the light of possible future inclusion of new indicators within the quality and outcomes framework, such as the management of falls.

● Patient choice of practitioner

Guidance

2.28 Although patients will, from 1 April 2004, register with a contractor rather than an individual GP, patients can still ask to be seen or treated by a particular practitioner. This could for example be the same GP for continuing care, or for a particular condition, or another GP who specialises in that area. When patients register with the contractor, contractors should ask patients if they want to name a preferred practitioner; for example, some women prefer to see a female GP. The general assumption would be that the GP with whom patients are currently registered will be the preferred GP but when patients attend they may wish to record an alternative preference which should then be recorded in the patient's medical record.

2.29 Choice of practitioner cannot be absolute; it also depends on availability, appropriateness and reasonableness. Where a patient asks to see a particular practitioner, the contractor must endeavour to meet these wishes and take into account the following:
   (i) the availability of the health professional. The patient may have to wait longer to see their preferred practitioner. In such a case, the delay would not count against achievement of the access targets measured in the access DES or access bonus points in the quality and outcomes framework

(ii) patients should bear in mind their general obligation not to unfairly discriminate for example by refusing to see a doctor of a particular ethnic minority

(iii) the practitioner would still be allowed the rights of reasonable refusal, such as in relation to violent patients (if the contractor does not have facilities to deal with such patients), or threats to, or fear for the personal safety of, any practice staff

(iv) the patient may be asked to accept an alternative if, for example, the service required was being delivered by another type of primary care professional. An example is if the contractor's protocol specifies that a service is nurse-led or therapist-led rather than doctor-led.

(ii) Information about choice of contractor

2.30 Patients can decide which contractor they want to apply to register with and will be helped in this by the proposed new PCT Guide to Primary Care Services. This will replace the Directory of Family Doctors. The Department will consult on the proposed content of the new guide in January 2004 and introduce regulations that set out what must be covered in the guide. The regulations will also make it a requirement for PCTs to have the guide available by 1 April 2004.

2.31 Patient choice is also supported by the requirement that all contractors produce a practice leaflet. The Contract Regulations set out what must be covered by the leaflet. The practice leaflet must be reviewed by the contractor at least annually. The contractor must also make any amendments needed to maintain its accuracy, and all contractors are advised to review and amend their patient leaflets in the light of the new arrangements by 1 April 2004. Key requirements include:

(i) names of clinical staff and partners

(ii) details of how to register, ability to specify a preferred practitioner, and a description of the practice area

(iii) the services available and PCT contact details (to obtain information about additional services that are not provided by the contractor), including home visits, checks for over-75s etc. as described in paragraph 2.23

(iv) the appointment system, where one exists, and normal surgery hours

(v) whether the practice premises have suitable access for disabled patients

(vi) the name and address of the nearest local walk-in centre

(vii) the method of obtaining repeat prescriptions

(viii) how to make complaints

(ix) action that may be taken where a patient is violent or abusive, and a reminder of the rights and responsibilities of the patient, including keeping appointments and respect for race, gender, disability.

2.32 Department of Health policy, as set out in the NHS Plan and supported in *Building the Best*, is for patients to be offered copies of clinicians' letters relating to them. PCTs will therefore wish to encourage contractors to include such information within patient leaflets. It is not, however, a contractual requirement. In addition, the leaflet could seek to promote effective use of services such as NHS Direct and pharmacies.

2.33 There are two key determinants of whether a patient can register with a contractor. First, the contractor's practice area, in other words its catchment area. The Contract Regulations specify that this must be agreed with the PCT as part of the contract agreement, just as it currently is. This should be discussed before the contract is provisionally agreed by the end of February 2004. The second key determinant is whether or not the contractor's list is open or closed.

Patient list – application for inclusion

Regulations

15.

(1) The contractor may, if its list of patients is open, accept an application for inclusion in its list of patients made by or on behalf of any person whether or not resident in its practice area or included, at the time of that application, in the list of patients of another contractor or provider of primary medical services.

(2) The contractor may, if its list of patients is closed, only accept an application for inclusion in its list of patients from a person who is an immediate family member of a registered patient whether or not resident in its practice area or included, at the time of that application, in the list of patients of another contractor or provider of primary medical services.

(3) Subject to sub-paragraph (4), an application for inclusion in a contractor's list of patients shall be made by delivering to the practice premises a medical card or an application signed (in either case) by the applicant or a person authorised by the applicant to sign on his behalf.

(4) An application may be made –
  (a) on behalf of any child –
    (i) by either parent, or in the absence of both parents, the guardian or other adult who has care of the child,

     (ii) by a person duly authorised by a local authority to whose care the child has been committed under the Children Act 1989[78], or

     (iii) by a person duly authorised by a voluntary organisation by which the child is being accommodated under the provisions of that Act; or

  (b) on behalf of any adult who is incapable of making such an application, or authorising such an application to be made on their behalf, by a relative or the primary carer of that person.

(5)   A contractor which accepts an application for inclusion in its list of patients shall notify the PCT in writing as soon as possible.

(6)   On receipt of a notice under sub-paragraph (5), the PCT shall –

  (a) include that person in the contractor's list of patients from the date on which the notice is received; and

  (b) notify the applicant (or, in the case of a child or incapable adult, the person making the application on their behalf) of the acceptance.

Patient list – cleaning

Regulations

List of patients

14.   The PCT shall prepare and keep up to date a list of the patients –

  (a) who have been accepted by the contractor for inclusion in its list of patients under paragraph 15 and who have not subsequently been removed from that list under paragraphs 19 to 27; and

  (b) who have been assigned to the contractor under paragraph 32 or 33 and whose assignment has not subsequently been rescinded.

Guidance

2.27   As under old GMS, the PCT is under a duty to keep and maintain a list of patients. It will be aided in this task by information provided by contractors to the registration systems. From 1 April 2004, lists will show individual patients as being registered with contractors rather than individual GPs. This change will happen automatically. Contractors will be under an obligation in the Statement of Financial Entitlements (SFE) to ensure that their lists of patients are accurate to the best of their knowledge, and that they provide timely notifications of patient registrations and removals. It is important they do this and ensure their lists are clean, not only to ensure accurate calculation of their global sum, but also because their global sum will – given the way in which all allocation formulas work – affect the weighted populations of other contractors. Contractors with ghost patients on their list will potentially be adversely affecting the income of other contractors.

Patient's preference of practitioner

Regulations

18. Patient preference of practitioner

(1) Where the contractor has accepted an application for inclusion in its list of patients, it shall –
   (a) notify the patient (or, in the case of a child or incapable adult, the person who made the application on their behalf) of the patient's right to express a preference to receive services from a particular performer or class of performer either generally or in relation to any particular condition; and
   (b) record in writing any such preference expressed by or on behalf of the patient.

(2) The contractor shall endeavour to comply with any reasonable preference expressed under sub-paragraph (1) but need not do so if the preferred performer –
   (a) has reasonable grounds for refusing to provide services to the patient; or
   (b) does not routinely perform the service in question within the practice.

Standard Contract

Patient preference of practitioner

184. Where the Contractor has accepted an application for inclusion in its list of patients, it shall –
   184.1 notify the patient (or, in the case of a *child* or incapable adult, the person making the application on their behalf) of the patient's

right to express a preference to receive services from a particular performer or class of performer either generally or in relation to any particular condition; and

184.2 record in writing any such preference expressed by or on behalf of the patient.

185. The Contractor shall endeavour to comply with any reasonable preference expressed under clause 184 but need not do so if the preferred performer has reasonable grounds for refusing to provide services to the patient, or does not routinely perform the service in question within the *practice.*

Patient records

Regulations

73. Patient records

(1) In this paragraph, "computerised records" means records created by way of entries on a computer.

(2) The contractor shall keep adequate records of its attendance on and treatment of its patients and shall do so –
   (a) on forms supplied to it for the purpose by the PCT; or
   (b) with the written consent of the PCT, by way of computerised records,
   or in a combination of those two ways.

(3) The contractor shall include in the records referred to in sub-paragraph (2) clinical reports sent in accordance with paragraph 7 of this Schedule or from any other health care professional who has provided clinical services to a person on its list of patients.

(4) The consent of the PCT required by sub-paragraph (2)(b) shall not be withheld or withdrawn provided the PCT is satisfied, and continues to be satisfied, that –
   (a) the computer system upon which the contractor proposes to keep the records has been accredited by the Secretary of State or another person on his behalf in accordance with "General Medical Practice Computer Systems – Requirements for Accreditation – RFA99" version 1.0, 1.1 or 1.2 (DTS/Nurse Prescribing);
   (b) the security measures, audit and system management functions incorporated into the computer system as accredited in accordance with paragraph (a) have been enabled; and

(c) the contractor is aware of, and has signed an undertaking that it will have regard to the guidelines contained in "Good Practice Guidelines for General Practice Electronic Patient Records" published on 26 September 2003.

(5) Where a patient's records are computerised records, the contractor shall, as soon as possible following a request from the PCT, allow the Trust to access the information recorded on the computer system on which those records are held by means of the audit function referred to in sub-paragraph (4)(b) to the extent necessary for the Trust to confirm that the audit function is enabled and functioning correctly.

(6) The contractor shall send the complete records relating to a patient to the PCT –
(a) where a person on its list dies, before the end of the period of 14 days beginning with the date on which it was informed by the PCT of the death, or (in any other case) before the end of the period of 1 month beginning with the date on which it learned of the death; or
(b) in any other case where the person is no longer registered with the contractor, as soon as possible at the request of the PCT.

(7) To the extent that a patient's records are computerised records, the contractor complies with sub-paragraph (6) if it sends to the PCT a copy of those records –
(a) in written form; or
(b) with the written consent of the PCT in any other form.

(8) The consent of the PCT to the transmission of information other than in written form for the purposes of sub-paragraph (7)(b) shall not be withheld or withdrawn provided it is satisfied, and continues to be satisfied, with the following matters –
(a) the contractor's proposals as to how the record will be transmitted;
(b) the contractor's proposals as to the format of the transmitted record;
(c) how the contractor will ensure that the record received by the PCT is identical to that transmitted; and
(d) how a written copy of the record can be produced by the PCT.

(9) A contractor whose patient records are computerised records shall not disable, or attempt to disable, either the security measures or the audit and system management functions referred to in sub-paragraph (4)(b).

Standard Contract

Patient records

425. In this part, "computerised records" means records created by way of entries on a computer.

426. The Contractor shall keep adequate records of its attendance on and treatment of its patients and shall do so –
426.1 on forms supplied to it for the purpose by the PCT; or
426.2 with the written consent of the PCT, by way of computerised records,
or in a combination of those two ways.

427. The Contractor shall include in the records referred to in clause 426 clinical reports sent in accordance with clause 38 or from any other *health care professional* who has provided clinical services to a person on its list of patients.

428. The consent of the PCT required by clause 426.2 shall not be withheld or, once given, withdrawn provided the PCT is satisfied, and continues to be satisfied, that –
428.1 the computer system upon which the Contractor proposes to keep the records has been accredited by *the Secretary of State* or another person on his behalf in accordance with "General Medical Practice Computer Systems – Requirements for Accreditation – RFA99" version 1.0, 1.1 or 1.2 (DTS/Nurse Prescribing) (RFA99 is published by the NHS Information Authority – copies are available on the NHS Information Authority's website at http://www.nhsia.nhs.uk/sat/specification/pages, or may also be obtained by writing to the NHS Information Authority, Systems Accreditation and testing team, Aqueous 2, Aston Cross, Rocky Lane, Birmingham B6 5RQ);
428.2 the security measures, audit and system management functions incorporated into the computer system as accredited in accordance with clause 428.1 have been enabled; and
428.3 the Contractor is aware of, and has signed an undertaking that it will have regard to the guidelines contained in "Good Practice Guidelines for General Practice Electronic Patient Records" published on 26 September 2003 (this document is available on the Department of Health's website at http://www.doh.gov.uk/pricare/computing, or a copy may be obtained by writing to the Department of Health, PCIT Branch, Room 1N06, Quarry House, Quarry Hill, Leeds LS2 7UE).

429. Where a patient's records are computerised records, the Contractor shall, as soon as possible following a request from the PCT, allow the PCT to access the information recorded on the computer system on which those records are held by means of the audit function referred to in clause 428.2 to the extent necessary for the PCT to check that the audit function is enabled and functioning correctly.

430. The Contractor shall send the complete records relating to a patient to the PCT –

430.1 where a person on its list dies, before the end of the period of 14 days beginning with the date on which it was informed by the PCT of the death, or (in any other case) before the end of the period of 1 month beginning with the date on which it learned of the death; or

430.2 in any other case where the person is no longer registered with the Contractor, as soon as possible at the request of the PCT, [and the Contractor's obligations pursuant to this clause, and clause 431 below shall survive the termination or expiry of the Contract].[42]

431. To the extent that a patient's records are computerised records, the Contractor complies with clause 430 if it sends to the PCT a copy of those records –

431.1 in written form; or

431.2 with the written consent of the PCT in any other form.

432. The consent of the PCT to the transmission of information other than in written form for the purposes of clause 431.2 shall not be withheld or withdrawn provided it is satisfied, and continues to be satisfied, with the following matters –

432.1 the Contractor's proposals as to how the record will be transmitted;

432.2 the Contractor's proposals as to the format of the transmitted record;

432.3 how the Contractor will ensure that the record received by the PCT is identical to that transmitted; and

432.4 how a written copy of the record can be produced by the PCT.

433. Where the Contractor's patient records are computerised records, the Contractor shall not disable, or attempt to disable, either the security measures or the audit and system management functions referred to in clause 428.2.

---

42   The words in square brackets are not mandatory but they are recommended to ensure that an obligation to provide patient records to the PCT continues to apply even where the Contract has ended.

Patient records – access for the purpose of the Quality Information Preparation Scheme

Regulations

74. (1) The contractor must provide access to its patient records on request to any appropriately qualified person with whom the PCT has made arrangements for the provision of the Quality Information Preparation Scheme referred to in section 7 of the GMS Statement of Financial Entitlements.

(2) The contractor shall not be obliged to grant access to a person referred to in sub-paragraph (1) unless he produces, on request, written evidence that he is authorised by the PCT to act on its behalf.

Standard Contract

434. The Contractor must provide access to its patient records on request to any appropriately qualified person with whom the PCT has made arrangements for the Quality Information Preparation Scheme referred to in section 7 of the *GMS Statement of Financial Entitlements.*

435. The Contractor shall not be obliged to grant access to a person referred to in clause 434 unless he produces, on request, written evidence that he is authorised by the PCT to act on its behalf.

Patients not seen within 3 years

Regulations

Patients not seen within 3 years

5. Where a registered patient who –
(a) has attained the age of 16 years but has not attained the age of 75 years; and

(b) has attended neither a consultation with, nor a clinic provided by, the contractor within the period of 3 years prior to the date of his request, requests a consultation the contractor shall, in addition and without prejudice to its other obligations in respect of that patient under the contract, provide such a consultation in the course of which it shall make such inquiries and undertake such examinations as appear to it to be appropriate in all the circumstances.

Standard Contract

34.   Where a *registered patient* who:

    34.1 has attained the age of 16 years but has not attained the age of 75 years; and

    34.2 has attended neither a consultation with, nor a clinic provided by, the Contractor within the period of 3 years prior to the date of his request,

requests a consultation the Contractor shall, in addition and without prejudice to its other obligations in respect of that patient under the Contract, provide such a consultation.

35.   Where the Contractor provides a consultation referred to in clause 34, the Contractor shall, in the course of that consultation, make such inquiries and undertake such examinations as appear to it to be appropriate in all the circumstances.

Guidance

2.23 (iii) the 3-year rule. In new GMS the obligation has been simplified. The contractor must, if a patient is 16 or over, provide a consultation if the patient requests it and has not had a consultation or attended a clinic provided by the contractor within 3 years

● Patients to whom services must be provided

Standard Contract

Persons to whom services are to be provided[43]

160. [Except where specifically stated otherwise in respect of particular services][44] the Contractor shall provide services under the Contract to:

160.1 *registered patients,*

160.2 *temporary residents,*

160.3 persons to whom the Contractor is required to provide immediately necessary treatment under clause 46.3 or 49,

160.4 any person for whom the Contractor is responsible under regulation 31 of *the Regulations*[45] [or article 20 of *the Transitional Order*];

160.5 any other person to whom the Contractor is responsible under arrangements made with another contractor of the kind referred to in clause 406; and

160.6 any other person to whom the Contractor has agreed to provide services under the Contract.

---

43   This provision is required by regulation 18(1)(c) of *the Regulations* which requires the Contract to specify to whom services under the Contract are to be provided.

44   The words in square brackets may be required where the Contractor is providing *additional services* not funded by the *global sum, enhanced services* or *out-of-hours services* only to specific categories of patients (and not all of the patients specified in clauses 160.1 to 160.5).

45   1.   Regulation 31 of *the Regulations* provides that if the Contract is with any of the persons specified in (a) to (c) below, the Contract must require the Contractor to continue providing *out-of-hours services* to patients of an exempt contractor where the Contractor is –

(a)   an individual medical practitioner who is, or was on 31 March 2004, responsible for providing services during all or part of the out-of-hours period to the patients of a medical practitioner who meets the requirements set out in paragraph 2 below ("exempt contractor");

(b)   two or more individuals practising in partnership at least one of whom was, or will be, on 31 March 2004, a medical practitioner responsible for providing such services; or

(c)   a company in which one or more of the shareholders was, or will be, on 31 March 2004, a medical practitioner responsible for providing such services,

and the Contractor must continue to provide such services until it has opted out of the provision of *out-of-hours services* in accordance with Part 10 of the Contract, or the PCT (or if it is different, the PCT with whom the exempt contractor holds its contract) has or have agreed in writing that the Contractor need no longer provide some or all of those services to some or all of those patients.

2.   The requirements are that-

(a)   the medical practitioner was relieved of responsibility for providing services to his patients under paragraph 18(2) of Schedule 2 to the National Health Service (General Medical Services) Regulations 1992; and

(b)   he –

- has entered or intends to enter into a contract which does not include *out-of-hours services* pursuant to paragraph 1(b) above,
- is one of two or more individuals practising in partnership who have entered or intends to enter into a contract which does not includes *out-of-hours services* pursuant to paragraph 1(b) above;
- is the owner of shares in a company which has entered or intends to enter into a contract which does not include *out-of-hours services* pursuant to paragraph 1(b) above.

Payment under the Contract

Regulations

Finance

22. (1) Subject to paragraph (2), the contract must contain a term which has
the effect of requiring the PCT to make payments to the contractor
under the contract promptly and in accordance with both the terms
of the contract and any other conditions relating to the payment
contained in directions given by the Secretary of State under
section 28T of the Act (GMS contracts: payments).
(2) The obligation referred to in paragraph (1) is subject to any right the
PCT may have to set off against any amount payable to the
contractor under the contract any amount –
(a) that is owed by the contractor to the PCT under the contract; or
(b) that the PCT may withhold from the contractor in accordance
with the terms of the contract or any other applicable provisions
contained in directions given by the Secretary of State under
section 28T of the Act.

23. The contract must contain a term to the effect that where, pursuant to
directions under section 17 (Secretary of State's directions: exercise of
functions) or 28T of the Act, a PCT is required to make a payment to a
contractor under a contract but subject to conditions, those conditions
are to be a term of the contract.

Standard Contract

472. The PCT shall make payments to the Contractor under the Contract
promptly and in accordance with both the terms of the Contract
(including, for the avoidance of doubt, any payment due pursuant to
clause 473), and any other conditions relating to the payment contained
in directions given by *the Secretary of State* under section 28T of *the Act*
subject to any right the PCT may have to set off against any amount
payable to the Contractor under the Contract any amount –
472.1 that is owed by the Contractor to the PCT under the Contract; or
472.2 that the PCT may withhold from the Contractor in accordance
with the terms of the Contract or any other applicable provisions
contained in directions given by *the Secretary of State* under section
28T of *the Act* (GMS contracts: payments).

473. [Subject to clause 474][46] The PCT shall make payments to the Contractor in such amount and in such manner as specified in any directions for the time being in force under section 17 or 28T of *the Act*. Where, pursuant to directions made under section 17 or 28T of *the Act*, the PCT is required to make a payment to the Contractor under the Contract but subject to conditions, those conditions are to be a term of the Contract.

474. [Payments to be made to the Contractor (and any relevant conditions to be met by the Contractor in relation to such payments) in respect of services where payments, or the amount of any such payments, are not specified in directions pursuant to clause 473, are set out in Schedule 7 to this Contract.][47]

[Payment provisions specific to a Contractor entering into the Contract following a *default contract* with the PCT

475. As a condition of entering into the Contract, the Contractor has surrendered all rights to further payments under the *default contract* to which the Contractor and the PCT were parties prior to entering into the Contract, and the Contractor acknowledges that any such rights were extinguished when the Contractor entered into the Contract.

476. For the purposes of payment under the Contract, the Contract shall be treated as if it commenced on 1 April 2004.

477. Any payment that has been made under the *default contract* to which the Contractor and the PCT were parties prior to entering into the Contract, that could have been made if the Contractor had entered into the Contract on or before 31 March 2004 –
  477.1 as a payment on account under the Contract, shall be treated as a payment on account under the Contract (and for these purposes any payment of one twelfth of a final *global sum* equivalent under that *default contract* shall be treated as a payment on account in respect of a payable *global sum* monthly payment);
  477.2 as a payment under the Contract, shall be treated as a payment under the Contract,

46   The words in square brackets only need to be included if clause 474 is to be included.

47   Clause 474 needs to be included if, pursuant to the Contract (Parts 8, 9 or 11), the Contractor is providing –
• *additional services* that are not funded by the *global sum* or *out-of-hours services*; and/or
• *enhanced services*
and in either case, the payments to be made in respect of such services, and the conditions upon which payment is to be made, are not specified in Directions made under section 17 or 28T of *the Act*. It will also need to be included if there are any other payments to be made, where the detail of such payments is not specified in directions, for example payments in respect of premises.

and accordingly any condition that attaches, or is to be attached, to such a payment when made under the Contract, by virtue of the *GMS Statement of Financial Entitlements* or any other relevant Directions given by *the Secretary of State*, is attached to that payment.

478. Any other payment that has been made under the *default contract* to which the Contractor and the PCT were parties prior to entering into the Contract, shall be set off, equitably, against any payment for equivalent services provided under the Contract.][48]

[Payment provisions specific to a Contractor entering into the Contract where the PCT has previously made payments to the Contractor under article 41(1) of *the Transitional Order*

479. As a condition of entering into the Contract, the Contractor has surrendered all rights to further payments from the PCT under article 41(1) of *the Transitional Order*, and the Contractor acknowledges that any such rights were extinguished when the Contractor entered into the Contract.

480. For the purposes of payment under the Contract, the Contract shall be treated as if it commenced on 1 April 2004.

481. Any payment that has been made under article 41(1) of *the Transitional Order* that could have been made –
    481.1 as a payment on account under the Contract, shall be treated as a payment on account under the Contract (and for these purposes any payment of one twelfth of a final *global sum* equivalent under article 41(1) shall be treated as a payment on account in respect of a payable *global sum* monthly payment);
    481.2 as a payment under the Contract, shall be treated as a payment under the Contract,
    and accordingly any condition that attaches, or is to be attached, to such a payment when made under the Contract, by virtue of the *GMS Statement of Financial Entitlements*, the National Health Service (General Medical Services – Premises Costs) (England) Directions 2004, or any other relevant Directions given by *the Secretary of State*, is attached to that payment.][49]

---

48 Clauses 475 to 478 are required by article 40 of *the Transitional Order* only where the Contractor has been a party to a *default contract* with the PCT and the Contract takes effect immediately after the *default contract* ceases to have effect.

49 Clauses 479 to 481 are required by article 41(2) of *the Transitional Order* only where payments have been made to the Contractor by the PCT pursuant to article 41(1) of *the Transitional Order* prior to the Contract being entered into.

PCT performance – management

Guidance

7.3   SHAs are responsible for supporting and monitoring the timely delivery
of contract implementation by PCTs. The SHA GMS contract leads have
drawn up a short list of key areas in which they will assess PCT progress
at six different key dates between January and early April 2004. Each PCT
will be asked to complete and send a standard *pro forma* to its SHA.
These should be signed off by a PCT board member. SHAs will in turn
collate responses and send summary sheets to the Department. The
purpose of this system is to help ensure that progress is on track, and that
support can be targeted where it is most needed. Table 18 sets out the key
assessment areas:

Table 18   **SHA assessment of PCT implementation**

Areas

1.   Planning to realise strategic benefits
2.   Effective local engagement
3.   PCT capacity
4.   PCT board engagement
5.   Dealing with movement between PMS and GMS
6.   Additional services planning and commissioning
7.   Out-of-hours planning and commissioning
8.   Enhanced services planning and commissioning
9.   Agreeing realistic quality aspiration points
10. Effective financial risk management
11. Completing indicative contractor budgets by the end of the first
     week in February 2004
12. Reaching provisional agreements with contractors by the end of
     February 2004
13. Signing contracts by the end of March 2004
14. Ensuring contractors get paid by the end of April 2004

Pensions

Guidance

4.17   GPs have been included in the NHS Pension Scheme since it was established in 1948. They automatically become members unless they decide not to join. As with other scheme members, their own contribution is based on 6% of their pensionable pay, and from 1 April 2004 the PCT which is treated as their employer contributes an amount equal to 14% of their pensionable pay. Chapter 5 describes how the increase in contributions will be funded by an increase in the global sum.

Calculation of pensionable pay

4.18   Chapter 5 of *Investing in General Practice* explained how the definition of NHS pensionable pay will be broadened. In broad terms pensionable pay will include all fees and regular remuneration, net of expenses and overtime, paid to practitioners in respect of the provision of primary medical services, and any other services that are treated as NHS work, but excluding all income derived from work undertaken on behalf of a commercial organisation. It will also include profits, net of expenses, for the practitioner in providing clinical placements for students undertaking a recognised course of healthcare learning and development. The Department is working with the GPC to set this out in regulations which will be made by the end of March 2004. This will be accompanied by further guidance which will be discussed with the GPC. This guidance will also set out the detail of the other pensions changes described in this section.

4.19   Future contributions paid by general practitioners as employees, and the employer's contribution paid on their behalf, will be assessed on practice profits. An estimated sum will normally be retained at PCT level from the global sum and paid to the NHS Pensions Agency monthly. PCTs and contractors will need to agree this sum during April 2004 following the March 2004 guidance and Regulations. At the end of the year the practice accountants will produce a certificate of NHS profits in a specified form, to be signed by GPs; this certificate will be included in the March 2004 guidance. The completed certificates will need to be agreed with the PCT and forwarded to the NHS Pensions Agency with any balance of payments. This will also inform the calculation of the uprating factor and also the final calculation of seniority pay. In future working commitment in relation to seniority will be calculated on the basis of average superannuable earnings.

Admission of non-GP partners to the NHS Pension Scheme

4.20 The existing right of non-GP practitioners in PMS to join the scheme is being extended to non-GP partners in GMS practices from 1 April 2004. They will be admitted on an officer basis; their eventual benefits will be assessed on the basis of final year salary, on the same basis of calculation as other officer members of the NHS superannuation scheme. Their contributions will be assessed on profit share.

Uprating factor

4.21 In the new contract, the uprating factor is based on the actual growth in GP pensionable earnings compared with the previous year. This will be adjusted by the Joint Health Departments/NHSC/GPC Technical Steering Committee to take account of the shift to less than full-time working. The exact figures cannot be known until after the end of the financial year, so the TSC will estimate an interim award to mitigate any short-term loss in benefits for newly retired doctors while the actual uprating factor for the year is assessed. The interim reward will be set at a level that avoids the need to make subsequent reductions or reclamation of pension or lump sum.

Flexibilities

4.22 The new contract introduces new flexibilities in the way that pensions are calculated for doctors who have worked in both general practice and other specialities. Doctors working in both general practice and hospital care, or who move between them, accrue benefits under both assessment regimes, and although the NHS Pension Scheme legislates specifically for these circumstances, the results may not always be optimal. To support doctors who pursue portfolio careers, four new pension flexibilities are being introduced. These complement existing rights by broadening the range of methods used to calculate final benefits where there is a mixture of GP and non-GP accrual. All options will be tested at retirement and the most favourable will be applied. Doctors currently working in the NHS will benefit automatically from the new flexibilities, and the impact will extend to their full scheme membership, not just that from the effective date of the regulations. All pension benefits will be automatically safeguarded when doctors move between GP and non-GP work.

4.23 The amending regulations came into force on 1 October 2003, and have retrospective effect from 1 April 2003. The new flexibilities are:
  (i) doctors who work in hospital care or as a GP Registrar for less than 10 years before becoming a Principal Practitioner will receive the most favourable of the following:

(a) a separate pension for hospital work using the non-GP formula plus a separate GP pension

(b) an addition to the practitioner pension pro rata to hospital work

(c) a GP pension for all work

(ii) doctors who work in hospital care for more than 10 years before becoming a Principal Practitioner will receive the most favourable of the following –

(a) a separate pension for hospital work using the non-GP formula plus a separate GP pension

(b) a GP pension for all work

(iii) doctors who work in general practice before moving to hospital care will receive a separate non-GP pension and the more favourable of the following:

(a) a GP pension plus pensions increases (linked to prices)

(b) a GP pension increased by uprating factors linked to pay up to retirement

(iv) doctors who work in both general practice and hospital care for more than 1 year at the same time will receive the more favourable of the following:

(a) a separate pension for hospital work using the non-GP formula plus a separate GP pension

(b) a GP pension for all work.

Performers list

Guidance

4.3   Chapter 7 of *Investing in General Practice* stated that the current medical, supplementary and PMS services lists would be rationalised into a single primary medical services performers list. This was enabled by the Health and Social Care (Community Health and Standards) Act 2003. It will come into force on 1 April 2004 through the NHS (Performer Lists) Regulations 2004. Detailed information on the regulation of individual GPs by PCTs using the list management arrangements can be found at http://www.doh.gov.uk/pclists.

4.4   Listing is mandatory for individual qualified doctors who personally perform NHS primary medical services for patients, or who intend to perform such services. There are a few exceptions:

(i)   certain clinicians employed by NHS trusts;

(ii)   certain provisionally registered Pre-Registration House Officers and Senior House Officers in training; and

    (iii) a limited easement which applies to GP registrars for the first 2 months of their training period. Providers of the services, whether or not they are doctors, are not entitled to be listed unless they personally perform, or intend to perform, the services.

Persons who perform services

Regulations

Qualifications of performers

53. (1) Subject to sub-paragraph (2), no medical practitioner shall perform medical services under the contract unless he is –
    (a) included in a medical performers list for a PCT in England;
    (b) not suspended from that list or from the Medical Register; and
    (c) not subject to interim suspension under section 41A of the Medical Act 1983 (interim orders).
  (2) Sub-paragraph (1)(a) shall not apply in the case of –
    (a) a medical practitioner employed by an NHS trust, an NHS foundation trust, (in Scotland) a Health Board, or (in Northern Ireland) a Health and Social Services Trust who is providing services other than primary medical services at the practice premises;
    (b) a person who is provisionally registered under section 15 (provisional registration), 15A (provisional registration for EEA nationals) or 21 (provisional registration) of the Medical Act 1983 acting in the course of his employment in a resident medical capacity in an approved medical practice; or
    (c) a GP Registrar during the first 2 months of his training period.

54. No health care professional other than one to whom paragraph 53 applies shall perform clinical services under the contract unless he is appropriately registered with his relevant professional body and his registration is not currently suspended.

55. Where the registration of a health care professional or, in the case of a medical practitioner, his inclusion in a primary care list is subject to conditions, the contractor shall ensure compliance with those conditions insofar as they are relevant to the contract.

56. No health care professional shall perform any clinical services unless he has such clinical experience and training as are necessary to enable him properly to perform such services.

Conditions for employment and engagement

57.　(1)　Subject to sub-paragraphs (2) and (3), a contractor shall not employ or engage a medical practitioner (other than one falling within paragraph 53(2)) unless –
    (a)　that practitioner has provided it with the name and address of the PCT on whose medical performers list he appears; and
    (b)　the contractor has checked that the practitioner meets the requirements in paragraph 53.

　　(2)　Where the employment or engagement of a medical practitioner is urgently needed and it is not possible for the contractor to check the matters referred to in paragraph 53 in accordance with sub-paragraph (1)(b) before employing or engaging him he may be employed or engaged on a temporary basis for a single period of up to 7 days whilst such checks are undertaken.

　　(3)　Where the prospective employee is a GP Registrar, the requirements set out in sub-paragraph (1) shall apply with the modifications that –
    (a)　the name and address provided under sub-paragraph (1) may be the name and address of the PCT on whose list he has applied for inclusion; and
    (b)　confirmation that his name appears on that list shall not be required until the end of the first 2 months of the Registrar's training period.

58.　(1)　A contractor shall not employ or engage –
    (a)　a health care professional other than one to whom paragraph 53 applies unless the contractor has checked that he meets the requirements in paragraph 54; or
    (b)　a health care professional to perform clinical services unless he has taken reasonable steps to satisfy himself that he meets the requirements in paragraph 56.

　　(2)　Where the employment or engagement of a health care professional is urgently needed and it is not possible to check the matters referred to in paragraph 54 in accordance with sub-paragraph (1) before employing or engaging him, he may be employed or engaged on a temporary basis for a single period of up to 7 days whilst such checks are undertaken.

　　(3)　When considering a health care professional's experience and training for the purposes of sub-paragraph (1)(b), the contractor shall have regard in particular to –
    (a)　any post-graduate or post-registration qualification held by the health care professional; and
    (b)　any relevant training undertaken by him and any relevant clinical experience gained by him.

59. (1) The contractor shall not employ or engage a health care professional to perform medical services under the contract unless –

    (a) that person has provided two clinical references, relating to two recent posts (which may include any current post) as a health care professional which lasted for 3 months without a significant break, or where this is not possible, a full explanation and alternative referees; and

    (b) the contractor has checked and is satisfied with the references.

(2) Where the employment or engagement of a health care professional is urgently needed and it is not possible to obtain and check the references in accordance with sub-paragraph (1)(b) before employing or engaging him, he may be employed or engaged on a temporary basis for a single period of up to 14 days whilst his references are checked and considered, and for an additional single period of a further 7 days if the contractor believes the person supplying those references is ill, on holiday or otherwise temporarily unavailable.

(3) Where the contractor employs or engages the same person on more than one occasion within a period of 3 months, it may rely on the references provided on the first occasion, provided that those references are not more than 12 months old.

60. (1) Before employing or engaging any person to assist it in the provision of services under the contract, the contractor shall take reasonable care to satisfy itself that the person in question is both suitably qualified and competent to discharge the duties for which he is to be employed or engaged.

(2) The duty imposed by sub-paragraph (1) is in addition to the duties imposed by paragraphs 57 to 59.

(3) When considering the competence and suitability of any person for the purpose of sub-paragraph (1), the contractor shall have regard, in particular, to –

    (a) that person's academic and vocational qualifications;

    (b) his education and training; and

    (c) his previous employment or work experience.

Training

61. The contractor shall ensure that for any health care professional who is –

(a) performing clinical services under the contract; or

(b) employed or engaged to assist in the performance of such services,

there are in place arrangements for the purpose of maintaining and updating his skills and knowledge in relation to the services which he is performing or assisting in performing.

62. The contractor shall afford to each employee reasonable opportunities to undertake appropriate training with a view to maintaining that employee's competence.

Terms and conditions

63. The contractor shall only offer employment to a general medical practitioner on terms and conditions which are no less favourable than those contained in the "Model terms and conditions of service for a salaried GP employed by a GMS practice" published by the British Medical Association and the NHS Confederation as item 1.2 of the supplementary documents to the new GMS contract 2003.

Arrangements for GP Registrars

64. (1) The contractor shall only employ a GP Registrar for the purpose of being trained by a GP Trainer with the agreement of the Secretary of State and subject to the conditions in sub-paragraph (2).

(2) The conditions referred to in sub-paragraph (1) are that the contractor shall not, by reason only of having employed or engaged a GP Registrar, reduce the total number of hours for which other medical practitioners perform primary medical services under the contract or for which other staff assist them in the performance of those services.

(3) A contractor which employs a GP Registrar shall –

(a) offer him terms of employment in accordance with the rates and subject to the conditions contained in any directions given by the Secretary of State to SHAs under section 17 of the Act (Secretary of State's directions: exercise of functions) concerning the grants, fees, travelling and other allowances payable to GP Registrars; and

(b) take into account any guidance issued by the Secretary of State in relation to the GP Registrar Scheme.

Independent nurse prescribers and supplementary prescribers

65. (1) Where –

(a) a contractor employs or engages a person who is an independent nurse prescriber or a supplementary prescriber whose functions will include prescribing;

(b) a party to the contract is an independent nurse prescriber or a supplementary prescriber whose functions will include prescribing; or

   (c) the functions of a person who is an independent nurse
       prescriber or a supplementary prescriber whom the contractor
       already employs or has already engaged are extended to include
       prescribing,
it shall notify the PCT in writing within the period of 7 days
beginning with the date on which the contractor employed or
engaged the person, the party became a party to the contract (unless
immediately before becoming such a party, he fell under paragraph
(a)), or the person's functions were extended, as the case may be.
(2) Where –
   (a) the contractor ceases to employ or engage a person who is an
       independent nurse prescriber or a supplementary prescriber
       whose functions included prescribing in its practice;
   (b) the party to the contract who is an independent nurse prescriber
       or a supplementary prescriber whose functions include
       prescribing, ceases to be a party to the contract;
   (c) the functions of a person who is an independent nurse
       prescriber or a supplementary prescriber whom the contractor
       employs or engages in its practice are changed so that they no
       longer include prescribing in its practice; or
   (d) the contractor becomes aware that a person who is an
       independent nurse prescriber or a supplementary prescriber
       whom it employs or engages has been removed or suspended
       from the relevant register,
it shall notify the PCT in writing by the end of the second working
day after the day when the event occurred.
(3) The contractor shall provide the following information when it
notifies the PCT in accordance with sub-paragraph (1) –
   (a) the person's full name;
   (b) his professional qualifications;
   (c) his identifying number which appears in the relevant register;
   (d) the date on which his entry in the relevant register was
       annotated to the effect that he was qualified to order drugs,
       medicines and appliances for patients;
   (e) the date on which –
       (i)   he was employed or engaged, if applicable,
       (ii) he became a party to the contract, if applicable, or
       (iii) one of his functions became to prescribe in its practice.
(4) The contractor shall provide the following information when it
notifies the PCT in accordance with sub-paragraph (2) –
   (a) the person's full name;
   (b) his professional qualifications;
   (c) his identifying number which appears in the relevant register;
   (d) the date –

(i)   he ceased to be employed or engaged in its practice,
(ii) he ceased to be a party to the contract,
(iii) his functions changed so as no longer to include prescribing, or
(iv) on which he was removed or suspended from the relevant register.

Signing of documents

66. (1) In addition to any other requirements relating to such documents whether in these regulations or otherwise, the contractor shall ensure that the documents specified in paragraph (2) include –
(a) the clinical profession of the health care professional who signed the document; and
(b) the name of the contractor on whose behalf it is signed.
(2) The documents referred to in sub-paragraph (1) are –
(a) certificates issued in accordance with regulation 21, unless regulations relating to particular certificates provide otherwise;
(b) prescription forms and repeatable prescriptions; and
(c) any other clinical documents.

Standard Contract

Qualifications of performers

339. Subject to clause 340, no medical practitioner shall perform medical services under the Contract unless he is –
339.1 included in a *medical performers list* for a PCT in England;
339.2 not suspended from that list or from the *Medical Register*; and
339.3 not subject to interim suspension under section 41A of the Medical Act 1983.

340. Clause 339.1 shall not apply in the case of –
340.1 a medical practitioner employed by an NHS trust, an NHS foundation trust, (in Scotland) a *Health Board*, or (in Northern Ireland) a *Health and Social Services Trust*, who is providing services other than primary medical services at the *practice premises*;
340.2 a person who is provisionally registered under section 15, 15A or 21 of the Medical Act 1983 acting in the course of his employment in a resident medical capacity in an approved medical practice; or
340.3 a *GP Registrar* during the first 2 months of his training period.

341. No *health care professional* other than one to whom clauses 339 and 340 apply shall perform clinical services under the Contract unless he is

registered with his relevant professional body and his registration is not currently suspended.

342. Where the registration of a *health care professional* or, in the case of a medical practitioner, his inclusion in a *primary care list* is subject to conditions, the Contractor shall ensure compliance with those conditions insofar as they are relevant to the Contract.

343. No *health care professional* shall perform any clinical services unless he has such clinical experience and training as are necessary to enable him properly to perform such services.

Conditions for employment and engagement

344. Subject to clauses 345 and 346, the Contractor shall not employ or engage a medical practitioner (other than one falling within clause 340.2) unless –
    344.1 that practitioner has provided it with the name and address of the PCT on whose *medical performers list* he appears; and
    344.2 the Contractor has checked that he meets the requirements in clause 339.

345. Where the employment or engagement of a medical practitioner is urgently needed and it is not possible to check the matters referred to in clause 339 in accordance with clause 344.1 before employing or engaging him, he may be employed or engaged on a temporary basis for a single period of up to 7 days whilst such checks are undertaken.

346. Where the prospective employee is a *GP Registrar*, the requirements set out in clause 344 shall apply with the modifications that –
    346.1 the name and address provided under 344.1 may be the name and address of the PCT on whose list he has applied for inclusion; and
    346.2 confirmation that his name appears on that list shall not be required until the end of the first 2 months of his training period.

347. The Contractor shall not employ or engage –
    347.1 a *health care professional* other than one to whom clauses 339 and 340 apply unless the Contractor has checked that he meets the requirements in clause 341; or
    347.2 a *health care professional* to perform clinical services unless he has taken reasonable steps to satisfy himself that he meets the requirements in clause 343.

348. Where the employment or engagement of a *health care professional* is urgently needed and it is not possible to check the matters referred to in clause 341 in accordance with clause 347 before employing or engaging him, he may be employed or engaged on a temporary basis for a single period of up to 7 days whilst such checks are undertaken.

349.   When considering a *health care professional's* experience and training pursuant to clause 347.2, the Contractor shall have regard to any post-graduate or post-registration qualification held by the *health care professional*, and any relevant training undertaken by him and any relevant clinical experience gained by him.

350.   The Contractor shall not employ or engage a *health care professional* to perform medical services under the Contract unless –
       350.1 that person has provided two clinical references, relating to two recent posts (which may include any current post) as a *health care professional* which lasted for 3 months without a significant break, or where this is not possible, a full explanation and alternative referees; and
       350.2 the Contractor has checked and is satisfied with the references.

351.   Where the employment or engagement of a *health care professional* is urgently needed and it is not possible to obtain and check the references in accordance with clause 350.2 before employing or engaging him, he may be employed or engaged on a temporary basis for a single period of up to 14 days whilst his references are checked and considered, and for an additional single period of a further 7 days if the Contractor believes the person supplying those references is ill, on holiday or otherwise temporarily unavailable.

352.   Where the Contractor employs or engages the same person on more than one occasion within a period of 3 months, he may rely on the references provided on the first occasion, provided that those references are not more than 12 months old.

353.   Before employing or engaging any person to assist it in the provision of services under the Contract, the Contractor shall take reasonable care to satisfy itself that the person in question is both suitably qualified and competent to discharge the duties for which he is to be employed or engaged.

354.   When considering the competence and suitability of any person for the purpose of clause 353, the Contractor shall have regard, in particular, to –
       354.1 that person's academic and vocational qualifications;
       354.2 education and training; and
       354.3 his previous employment or work experience.

Training

355.   The Contractor shall ensure that for any *health care professional* who is –
       355.1 performing clinical services under the Contract; or
       355.2 employed or engaged to assist in the performance of such services

there are in place arrangements for the purpose of maintaining and updating his skills and knowledge in relation to the services which he is providing or assisting in performing.

356. The Contractor shall afford to each employee reasonable opportunities to undertake appropriate training with a view to maintaining that employee's competence.

Terms and conditions

357. The Contractor shall only offer employment to a general medical practitioner on terms and conditions which are no less favourable than those contained in the "Model terms and conditions of service for a salaried general practitioner employed by a GMS practice" published by the British Medical Association and the NHS Confederation as item 1.2 of the supplementary documents to the new GMS contract 2003 (this document is available on the Department of Health's website at http://www.doh.gov.uk/gmscontract/supportingdocs.htm, or a copy may be obtained by writing to the NHS Confederation, 1 Warwick Row, London SW1E 5ER).

Arrangements for *GP Registrars*

358. The Contractor shall only employ a *GP Registrar* for the purpose of being trained by a *GP Trainer* with the agreement of *the Secretary of State* and subject to the conditions in clause 359.

359. The conditions referred to in clause 358 are that the Contractor shall not, by reason only of having employed or engaged a *GP Registrar*, reduce the total number of hours for which other medical practitioners perform primary medical services under the contract or for which other staff assist them in the performance of those services.

360. Where the Contractor employs a *GP Registrar*, the Contractor shall –
   360.1 offer him terms of employment in accordance with the rates and subject to the conditions contained in any directions given by *the Secretary of State* to SHAs under section 17 of *the Act* concerning the grants, fees, travelling and other allowances payable to *GP Registrars*; and
   360.2 take into account any guidance issued by *the Secretary of State* in relation to the GP Registrar scheme.

Independent nurse prescribers and supplementary prescribers

361. Where –
   361.1 the Contractor employs or engages a person who is an *independent*

nurse prescriber or a *supplementary prescriber* whose functions will include prescribing;

361.2 a party to the Contract is an *independent nurse prescriber* or a *supplementary prescriber* whose functions will include prescribing; or

361.3 the functions of a nurse who is an *independent nurse prescriber* a *supplementary prescriber* whom the Contractor already employs or has already engaged are extended to include prescribing,

it shall notify the PCT within the period of 7 days beginning with the date on which the Contractor employed or engaged the person, the party became a party to the Contract (unless, immediately before becoming such a party, he fell under clause 361.1) or the person's functions were extended, as the case may be.

362. Where –

362.1 the Contractor ceases to employ or engage a person who is an *independent nurse prescriber* or a *supplementary prescriber* whose functions included prescribing in its practice;

362.2 the party to the Contract who is an *independent nurse prescriber* or a *supplementary prescriber* whose functions include prescribing, ceases to be a party to the Contract;

362.3 the functions of a person who is an *independent nurse prescriber* or a *supplementary prescriber* whom the Contractor employs or engages in its practice are changed so that they no longer include prescribing in its practice; or

362.4 the Contractor becomes aware that a person who is an *independent nurse prescriber* or a *supplementary prescriber* whom it employs or engages has been removed or suspended from the *relevant register*,

it shall notify the PCT by the end of the second working day after the day when the event occurred.

363. The Contractor shall provide the following information when it notifies the PCT in accordance with clause 361 –

363.1 the person's full name;

363.2 his professional qualifications;

363.3 his identifying number which appears in the relevant register;

363.4 the date on which his entry in the relevant register was annotated to the effect that he was qualified to order drugs, medicines and appliances for patients;

363.5 the date on which –

363.5.1 he was employed or engaged, if applicable,

363.5.2 he became a party to the Contract, if applicable, or

363.5.3 one of his functions became to prescribe in its *practice*.

364. The Contractor shall provide the following information when it notifies the PCT in accordance with clause 362 –

364.1 the person's full name;

364.2 his professional qualifications;

364.3 his identifying number which appears in the *relevant register*;

364.4 the date –

364.4.1 he ceased to be employed or engaged in its practice,

364.4.2 he ceased to be a party to the Contract,

364.4.3 his functions changed so as no longer to include prescribing, or

364.4.4 on which he was removed or suspended from the *relevant register*.

Signing of documents

365.   In addition to any other requirements relating to such documents whether in this Contract or otherwise, the Contractor shall ensure that the documents specified in clause 366 include –

365.1 the clinical profession of that *health care professional* who signed the document; and

365.2 the name of the Contractor on whose behalf it is signed.

366.   The documents referred to in clause 365 are –

366.1 certificates issued in accordance with clause 470 unless regulations relating to a particular certificate provide otherwise;

366.2 *prescription forms* and *repeatable prescriptions*; and

366.3 any other clinical documents.

● Practice area

Standard Contract

Patient registration area

161.   The area in respect of which persons resident in it will, subject to any other terms of the Contract relating to patient registration, be entitled to register with the Contractor, or seek acceptance by the Contractor as a *temporary resident*, is [...].[50]

---

50   The *practice area* needs to be specified here – this is required by regulation 18(1)(d) of *the Regulations*.

Practice leaflet

Regulations

Practice leaflet

76. The contractor shall –
 (a) compile a document (in this paragraph called a practice leaflet) which shall include the information specified in Schedule 10;
 (b) review its practice leaflet at least once in every period of 12 months and make any amendments necessary to maintain its accuracy; and
 (c) make available a copy of the leaflet, and any subsequent updates, to its patients and prospective patients.

Standard Contract

Practice leaflet

437. The Contractor shall –
 437.1 compile a *practice leaflet* which shall include the information specified in Schedule 3;
 437.2 review its *practice leaflet* at least once in every period of 12 months and make any amendments necessary to maintain its accuracy; and
 437.3 make available a copy of the leaflet, and any subsequent updates, to its patients and prospective patients.

ANNEX 3 OF STANDARD CONTRACT

Information to be included in practice leaflets

A practice leaflet shall include –

1. The name of the Contractor.

2. In the case of a Contract with a partnership –
 (a) whether or not it is a *limited partnership*; and
 (b) the names of all the partners and, in the case of a *limited partnership*, their status as a general or limited partner.

3. In the case of a Contract with a company –
 (a) the names of the directors, the company secretary and the shareholders of that company; and
 (b) the address of the company's registered office.

4. The full name of each person performing services under the Contract.

5. In the case of each *health care professional* performing services under the Contract his professional qualifications.

6. Whether the Contractor undertakes the teaching or training of *health care professionals* or persons intending to become *health care professionals*.

7. The contractor's *practice area*, by reference to a sketch diagram, plan or postcode.

8. The address of each of the *practice premises*.

9. The Contractor's telephone and fax numbers and the address of its website (if any).

10. Whether the *practice premises* have suitable access for all disabled patients and, if not, the alternative arrangements for providing services to such patients.

11. How to register as a patient.

12. The right of patients to express a preference of practitioner in accordance with clause 184 and the means of expressing such a preference.

13. The services available under the Contract.

14. The opening hours of the *practice premises* and the method of obtaining access to services throughout the *core hours*.

15. The criteria for home visits and the method of obtaining such a visit.

16. The consultations available to patients under clauses 34 and 35, and 36 and 37.

17. The arrangements for services in the *out-of-hours period* and how the patient may contact such services.

18. If the services in paragraph 17 are not provided by the Contractor, the fact that the PCT referred to in paragraph 28 is responsible for commissioning the services.

19. The name and address of any local *walk-in centre*.

20. The telephone number of NHS Direct and details of NHS Direct online.

21. The method by which patients are to obtain repeat prescriptions.

22. If the Contractor offers repeatable prescribing services, the arrangements for providing such services.

23. If the Contractor is a dispensing contractor the arrangements for dispensing prescriptions.

24. How patients may make a complaint or comment on the provision of service.

25. The rights and responsibilities of the patient, including keeping appointments.

26. The action that may be taken where a patient is violent or abusive to the Contractor, its staff or other persons present on the *practice premises* or in the place where treatment is provided under the Contract or other persons specified in clause 202.

27. Details of who has access to patient information (including information from which the identity of the individual can be ascertained) and the patient's rights in relation to disclosure of such information.

28. The name, address and telephone number of the PCT and from whom details of primary medical services in the area may be obtained.

Practice lists – open/closed

Standard Contract

List of patients

162. The Contractor's list of patients is [open/closed].[51]

163. [The Contractor's list of patients shall remain closed for the period of 12 months from the date on which the Contract comes into force unless the Contractor notifies the PCT in writing of its intention to re-open the list before the end of that period and of the date on which it will re-open: if the Contractor does re-open its list before the end of the 12 month period, it shall not be entitled to close it again during that period except in accordance with clauses 229 to239].[52]

164. The period of time for which the Contractor's list of patients will be closed is [please specify a period of time, which may not exceed 12 months]. The current number of the Contractor's *registered patients* is [please specify]. The number of *registered patients* (lower than the current number of such patients and expressed either in absolute terms or as a percentage of the current number of patients) which if that number were reached would trigger the re-opening of the Contractor's list of patients is [please specify]. The number of *registered patients* (expressed either in absolute terms or as a percentage of the number of

current patients) which, if that number were reached, would trigger the re-closure of the Contractor's list of patients is [please specify].[53]

165. The PCT shall prepare and keep up to date a list of the patients –
    165.1 who have been accepted by the Contractor for inclusion in its list of patients under clauses 170 to 175 and who have not subsequently been removed from that list under clauses 186 to 223; and
    165.2 who have been assigned to the Contractor under clauses 253 and 254, or clauses 255 and 256 and whose assignment has not subsequently been rescinded.

166. [The PCT shall also include in the Contractor's list of patients –
    166.1 those patients who, on 31 March 2004, were recorded by the PCT pursuant to regulation 19 of the National Health Service (General Medical Services) Regulations 1992 as being on the list of –
        166.1.1 the Contractor, if the Contractor is an individual medical practitioner,

51   The Contract must specify whether, at the date the Contract comes into force, the Contractor's list of patients will be *open* or *closed*. Please delete as appropriate. This clause is required by regulation 18(1)(e) of *the Regulations*. However, pursuant to article 32 of *the Transitional Order*, if a medical practitioner was on 31 March 2004, providing general medical services under section 29 of *the Act* and, on or before 31 March 2004, he enters into a *general medical services contract*, whether as an individual medical practitioner or as one of two or more persons practising in partnership, or he is a legal and beneficial shareholder in a company which enters into a *general medical services contract* on or before 31 March 2004, the Contractor's list of patients must be open to applications in accordance with the provisions of the Contract on the date the Contract comes into force unless –
• on 31 March 2004, or on the date on which the Contract is signed if earlier-
  – if the Contract is with an individual medical practitioner, that practitioner is or was exempt from the liability to have persons (other than a specified person) assigned to him under regulation 4(8) of the National Health Service (Choice of Medical Practitioner) Regulations 1998;
  – if the Contract is with a partnership, all those individuals who are medical practitioners are or were exempt from such liability; or
  – if the contract is with a company, all of the medical practitioners who are legal and beneficial shareholders in that company are exempt from such liability; and
• the PCT has determined, in the light of the circumstances in which it granted the exemption or exemptions referred to above, that the Contractor's list of patients should, from the commencement of the Contract, be closed to applications for inclusion in the list other than from the *immediate family members* of registered patients.
If the Contractor falls within one of these exceptions, the words 'closed' should be selected, clause 163 should be included and clause 164 should be deleted.

52   This clause should only be included if clause 162 states that the Contractor's list is *closed* because, pursuant to article 32 of *the Transitional Order*, the Contractor is entitled to have a *closed* list at the date the Contract comes into force.

53   This clause is only required if the Contract specifies in accordance with clause 162 that the Contractor's list of patients is *closed*: see regulation 18(4) of *the Regulations*. The parties are required to incorporate the information indicated in square brackets.

166.1.2 any of the two or more medical practitioners practising in partnership who have entered into the contract, if the Contractor is a partnership, or

166.1.3 any of the medical practitioners who are legal and beneficial shareholders in the company which has entered into the contract,

unless the patient lives outside the *practice area*, and that patient was included on that medical practitioner's list other than by virtue of an assignment under regulation 4 of the National Health Service (Choice of Medical Practitioner) Regulations 1998; and

166.2 any patient who, on or before 31 March 2004, had been assigned to the Contractor, or any one of the persons specified in clause 166.1.2 or 166.1.3 or, under regulation 4 of the National Health Service (Choice of Medical Practitioner) Regulations 1998 but not yet included in the list of the Contractor referred to in clause 166.1.]⁵⁴

167. [The PCT shall also include in the Contractor's list of patients –

167.1 all the patients who, on the date immediately before the coming into force of the *general medical services contract* were on the Contractor's list of patients for the purposes of a *default contract* with the PCT, unless the patient lives outside the *practice area*, and that patient was included on the Contractor's list other than by virtue of an assignment under regulation 4 of the National Health Service (Choice of Medical Practitioner) Regulations 1998 or under the *default contract*; and

167.2 any patient who had been assigned to the Contractor when he was a party to that *default contract* in accordance with the terms of that contract but not yet included in the list referred to in clause 167.1.]⁵⁵

168. [The PCT shall also include in the Contractor's list of patients all of the patients who, on the date on which temporary arrangements under regulation 25(2) or (6) of the National Health Service (General Medical Services) Regulations 1992 came to an end, were –

54 Clause 166 should be included if the Contract is entered into with a medical practitioner who, on 31 March 2004, is providing general medical services under section 29 of *the Act* and on or before 31 March 2004 he enters into a *general medical services contract* whether as an individual medical practitioner or as one of two or more individuals practising in partnership, or he is a legal and beneficial shareholder in a company which enters into a *general medical services contract* on or before 31 March 2004: see article 28 of *the Transitional Order* which contains the requirement. If this clause is not applicable to the Contractor, it should be deleted.

55 This clause should only be included if the Contract with the PCT is being entered into with a Contractor who was a party to a *default contract* with the PCT immediately before the coming into force of the Contract: see article 29 of *the Transitional Order*. If the clause does not apply, it should be deleted.

168.1 temporarily re-assigned to other medical practitioners under
paragraph (14A) of regulation 25; or

168.2 included on the list of the medical practitioner for whom the
temporary arrangements were in place

unless the patient lives outside the *practice area* and that patient became
registered with either the medical practitioner for whom the temporary
arrangements are in place or the medical practitioner or practitioners
providing the temporary arrangements otherwise than as a result of an
assignment under regulation 4 of the National Health Service (Choice of
Medical Practitioner) Regulations 1998.][56]

169.   [The PCT shall also include in the Contractor's list of patients, all of the
patients who were, on the date on which contractual arrangements under
article 15 of *the Transitional Order* in respect of the Contractor's patients
came to an end, on the list or lists of patients prepared and maintained
by the PCT for the purpose of those contractual arrangements, unless the
patient lives outside the *practice area* and that patient's inclusion in the
list of patients did not result from an assignment under regulation 4 of
the National Health Service (Choice of Medical Practitioner) Regulations
1998 or under the contractual arrangements under article 15].[57]

Application for inclusion in a list of patients

170.   The Contractor may, if its list of patients is *open*, accept an application
for inclusion in its list of patients made by or on behalf of any person,
whether or not resident in its *practice area* or included, at the time of that
application, in the list of patients of another contractor or provider of
primary medical services.

171.   The Contractor may, if its list of patients is *closed*, only accept an
application for inclusion in its list of patients from a person who is an
immediate family member of a *registered patient* whether or not resident in
its *practice area* or included, at the time of that application, in the list of
patients of another contractor or provider of primary medical services.

56   This clause is required by article 30(1) of *the Transitional Order* if the Contractor is an
individual medical practitioner for whom, immediately before the Contract commences, the PCT
had in place temporary arrangements under regulation 25(2) or (6) of the National Health Service
(General Medical Services) Regulations 1992: if the Contractor is not such a person, this clause
should be deleted.

57   Clause 169 is required by article 30(2) of *the Transitional Order* if the Contractor is an
individual medical practitioner for whom, immediately before the Contract commences, the PCT
had in place contractual arrangements under article 15 of *the Transitional Order*. If the Contractor is
not such a person, this clause should be deleted.

172.   Subject to clause 173, an application for inclusion in the Contractor's list of patients shall be made by delivering to the *practice premises* a *medical card* or an application signed (in either case) by the applicant or a person authorised by the applicant to sign on his behalf.

173.   An application may be made –
173.1 on behalf of any *child* –
173.1.1 by either *parent*, or in the absence of both *parents*, the guardian or other adult who has care of the *child*,
173.1.2 by a person duly authorised by a local authority to whose care the *child* has been committed under the Children Act 1989, or
173.1.3 by a person duly authorised by a voluntary organisation by which the *child* is being accommodated under the provisions of that Act;
173.2 on behalf of any adult who is incapable of making such an application or authorising such an application to be made on their behalf, by a relative or *primary carer* of that person.

174.   Where the Contractor accepts an application for inclusion in its list of patients, the Contractor shall notify the PCT in writing as soon as possible.

175.   On receipt of a notice under clause 174, the PCT shall include that person in the Contractor's list of patients from the date on which the notice is received, and shall notify the applicant (or, in the case of a *child* or incapable adult, the person making the application on their behalf) in writing of the acceptance.

Temporary residents

176.   The Contractor may if its list of patients is *open* accept a person as a *temporary resident* provided it is satisfied that the person is –
176.1 temporarily resident away from his normal place of residence and is not being provided with *essential services* under any other arrangement in the locality where he is temporarily residing; or
176.2 moving from place to place and not for the time being resident in any place.

177.   For the purposes of clause 176, a person shall be regarded as temporarily resident in a place if, when he arrives in that place, he intends to stay there for more than 24 hours but not more than 3 months.

178.   Where the Contractor wishes to terminate its responsibility for a person accepted as a *temporary resident* before the end of 3 months or such shorter period for which it had agreed to accept him as a patient, the Contractor shall notify the patient either orally or in writing and its responsibility for that person shall cease 7 days after the date on which the notification was given.

Pre-contract disputes

Regulations

9. Pre-contract disputes

(1) Except where both parties to the prospective contract are health service bodies (in which case section 4(4) of the 1990 Act (NHS contracts) applies), if, in the course of negotiations intending to lead to a contract, the prospective parties to that contract are unable to agree on a particular term of the contract, either party may refer the dispute to the Secretary of State to consider and determine the matter.

(2) Disputes referred to the Secretary of State in accordance with paragraph (1), or section 4(4) of the 1990 Act, shall be considered and determined in accordance with the provisions of paragraphs 101(3) to (14) and 102(1) of Schedule 6, and paragraph (3) (where it applies) of this regulation.

(3) In the case of a dispute referred to the Secretary of State under paragraph (1), the determination –
(a) may specify terms to be included in the proposed contract;
(b) may require the PCT to proceed with the proposed contract, but may not require the proposed contractor to proceed with the proposed contract; and
(c) shall be binding upon the prospective parties to the contract.

Guidance

6.15 One of the main reasons why the process of agreeing provisional contracts could potentially be delayed beyond the end of February 2004 is a pre-contract dispute. The new arrangements have been designed to keep these disputes to a minimum:
(i) disputes over aspiration levels should be resolved in line with the guidance in chapter 3
(ii) disputes about what additional services should be provided will be minimised because the formal opt-out rules and procedures do not start until 1 April 2004
(iii) disputes about open or closed list status should be minimised because contractors will have recourse to the new procedures from 1 April 2004

(iv) disputes about what enhanced services are to be provided will be minimised because the SFE makes clear what enhanced services contractors have a right to provide (access, quality information, and childhood vaccinations and immunisations if they are also providing the additional service). Other enhanced services are commissioned from contractors at the discretion of the PCT

(v) disputes about premises, IM&T funding and PCT-administered funding items should similarly be kept to a minimum because the SFE and premises Directions are clear about contractor entitlements.

It does not make sense for concerns about the interim global sum or MPIG figures to delay the contract being signed. The GPC, the NHS Confederation and the Department of Health all strongly advise contractors and PCTs to defer potential disputes on the global sum and MPIG until actual figures are known following the introduction of the revised Exeter system. It is important for PCTs and contractors to note that by signing the contract, neither side is indicating its agreement to the final global sum and MPIG payments.

6.16   Despite these considerations, if in the course of negotiations intending to lead to a GMS contract, the prospective parties are unable to reach agreement on a particular term, either party may refer the dispute for consideration and determination by the Family Health Service Appeals Authority (Special Health Authority) (FHSAA (SHA)) or, where appropriate, the SHA.

6.17   All such disputes will be considered and determined in accordance with the procedure set out in regulations 9 and paragraphs 100(3) to 100(13) of Schedule 6 to the GMS Contract Regulations. This pre-contract dispute mechanism will take effect from the date that the Contract Regulations take effect, which is expected to be in February 2004. However, PCTs and contractors should note that in practice there would almost certainly not be sufficient time for such formal disputes to be resolved before 31 March 2004. Where a formal dispute has not been resolved by 1 April 2004 the contract will come into effect subject to the later determination of the disputed issue(s). In some cases the parties may wish to make use of the local implementation protocol agreed between the NHS Confederation, GPC and Department of Health but this may not be appropriate for routine local issues. A copy of the protocol is attached at annex E.

6.18   At the end of 3 months, or on such earlier date as its responsibility for the patient has come to an end, the Contractor shall notify the PCT in writing of any person whom it accepted as a *temporary resident*.

Preferred provider status

Guidance

2.81   GMS contractors have preferred provider status for three DESs: access, quality information preparation, and childhood vaccinations and immunisation target payments if that contractor is providing the additional service. PCTs must offer these services to GMS contractors, using the DES specifications and prices which are set out in the SFE. They will want to do so, and reach agreement with contractors, before GMS contracts are provisionally agreed by the end of February 2004. Contractors do not have preferred provider status for other enhanced services newly commissioned by the PCT but pre-existing arrangements for enhanced services would continue for the duration of those contracts.

Premises

Regulations

1.   Subject to any plan which is included in the contract pursuant to regulation 18(3), the contractor shall ensure that the premises used for the provision of services under the contract are –
(a) suitable for the delivery of those services; and
(b) sufficient to meet the reasonable needs of the contractor's patients.

Standard Contract

25.   The address of each of the premises to be used by the Contractor or any sub-contractor for the provision of services under the Contract is as follows: [...].[58]

26.   Subject to any plan which is included in the Contract pursuant to clause 27, the Contractor shall ensure that premises used for the provision of services under the Contract are:
26.1 suitable for the delivery of those services; and
26.2 sufficient to meet the reasonable needs of the Contractor's patients.

27.   Where, on the date on which the Contract was signed, the PCT is not satisfied that all or any of the premises specified in clause 26 met the

requirements set out in clause 26 and consequently the PCT and the Contractor have together drawn up a plan (contained in Schedule 6 to this Contract) which specifies –

27.1 the steps to be taken by the Contractor to bring the premises up to the relevant standard;

27.2 any financial support that is available from the PCT; and

27.3 the timescale in which such steps will be taken.[59]

28. The Contractor shall comply with the plan specified in clause 27 and contained in Schedule 6 to this Contract as regards the steps to be taken by the Contractor to meet the requirements in clause 26 and the timescale in which those steps will be taken.

---

58   All relevant addresses from which services under the Contract will be provided by the Contractor or any sub-contractor must be included here. It does not include the homes of patients or any other premises where services are provided on an emergency basis. This clause is required by regulation 18(1)(b) of *the Regulations*, together with regulation 18(2).

However, where a medical practitioner who, on 31 March 2004, is providing general medical services under section 29 of *the Act*, enters into a *general medical services* contract on or before 31 March 2004 whether as an individual medical practitioner, as one or two or more individuals practising in partnership, or if that person is a legal and beneficial shareholder in a company which enters into a general medical services contract on or before 31 March 2004, *the practice* premises specified in the Contract at its commencement must, unless the PCT agrees otherwise in writing, be –

• if the Contractor is an individual medical practitioner, all the premises which, on 31 March 2004 (or on the date on which the contract is signed, if earlier), were approved (whether with or without conditions) by the PCT or *the Secretary of State* under paragraph 29 or 29A of Schedule 2 to the National Health Service (General Medical Services) Regulations 1992 in respect of that practitioner and whose approval had not been withdrawn;

• if the Contractor is a partnership, all the premises which, on 31 March 2004 (or on the date on which the contract is signed, if earlier), were approved (whether with or without conditions) by the PCT or *the Secretary of State* under paragraph 29 or 29A of Schedule 2 to the National Health Service (General Medical Services) Regulations 1992 in respect of any of those practitioners and whose approval had not been withdrawn; or

• if the Contractor is a company, all the premises which, on 31 March 2004 (or on the date on which the Contract is signed if earlier), were approved (whether with or without conditions) by the PCT or *the Secretary of State* under paragraph 29 or 29A of Schedule 2 to the National Health Service (General Medical Services) Regulations 1992 in respect of any of the medical practitioners who are legal and beneficial shareholders in that company and whose approval had not been withdrawn.

This is a requirement of article 26 of *the Transitional Order*. The applicability of article 26 of *the Transitional Order* does not prevent the inclusion of a plan pursuant to clause 27 where the PCT does not consider that all or any one of the premises meets the standards in clause 26.

59   Clause 27, clause 28 and Schedule 6 need only be included in the Contract if the PCT is not satisfied that any or all of the premises at which services are to be provided meet the standards set out in clause 26 at the date the Contract is signed. If the premises do meet the standards, these clauses can be deleted.

Guidance

4.24 The contract allows PCTs to agree to the extent of reasonable premises costs they incur and the nature and level of payments to be made. Where premises are used to provide services other than general medical services, payments will be reduced proportionately. This will be a matter for agreement under the contract. PCTs will need to comply with the payment arrangements, which will be set out in Directions to be published in draft in January 2004. The new funding arrangements for PCTs are described in chapter 5.

4.25 Contractors whose premises were approved for payment at 31 March 2004 need not seek confirmation of that approval in order to continue receiving payments calculated under the arrangements that existed on that date. The arrangements set out in the rest of this section will come into operation in respect of any changes made to existing premises, when new premises agreed in the contract are brought into use or any of the payment mechanisms outlined in this guidance are effected.

4.26 PCTs should be satisfied that new premises development or refurbishment demonstrates value for money. In so doing, PCTs, in consultation with the District Valuer, shall have regard to the standards provided in *Primary and Social Care Premises – Planning and Design Guidance*, available at http://www.primarycare.nhsestates.gov.uk. There may be occasions where, for example, because of the physical nature of the building/site, full compliance with those standards is not possible for an otherwise suitable site or building. In such cases, the PCT should be satisfied that any reduction of or enhancement to those standards is reasonable and demonstrates value for money. Where a contractor does not agree with a PCT decision not to accept premises or disputes the level of funding offered by the PCT, the matter will be resolved through the dispute resolution arrangements described in chapter 6.

Minimum standards

4.27 Chapter 4 of *Investing in Primary Care* set new quality standards for premises to be used for the delivery of general medical services. It also set out actions to be taken should any premises not meet those standards. Details are available at http://www.nhsestates.gov.uk/primary_care/index.asp.

Premises – entry and inspection by the PCT

Standard Contract

465.   Subject to the conditions in clause 466, the Contractor shall allow persons authorised in writing by the PCT to enter and inspect the *practice premises* at any reasonable time.

466.   The conditions referred to in clause 465 are that –
466.1 reasonable notice of the intended entry has been given;
466.2 written evidence of the authority of the person seeking entry is produced to the Contractor on request; and
466.3 entry is not made to any premises or part of the premises used as residential accommodation without the consent of the resident.

467.   Either the Contractor or the PCT may, if it wishes to do so, invite the *Local Medical Committee* for the area of the PCT to be present at an inspection of the *practice premises* which takes place under clause 465.

Entry and inspection by members of PCT Patients' Forums

468.   The Contractor shall allow members of a PCT Patients' Forum authorised by or under regulation 3 of the Patients' Forums (Functions) Regulations 2003 to enter and inspect the *practice premises* for the purpose of any of the Forum's functions in accordance with the requirements of that regulation.

Entry and inspection by the Commission for Healthcare Audit and Inspection

469.   The Contractor shall allow persons authorised by the Commission for Healthcare Audit and Inspection to enter and inspect the premises in accordance with section 66 of the Health and Social Care (Community Health and Standards) Act 2003.

Premises – payments

Guidance

4.28   This section sets out the arrangements by which recurrent payments for new or substantially refurbished premises should be calculated. PCTs should seek advice from the District Valuer on matters relating to current market rent and open market valuation. Contractors may receive, at the PCT's discretion, payments towards for example, costs to improve practice premises, overcome barriers to capital investment or assist moves from poor premises into modern replacements. The main arrangements are set out in Table 12.

Table 12 **Premises payments**	
Arrangement	Description
1. Owner-occupier borrowing costs	1. The appointment of a firm to undertake construction works should be subject to at least three written quotes following an open competitive tendering exercise. The GMS Contractor and the PCT should agree which quote represents best value for money.
	2. A prescribed percentage should be applied to the necessary level of loan incurred to meet the aggregated cost elements. Costs can include: site purchase, building works, reasonable professional fees agreed in advance with the PCT, any rolled-up interest incurred on loans taken to procure the premises, necessary local authority and planning application fees, VAT where properly applied and agreed levels of furnishing, fitting and equipping.
	3. The prescribed percentage for fixed interest rate loans is equivalent to the 20 high year gilt rate issued by the Bank of England plus 1.5%. Details of the Gilt rate are at *Gilts Yield*.
	4. The variable prescribed percentage, which should be recalculated annually, is the Bank of England Base Interest Rate plus 1%. Details of Base Rates are at *Base Rate*.
	Continued

Table 12 – continued	
Arrangement	**Description**
2. Subsequent changes	1. Borrowing cost payments arrangements may transfer when an outgoing practitioner sells his or her equity interest in the premises to an incoming practitioner at the outstanding level of borrowing required to purchase the premises.
	2. Where the practitioner is financing the scheme wholly or mainly from his or her own money, ie any loan is for the lesser part of the total cost, the prescribed percentage will be that agreed by the PCT as representing best value for money.
	3. Contractors in receipt of a fixed interest rate loan should advise their PCT of any change of lender or any reduction in the level of interest charged to their loan.
	4. From 1 April 2004, where a practitioner changes lender and/or re-negotiates lower loan costs, the cost rent reimbursement level shall be recalculated using the appropriate prescribed percentage in force at the time that the changed loan arrangements came into effect.
	5. From 1 April 2004, when a practitioner has repaid his or her loan, entitlement to borrowing cost payments shall cease and be replaced with notional rent payments.
	6. PCTs should also conduct an annual enquiry of Contractors to confirm what borrowing arrangements are in place. PCTs should recover any overpayments made to practitioners after 1 April 2004.
3. Rental costs for leasehold premises	1. Payments for all rented premises will initially be based on the current market

Table 12 – continued	
Arrangement	**Description**
	rent (CMR) or the actual rent whichever is the less. The CMR will be set having regard to the terms of the lease on offer adjusted, if necessary, to a tenant's internal repairing basis. The CMR will be reviewed to take account of periodic landlord reviews of the rent. The exception is where the landlord review results in no change to the rent charged or to the lease itself. 2. For leases where landlord reviews are linked to an index (e.g. RPI), the level of rental payment will be adjusted in accordance with the arrangements set out in the lease. PCTs should receive a copy of the lease being offered and obtain advice from the District Valuer as to the appropriateness of the terms and the initial rent being offered. 3. In all cases, VAT should be added where this is properly charged by the landlord.
4. Notional – rented premises	1. Contractors which owner-occupy their premises may opt to change from payments based on their borrowing costs and receive a notional rent. Payments will be calculated using the CMR assumptions contained in the notional lease and be reviewed 3-yearly after the first payment has been made. Only in the event of a change in the purpose for which the premises are to be used or as a result of further capital investment in the premises agreed in the contract will a subsequent assessment be made earlier than the normal 3-yearly review date.

Continued

Table 12 – continued	
Arrangement	**Description**
	2. Full notional rent will be equivalent to the current market rent assessment. Where NHS capital has contributed to the cost of the work completed the full notional rent will be abated in proportion to the total cost of the work carried out. On completion of the development, the abated notional rent payable should be calculated in accordance with the details to be found at http://www.nhsestates.gov.uk/primary_care/index.asp. The abated notional rent will be paid to the Contractor for a period of 10 years, after which full notional rent will become payable.
5. Temporary premises costs	Occasions arise whereby premises are to be wholly replaced on the existing site or extension work may require the practice to move to temporary premises. Where agreed in the contract, PCTs may provide a grant and/or recurrent funding to meet associated set-up and rental costs.
6. Improvement grants	At the PCT's discretion, contractors may receive a grant of between 33% and 66% towards costs incurred to improve their premises to provide GMS. Examples include reconfiguration of the internal layout, adding an extension, DDA compliance and improved security.
7. Uplift to current market rents	Current market rent levels in some areas of deprivation may be too low to provide sufficient returns to support new capital investment in practice premises or provide sufficient support for existing premises that meet minimum standards. Where this is the case, CMR may be increased by applying

Table 12 – continued	
Arrangement	**Description**
	an uplifting factor held by the PCT. The resulting level of reimbursement will remain in payment until it is overtaken by the naturally occurring current market rent.
8. **Notional rent and leasehold premises**	Notional rent may be paid in respect of tenant improvements agreed in the contract carried out by practitioners on their leasehold premises to the extent the improvement is not reflected in the rent charged by the landlord.
9. **Combined borrowing cost and notional rent payments**	Notional rent may be paid also to practitioners in addition to borrowing cost payments when further capital investment still results in a CMR on the whole premises which is lower than the existing borrowing cost payments being made.
10. **Reconversion of former residential premises**	PCTs may award a grant to re-convert former residential premises to their former use.
11. **Guaranteed minimum sale price for redundant owner-occupied premises**	To overcome any lack of surety on the sale price of redundant practice premises, PCTs may provide a grant to ensure a guaranteed minimum sale price to enable a contractor to move to modern alternative premises to improve the range of services provided to patients.
12. **Legal and other professional fees for new purpose-built premises**	PCTs may agree to pay a grant towards legal and other professional fees incurred by Contractors who occupy new leasehold premises or new owner-occupied premises built or significantly improved under notional rented premises payment arrangements.

Continued

Table 12 – continued	
Arrangement	**Description**
13. Reimbursement of equipment leasing costs in new leasehold premises	PCTs may meet reasonable costs of lease arrangements to furnish, fit and equip new practice premises.
14. Grant to meet mortgage deficit and/or redemption costs	PCTs may meet all or a proportion of mortgage deficit and early redemption penalty costs in respect of contractors which move from old premises to modern alternatives.

Premises – payments for existing commitments

Statement of Financial Entitlement

Existing commitments

19.1   Where PCTs have already committed themselves, prior to 1 April 2004, to provide financial assistance in the financial year 2004/05 –

(a) towards the building of new premises to be used for providing medical services;

(b) towards the purchase of premises to be used for providing medical services;

(c) towards the development of premises which are used or are to be used for providing medical services; or

(d) in the form of premises improvement grants,

in accordance with the arrangements for funding capital investment in premises set out in the Red Book, then subject to the provisions of this Section, those commitments are to be met.

19.2   As regards any such capital investment project, a PCT must pay to a contractor under its GMS contract any amount that the PCT agreed before 1 April 2004 to pay to the contractor (or to the practice for which the contractor is now responsible) during the financial year 2004/05, subject to the following conditions –

(a) the contractor must comply with any conditions to which the agreement to make the payment was subject. For these purposes, it shall be deemed that the specifications for the project which are set out in the project proposal, and any standards to be met during construction or development work which are set out in the project proposal, are all conditions of the agreement to make the payment; and

(b) the project must not change significantly (in the PCT's view) from the version of the project in respect of which the PCT agreed to make the payments.

19.3   If any of these conditions are breached, the PCT may in appropriate circumstances withhold payment of any or any part of any payment that is otherwise payable under paragraph 19.2. If the breach arises because the project has changed significantly, and additional costs will be incurred as a consequence, any claim for PCT funding in respect of those additional costs is to be determined in accordance with the arrangements for funding new capital investment set out in the Primary Medical Services (Premises Costs) (England) Directions 2004.

19.4   If it was agreed before 1 April 2004 that the amount of payments payable in respect of the project plan would be reviewed in the financial year 2004/05, the payments payable under this Section are subject to the outcome of that review and any revised amount agreed in accordance with that review becomes the amount payable under this Section. If a dispute as to the amounts payable arises as a result of that review, that dispute shall be resolved in accordance with –

(a) any dispute resolution procedure (for resolution of disputes between the PCT and the contractor) agreed in respect of the project plan; or

(b) if no such procedure was agreed, the NHS dispute resolution procedures – or by the courts (see Part 7 of Schedule 6 to the 2004 Regulations).

Prescribing

Regulations

Prescribing

38.   The contractor shall ensure that any prescription form or repeatable prescription for drugs, medicines or appliances issued by a prescriber complies as appropriate with the requirements in paragraphs 39 and 41 to 44.

39. (1) Subject to paragraphs 42 and 43, a prescriber shall order any drugs, medicines or appliances which are needed for the treatment of any patient who is receiving treatment under the contract by issuing to that patient a prescription form or a repeatable prescription and such a prescription form or repeatable prescription shall not be used in any other circumstances.

(2) A prescriber may order drugs, medicines or appliances on a repeatable prescription only where the drugs, medicines or appliances are to be provided more than once.

(3) In issuing any such prescription form or repeatable prescription the prescriber shall himself sign the prescription form or repeatable prescription in ink with his initials, or forenames, and surname in his own handwriting and not by means of a stamp and shall so sign only after particulars of the order have been inserted in the prescription form or repeatable prescription, and –
 (a) the prescription form or repeatable prescription shall not refer to any previous prescription form or repeatable prescription; and
 (b) a separate prescription form or repeatable prescription shall be used for each patient, except where a bulk prescription is issued for a school or institution under paragraph 44.

(4) Where a prescriber orders the drug buprenorphine or a drug specified in Schedule 2 to the Misuse of Drugs Regulations 2001 (controlled drugs to which regulations 14, 15, 16, 18, 19, 20, 21, 23, 26 and 27 of those Regulations apply) for supply by instalments for treating addiction to any drug specified in that Schedule, he shall –
 (a) use only the prescription form provided specially for the purposes of supply by instalments;
 (b) specify the number of instalments to be dispensed and the interval between each instalment; and
 (c) order only such quantity of the drug as will provide treatment for a period not exceeding 14 days.

(5) The prescription form provided specially for the purpose of supply by instalments shall not be used for any purpose other than ordering drugs in accordance with sub-paragraph (4).

(6) In a case of urgency a prescriber may request a chemist to dispense a drug or medicine before a prescription form or repeatable prescription is issued, only if –
 (a) that drug or medicine is not a Scheduled drug;
 (b) that drug is not a controlled drug within the meaning of the Misuse of Drugs Act 1971, other than a drug which is for the time being specified in Schedules 4 or 5 to the Misuse of Drugs Regulations 2001; and

(c) he undertakes to furnish the chemist, within 72 hours, with a prescription form or repeatable prescription completed in accordance with sub-paragraph (3).

(7) In a case of urgency a prescriber may request a chemist to dispense an appliance before a prescription form or repeatable prescription is issued only if –
   (a) that appliance does not contain a Scheduled drug or a controlled drug within the meaning of the Misuse of Drugs Act 1971, other than a drug which is for the time being specified in Schedule 5 to the Misuse of Drugs Regulations 2001;
   (b) in the case of a restricted availability appliance, the patient is a person, or it is for a purpose, specified in the Drug Tariff; and
   (c) he undertakes to furnish the chemist, within 72 hours, with a prescription form or repeatable prescription completed in accordance with sub-paragraph (3).

40. Repeatable prescribing services

(1) The contractor may only provide repeatable prescribing services to any person on its list of patients if it –
   (a) satisfies the conditions in sub-paragraph (2); and
   (b) has notified the PCT of its intention to provide repeatable prescribing services in accordance with sub-paragraphs (3) and (4).

(2) The conditions referred to in sub-paragraph (1)(a) are –
   (a) the contractor holds a contract with a PCT specified in Schedule 9;
   (b) the contractor has access to computer systems and software which enable it to issue repeatable prescriptions and batch issues; and
   (c) the practice premises at which the repeatable prescribing services are to be provided are located in an area of the PCT in which there is also located the premises of at least one chemist who has undertaken to provide, or has entered into an arrangement to provide, repeat dispensing services.

(3) The notification referred to in sub-paragraph (1)(b) is a notification, in writing, by the contractor to the PCT that it –
   (a) wishes to provide repeatable prescribing services; and
   (b) intends to begin to provide those services from a specified date; and
   (c) satisfies the conditions in paragraph (2).

(4) The date specified by the contractor pursuant to sub-paragraph (3)(b) must be at least 10 days after the date on which the notification specified in sub-paragraph (1) is given.

(5) Nothing in this paragraph requires a contractor or prescriber to provide repeatable prescribing services to any person.

(6) A prescriber may only provide repeatable prescribing services to a person
on a particular occasion if –
(a) that person has agreed to receive such services on that occasion; and
(b) the prescriber considers that it is clinically appropriate to provide
such services to that person on that occasion.

(7) The contractor may not provide repeatable prescribing services to any
patient of its to whom –
(a) it is authorised or required by the PCT to provide dispensing services
under paragraph 47 or 49; or
(b) any of the persons specified in sub-paragraph (8) is authorised or
required by the PCT under regulation 20 of the Pharmaceutical
Regulations to provide pharmaceutical services.

(8) The persons referred to in sub-paragraph (7) are –
(a) in the case of a contract with an individual medical practitioner, that
medical practitioner;
(b) in the case of a contract with two or more individuals practising in
partnership, any medical practitioner who is a partner;
(c) in the case of a contract with a company, any medical practitioner
who is a legal and beneficial shareholder in that company; or
(d) any medical practitioner employed by the contractor.

41. Repeatable prescriptions

(1) A prescriber who issues a repeatable prescription must at the same time
issue the appropriate number of batch issues.

(2) A prescriber who has provided repeatable prescribing services to a person
must, as soon as is practicable, notify that person, and make reasonable
efforts to contact the chemist providing repeat dispensing services to that
person, if –
(a) he makes any change to the type, quantity, strength or dosage of
drugs, medicines or appliances ordered on that person's repeatable
prescription; or
(b) he considers that it is no longer appropriate or safe for that person to
receive the drugs, medicines or appliances ordered on his repeatable
prescription, or no longer appropriate or safe for him to continue to
receive repeatable prescribing services.

(3) If a prescriber provides repeatable prescribing services to a person in
respect of whom he has previously issued a repeatable prescription which
has not yet expired (for example, because that person wishes to obtain
the drugs, medicines or appliances from a different chemist), the
prescriber must make reasonable efforts to notify the chemist which has
in its possession the repeatable prescription which is no longer required.

(4)   If a prescriber has issued a repeatable prescription in respect of a person, and (before the expiry of that repeatable prescription) it comes to his notice that that person has been removed from the list of patients of the contractor on whose behalf the prescription was issued, that prescriber must –
(a) notify that person; and
(b) make reasonable efforts to notify the chemist who has been providing repeat dispensing services to that person,
that the repeatable prescription should no longer be used to obtain or provide repeat dispensing services.

42.   Restrictions on prescribing by medical practitioners

(1)   In the course of treating a patient to whom he is providing treatment under the contract, a medical practitioner shall not order on a prescription form or repeatable prescription a drug, medicine or other substance specified in any directions given by the Secretary of State under section 28U of the Act (GMS contracts: prescription of drugs etc.) as being drugs, medicines or other substances which may not be ordered for patients in the provision of medical services under the contract but may, subject to regulation 24(2)(b), prescribe such a drug, medicine or other substance for that patient in the course of that treatment under a private arrangement.

(2)   In the course of treating a patient to whom he is providing treatment under the contract, a medical practitioner shall not order on a prescription form or repeatable prescription a drug, medicine or other substance specified in any directions given by the Secretary of State under section 28U of the Act as being a drug, medicine or other substance which can only be ordered for specified patients and specified purposes unless –
(a) that patient is a person of the specified description;
(b) that drug, medicine or other substance is prescribed for that patient only for the specified purpose; and
(c) the practitioner endorses the form with the reference "SLS",
but may, subject to regulation 24(2)(b), prescribe such a drug, medicine or other substance for that patient in the course of that treatment under a private arrangement.

(3)   In the course of treating a patient to whom he is providing treatment under the contract, a medical practitioner shall not order on a prescription form or repeatable prescription a restricted availability appliance unless –
(a) the patient is a person, or it is for a purpose, specified in the Drug Tariff; and

(b) the practitioner endorses the face of the form with the reference "SLS", but may, subject to regulation 24(2)(b), prescribe such an appliance for that patient in the course of that treatment under a private arrangement.

(4) In the course of treating a patient to whom he is providing treatment under the contract, a medical practitioner shall not order on a repeatable prescription a controlled drug within the meaning of the Misuse of Drugs Act 1971, other than a drug which is for the time being specified in Schedule 4 or 5 to the Misuse of Drugs Regulations 2001, but may, subject to regulation 24(2)(b), prescribe such a drug for that patient in the course of that treatment under a private arrangement.

43. Restrictions on prescribing by supplementary prescribers

(1) The contractor shall have arrangements in place to secure that a supplementary prescriber will –
(a) give a prescription for a prescription only medicine;
(b) administer a prescription only medicine for parenteral administration; or
(c) give directions for the administration of a prescription only medicine for parenteral administration,
as a supplementary prescriber only under the conditions set out in sub-paragraph (2).

(2) The conditions referred to in sub-paragraph (1) are that –
(a) the person satisfies the applicable conditions set out in article 3B(3) of the POM Order (prescribing and administration by supplementary prescribers), unless those conditions do not apply by virtue of any of the exemptions set out in the subsequent provisions of that Order;
(b) the medicine is not a controlled drug within the meaning of the Misuse of Drugs Act 1971;
(c) the drug, medicine or other substance is not specified in any directions given by the Secretary of State under section 28U of the Act as being a drug, medicine or other substance which may not be ordered for patients in the provision of medical services under the contract;
(d) the drug, medicine or other substance is not specified in any directions given by the Secretary of State under section 28U of the Act as being a drug, medicine or other substance which can only be ordered for specified patients and specified purposes unless –
(i) the patient is a person of the specified description,
(ii) the medicine is prescribed for that patient only for the specified purposes, and
(iii) if the supplementary prescriber is giving a prescription, he endorses the face of the form with the reference "SLS".

(3) Where the functions of supplementary prescriber include prescribing, the contractor shall have arrangements in place to secure that that person will only give a prescription for –
(a) an appliance; or
(b) a medicine which is not a prescription only medicine,
   as a supplementary prescriber under the conditions set out in sub-paragraph (4).

(4) The conditions referred to in sub-paragraph (3) are that –
(a) the supplementary prescriber acts in accordance with a clinical management plan which is in effect at the time he acts and which contains the following particulars –
   (i)   the name of the patient to whom the plan relates,
   (ii)   the illness or conditions which may be treated by the supplementary prescriber,
   (iii) the date on which the plan is to take effect, and when it is to be reviewed by the medical practitioner or dentist who is a party to the plan,
   (iv)   reference to the class or description of medicines or types of appliances which may be prescribed or administered under the plan,
   (v)   any restrictions or limitations as to the strength or dose of any medicine which may be prescribed or administered under the plan, and any period of administration or use of any medicine or appliance which may be prescribed or administered under the plan,
   (vi)   relevant warnings about known sensitivities of the patient to, or known difficulties of the patient with, particular medicines or appliances,
   (vii) the arrangements for notification of –
      (aa) suspected or known adverse reactions to any medicine which may be prescribed or administered under the plan, and suspected or known adverse reactions to any other medicine taken at the same time as any medicine prescribed or administered under the plan,
      (bb) incidents occurring with the appliance which might lead, might have led or has led to the death or serious deterioration of state of health of the patient, and
   (viii) the circumstances in which the supplementary prescriber should refer to, or seek the advice of, the medical practitioner or dentist who is a party to the plan;
(b) he has access to the health records of the patient to whom the plan relates which are used by any medical practitioner or dentist who is a party to the plan;

(c) if it is a prescription for a medicine, the medicine is not a controlled drug within the meaning of the Misuse of Drugs Act 1971;

(d) if it is a prescription for a drug, medicine or other substance, that drug, medicine or other substance is not specified in any directions given by the Secretary of State under section 28U of the Act as being a drug, medicine or other substance which may not be ordered for patients in the provision of medical services under the contract;

(e) if it is a prescription for a drug, medicine or other substance, that drug, medicine or other substance is not specified in any directions given by the Secretary of State under section 28U of the Act as being a drug, medicine or other substance which can only be ordered for specified patients and specified purposes unless –

  (i) the patient is a person of the specified description,

  (ii) the medicine is prescribed for that patient only for the specified purposes, and

  (iii) when giving the prescription, he endorses the face of the form with the reference "SLS";

(f) if it is a prescription for a medicine –

  (i) the medicine is the subject of a product licence, a marketing authorisation or a homeopathic certificate of registration granted by the licensing authority or the European Commission, or

  (ii) subject to paragraph (6), the use of the medicine is for the purposes of a clinical trial, and –

    (aa) that trial is the subject of a clinical trial certificate issued in accordance with the Medicines Act 1968, or

    (bb) a clinical trial certificate is not needed in respect of that trial by virtue of any exemption conferred by or under that Act;

(g) if it is a prescription for an appliance, the appliance is listed in Part IX of the Drug Tariff; and

(h) if it is a prescription for a restricted availability appliance –

  (i) the patient is a person of a description mentioned in the entry in Part IX of the Drug Tariff in respect of that appliance,

  (ii) the appliance is prescribed only for the purposes specified in respect of that person in that entry, and

  (iii) when giving the prescription, he endorses the face of the form with the reference "SLS".

(5) In sub-paragraph (4)(a), "clinical management plan" means a written plan (which may be amended from time to time) relating to the treatment of an individual patient agreed by –

(a) the patient to whom the plan relates;

(b) the medical practitioner or dentist who is a party to the plan; and

(c) any supplementary prescriber who is to prescribe, give directions for administration or administer under the plan.

(6) In relation to any time from the coming into force of any regulations made by the Secretary of State under section 2(2) of the European Communities Act 1972 (general implementation of treaties) to implement Directive 2001/83/EC on the Community code relating to medicinal products for human use, sub-paragraph (4)(f)(ii) shall be read as if it referred to a clinical trial which has been authorised, or sis treated as having been authorised by the licensing authority for the purposes of those Regulations.

44. Bulk prescribing

(1) Where –
(a) a contractor is responsible under the contract for the treatment of 10 or more persons in a school or other institution in which at least 20 persons normally reside; and
(b) a prescriber orders, for any two or more of those persons for whose treatment the contractor is responsible, drugs, medicines or appliances to which this paragraph applies,
the prescriber may use a single prescription form for the purpose.

(2) Where a prescriber uses a single prescription form for the purpose mentioned in sub-paragraph (1)(b), he shall (instead of entering on the form the names of the persons for whom the drugs, medicines or appliances are ordered) enter on the form –
(a) the name of the school or institution in which those persons reside; and
(b) the number of persons residing there for whose treatment the contractor is responsible.

(3) This paragraph applies to any drug, medicine or appliance which can be supplied as part of pharmaceutical services or local pharmaceutical services and which –
(a) in the case of a drug or medicine, is not a product of a description or class which is for the time being specified in an order made under section 58(1) of the Medicines Act 1968 (medicinal products on prescription only); or
(b) in the case of an appliance, does not contain such a product.

45. Interpretation of paragraphs 38, 39 and 41 to 44

For the purposes of paragraphs 38, 39 and 41 to 44 in their application to a contractor whose contract includes the provision of contraceptive services, drugs includes contraceptive substances and appliances includes contraceptive appliances.

46. Excessive prescribing

(1) The contractor shall not prescribe drugs, medicines or appliances whose cost or quantity, in relation to any patient, is, by reason of the character of the drug, medicine or appliance in question in excess of that which was reasonably necessary for the proper treatment of that patient.

(2) In considering whether a contractor has breached its obligations under sub-paragraph (1) the PCT shall seek the views of the Local Medical Committee (if any) for its area.

Standard Contract

268. The Contractor shall comply with any directions given by *the Secretary of State* for the purposes of section 28U of *the Act* as to the drugs, medicines or other substances which may or may not be ordered for patients in the provision of medical services under the Contract.[60]

Prescribing

269. The Contractor shall ensure that any *prescription form* or *repeatable prescription* for drugs, medicines or appliances issued by a *prescriber* complies as appropriate with the requirements in clauses 270 to 276 and clauses 284 to 301.

270. Subject to clauses 289 to 297, a *prescriber* shall order any drugs, medicines or appliances which are needed for the treatment of any patient who is receiving treatment under the contract by issuing to that patient a *prescription form* or a *repeatable prescription* and such a *prescription form* or *repeatable prescription* shall not be used in any other circumstances.

271. A *prescriber* may order drugs, medicines or appliances on a *repeatable prescription* only where the drugs, medicines or appliances are to be provided more than once.

272. In issuing any *prescription form* or *repeatable prescription* the *prescriber* shall sign the *prescription form* or *repeatable prescription* in ink with his initials and surname, or forenames, and surname in his own handwriting

---

60   This clause is required by section 28U(1) of *the Act*.

and not by means of a stamp, and shall so sign only after particulars of the order have been inserted in the *prescription form* or *repeatable prescription*, and –

272.1 the *prescription form* or *repeatable prescription* shall not refer to any previous *prescription form* or *repeatable prescription*; and

272.2 a separate *prescription form* shall be used for each patient, except where a bulk prescription is issued for a school or institution under clauses 299 to 302.

273.   Where a *prescriber* orders the drug buprenorphine or a drug specified in Schedule 2 to the Misuse of Drugs Regulations 2001 (controlled drugs to which regulations 14, 15, 16, 18, 19, 20, 21, 23, 26 and 27 of those Regulations apply) for supply by instalments for treating addiction to any drug specified in that Schedule, he shall –

273.1 use only the *prescription form* provided specially for the purposes of supply by instalments;

273.2 specify the number of instalments to be dispensed and the interval between each instalment; and

273.3 order only such quantity of the drug as will provide treatment for a period not exceeding 14 days.

274.   The *prescription form* provided specially for the purpose of supply by instalments shall not be used for any purpose other than ordering drugs in accordance with clause 273.

275.   In a case of urgency a *prescriber* may request a *chemist* to dispense a drug or medicine before a *prescription form* or *repeatable prescription* is issued, but only if:

275.1 that drug or medicine is not a *Scheduled drug*;

275.2 that drug is not a controlled drug within the meaning of the Misuse of Drugs Act 1971, other than a drug which is for the time being specified in Schedules 4 or 5 to the Misuse of Drugs Regulations 2001; and

275.3 he undertakes to furnish the *chemist*, within 72 hours, with a *prescription form* or *repeatable prescription* completed in accordance with clause 272.

276.   In a case of urgency a *prescriber* may request a *chemist* to dispense an appliance before a *prescription form* or *repeatable prescription* is issued, but only if –

276.1 that appliance does not contain a *Scheduled drug* or a controlled drug within the meaning of the Misuse of Drugs Act 1971, other than a drug which is for the time being specified in Schedule 5 to the Misuse of Drugs Regulations 2001;

276.2 in the case of a *restricted availability appliance*, the patient is a person, or it is for a purpose, specified in the *Drug Tariff*; and

276.3 he undertakes to furnish the *chemist*, within 72 hours, with a *prescription form* or *repeatable prescription* completed in accordance with clause 272.

Repeatable prescribing services

277. The Contractor may only provide *repeatable prescribing services* to any person on its list of patients if it –
277.1 satisfies the conditions in clause 278; and
277.2 has notified the PCT of its intention to provide repeatable prescribing in accordance with clauses 279 and 280.

278. The conditions referred to in clause 277.1 are –
278.1 the PCT is specified in Schedule 9 to *the Regulations*; and
278.2 the Contractor has access to computer systems and software which enable it to issue *repeatable prescriptions* and *batch issues*; and
278.3 the *practice premises* at which the *repeatable prescribing services* are to be provided are located in an area of the PCT in which there is also located the premises of at least one *chemist* who has undertaken to provide, or has entered into an arrangement to provide, *repeat dispensing services*.

279. The notification referred to in clause 277.2 is a notification, in writing, by the Contractor to the PCT that it –
279.1 wishes to provide *repeatable prescribing services*; and
279.2 intends to begin to provide those services from a specified date; and
279.3 satisfies the conditions in clause 278.

280. The date specified by the Contractor pursuant to clause 279.2 must be at least 10 days after the date on which the notification specified in clause 277.2 is given.

281. Nothing in clauses 277 to 288 requires the Contractor or *prescriber* to provide *repeatable prescribing services* to any person.

282. A *prescriber* may only provide *repeatable prescribing services* to a person on a particular occasion if –
282.1 that person has agreed to receive such services on that occasion; and
282.2 the *prescriber* considers that it is clinically appropriate to provide such services to that person on that occasion.

283. The Contractor may not provide *repeatable prescribing services* to any patient of its to whom –
283.1 it is authorised or required by the PCT to provide *dispensing services* under clauses 305 to 314 and clauses 321 to 325; or
283.2 any of the persons specified in clause 284 is authorised or required by the PCT under regulation 20 of the *Pharmaceutical Regulations* to provide pharmaceutical services.

284. The persons referred to in clause 283 are –
    284.1 if the Contract is with an individual medical practitioner, that medical practitioner;
    284.2 if the Contract is with a partnership, any medical practitioner who is a partner;
    284.3 if the Contract is with a company, any medical practitioner who is a legal and beneficial shareholder in that company; or
    284.4 any medical practitioner employed by the Contractor.

285. A *prescriber* who issues a *repeatable prescription* must at the same time issue the appropriate number of *batch issues*.

286. A *prescriber* who has provided *repeatable prescribing services* to a person must, as soon as is practicable, notify that person, and make reasonable efforts to contact the *chemist* providing *repeat dispensing services* to that person, if –
    286.1 he makes any change to the type, quantity, strength or dosage of drugs, medicines or appliances ordered on that person's *repeatable prescription*; or
    286.2 he considers that it is no longer appropriate or safe for that person to receive the drugs, medicines or appliances ordered on his *repeatable prescription*, or no longer appropriate or safe for him to continue to receive *repeatable prescribing services*.

287. If a *prescriber* provides *repeatable prescribing services* to a person in respect of whom he has previously issued a *repeatable prescription* which has not yet expired (for example, because that person wishes to obtain the drugs, medicines or appliances from a different *chemist*), the prescriber must make reasonable efforts to notify the *chemist* which has in its possession the *repeatable prescription* which is no longer required.

288. If a *prescriber* has issued a *repeatable prescription* in respect of a person, and (before the expiry of that *repeatable prescription*) that person is removed from the list of patients of the Contractor on whose behalf the prescription was issued, that *prescriber* must –
    288.1 notify that person; and
    288.2 make reasonable efforts to notify the *chemist* who has been providing *repeat dispensing services* to that person,
    that the *repeatable prescription* should no longer be used to obtain or provide *repeat dispensing services*.

Restrictions on prescribing by medical practitioners

289. In the course of treating a patient to whom he is providing treatment under the Contract, a medical practitioner shall not order on a *prescription form* or *repeatable prescription* a drug, medicine or other

substance specified in any directions given by *the Secretary of State* under section 28U of *the Act* as being drugs, medicines or other substances which may not be ordered for patients in the provision of medical services under the Contract but may, subject to clause 482, prescribe such a drug, medicine or other substance for that patient in the course of that treatment under a private arrangement.

290. In the course of treating a patient to whom he is providing treatment under the Contract, a medical practitioner shall not order on a *prescription form* or *repeatable prescription* a drug, medicines or other substance specified in any directions given by *the Secretary of State* under section 28U of *the Act* as being a drug, medicine or other substance which can only be ordered for specified patients and specified purposes unless –

290.1 that patient is a person of the specified description;

290.2 that drug, medicine or other substance is prescribed for that patient only for the specified purpose; and

290.3 the practitioner endorses the form with the reference "SLS",

but may, subject to clause 482, prescribe such a drug, medicine or other substance for that patient in the course of that treatment under a private arrangement.

291. In the course of treating a patient to whom he is providing treatment under the Contract, a medical practitioner shall not order on a *prescription form* or *repeatable prescription* a *restricted availability appliance* unless –

291.1 the patient is a person, or it is for a purpose, specified in the *Drug Tariff*; and

291.2 the practitioner endorses the face of the form with the reference "SLS",

but may, subject to clause 482, prescribe such an appliance for that patient in the course of that treatment under a private arrangement.

292. In the course of treating a patient to whom he is providing treatment under the Contract, a medical practitioner shall not order on a *repeatable prescription* a controlled drug within the meaning of the Misuse of Drugs Act 1971, other than a drug which is for the time being specified in Schedule 4 or 5 to the Misuse of Drugs Regulations 2001, but may, subject to clause 482, prescribe such a drug for that patient in the course of that treatment under a private arrangement.

Restrictions on prescribing by *supplementary prescribers*

293. Where the Contractor employs or engages a *supplementary prescriber* and that person's functions include prescribing, the Contractor shall have arrangements in place to secure that a *supplementary prescriber* will –

293.1 give a prescription for a *prescription only medicine*;

293.2 administer a *prescription only medicine* for parenteral administration; or

293.3 give directions for the administration of a *prescription only medicine* for parenteral administration,

as a *supplementary prescriber* only under the conditions set out in clause 294.

294. The conditions referred to in clause 293 are that –

294.1 the person satisfies the applicable conditions set out in article 3B(3) of *the POM Order* (prescribing and administration by *supplementary prescribers*), unless those conditions do not apply by virtue of any of the exemptions set out in the subsequent provisions of that Order;

294.2 the medicine is not a controlled drug within the meaning of the Misuse of Drugs Act 1971;

294.3 the drug, medicine or other substance is not specified in any directions given by *the Secretary of State* under section 28U of *the Act* as being a drug, medicine or other substance which may not be ordered for patients in the provision of medical services under the Contract;

294.4 the drug, medicine or other substance is not specified in any directions given by *the Secretary of State* under section 28U of *the Act* as being a drug, medicine or other substance which can only be ordered for specified patients and specified purposes unless –

294.4.1 the patient is a person of the specified description,

294.4.2 the medicine is prescribed for that patient only for the specified purposes, and

294.4.3 if the *supplementary prescriber* is giving a prescription, he endorses the face of the form with the reference "SLS".

295. Where the functions of a *supplementary prescriber* include prescribing, the Contractor shall have arrangements in place to secure that that person will only give a prescription for –

295.1 an appliance; or

295.2 a medicine which is not a *prescription only medicine*,

as a *supplementary prescriber* under the conditions set out in clause 296.

296. The conditions referred to in clause 295 are that –

296.1 the *supplementary prescriber* acts in accordance with a clinical management plan which is in effect at the time he acts and which contains the following particulars –

296.1.1 the name of the patient to whom the plan relates,

296.1.2 the illness or conditions which may be treated by the *supplementary prescriber*,

296.1.3 the date on which the plan is to take effect, and when it is to be reviewed by the medical practitioner or dentist who is a party to the plan,

296.1.4 reference to the class or description of medicines or types of appliances which may be prescribed or administered under the plan,

296.1.5 any restrictions or limitations as to the strength or dose of any medicine which may be prescribed or administered under the plan, and any period of administration or use of any medicine or appliance which may be prescribed or administered under the plan,

296.1.6 relevant warnings about known sensitivities of the patient to, or known difficulties of the patient with, particular medicines or appliances,

296.1.7 the arrangements for notification of –

296.1.7.1 suspected or known adverse reactions to any medicine which may be prescribed or administered under the plan, and suspected or known adverse reactions to any other medicine taken at the same time as any medicine prescribed or administered under the plan,

296.1.7.2 incidents occurring with the appliance which might lead, might have led or has led to the death or serious deterioration of state of health of the patient, and

296.1.7.3 the circumstances in which the *supplementary prescriber* should refer to, or seek the advice of, the medical practitioner or dentist who is a party to the plan;

296.2 he has access to the health records of the patient to whom the plan relates which are used by any medical practitioner or dentist who is a party to the plan;

296.3 if it is a prescription for a medicine, the medicine is not a controlled drug within the meaning of the Misuse of Drugs Act 1971;

296.4 if it is a prescription for a drug, medicine or other substance, that drug, medicine or other substance is not specified in any directions given by *the Secretary of State* under section 28U of *the Act* as being a drug, medicine or other substance which may not be ordered for patients in the provision of medical services under the Contract;

296.5 if it is a prescription for a drug, medicine or other substance, that drug, medicine or other substance is not specified in any directions given by *the Secretary of State* under section 28U of *the Act* as being a drug, medicine or other substance which can only be ordered for specified patients and specified purposes unless –

296.5.1 the patient is a person of the specified description,

296.5.2 the medicine is prescribed for that patient only for the specified purposes, and

296.5.3 when giving the prescription, he endorses the face of the form with the reference "SLS";

296.6 if it is a prescription for a medicine –

296.6.1 the medicine is the subject of a product licence, a marketing authorisation or a homeopathic certificate of registration granted by the licensing authority or the European Commission, or

296.6.2 subject to clause 298, the use of the medicine is for the purposes of a clinical trial, and either that trial is the subject of a clinical trial certificate issued in accordance with the Medicines Act 1968, or a clinical trial certificate is not needed in respect of that trial by virtue of any exemption conferred by or under that Act,

296.7 if it is a prescription for an appliance, the appliance is listed in Part IX of the *Drug Tariff*; and

296.8 if it is a prescription for a *restricted availability appliance* –

296.8.1 the patient is a person of a description mentioned in the entry in Part IX of the *Drug Tariff* in respect of that appliance,

296.8.2 the appliance is prescribed only for the purposes specified in respect of that person in that entry, and

296.8.3 when giving the prescription, he endorses the face of the form with the reference "SLS".

297. In clause 221.1, "clinical management plan" means a written plan (which may be amended from time to time) relating to the treatment of an individual patient agreed by –

297.1 the patient to whom the plan relates;

297.2 the medical practitioner or dentist who is a party to the plan; and

297.3 any *supplementary prescriber* who is to prescribe, give directions for administration or administer under the plan.

298. In relation to any time from the coming into force of any regulations made by *the Secretary of State* under section 2(2) of the European Communities Act 1972 to implement Directive 2001/83/EC on the Community code relating to medicinal products for human use, clause 296.6.2 shall be read as if it referred to a clinical trial which has been authorised, or is treated as having been authorised by the *licensing authority* for the purposes of those Regulations.

Bulk prescribing

299.   Where the Contractor is responsible under the Contract for the treatment of 10 or more persons in a school or other institution in which at least 20 persons normally reside, and a *prescriber* orders, for any two or more of those persons for whose treatment the Contractor is responsible, drugs, medicines or appliances to which this clause to clause 302 apply, the *prescriber* may use a single *prescription form* for the purpose.

300.   Where a *prescriber* uses a single *prescription form* for the purpose mentioned in clause 299, he shall (instead of entering on the form the names of the persons for whom the drugs, medicines or appliances are ordered) enter on the form –
300.1 the name of the school or institution in which those persons reside; and
300.2 the number of persons residing there for whose treatment the Contractor is responsible.

301.   Clauses 299 and 300 apply to any drug, medicine or appliance which can be supplied as part of pharmaceutical services or local pharmaceutical services and which –
301.1 in the case of a drug or medicine, is not a product of a description or class which is for the time being specified in an order made under section 58(1) of the Medicines Act 1968; or
301.2 in the case of an appliance, does not contain such a product.

302.   For the purposes of clauses 299 to 301, if the Contractor has contracted to provide *contraceptive services*, drugs include contraceptive substances and appliances include contraceptive appliances.

Excessive prescribing

303.   The Contractor shall not prescribe drugs, medicines or appliances whose cost or quantity, in relation to any patient, is, by reason of the character of the drug, medicine or appliance in question, in excess of that which was reasonably necessary for the proper treatment of that *patient*. In considering whether the Contractor has breached its obligations under this clause, the PCT shall seek the views of the *Local Medical Committee* (if any) for its area.

Provision of drugs, medicines and appliances for immediate treatment or personal administration

339.   The Contractor –
339.1 shall provide to a patient any drug, medicine or appliance, not being a *Scheduled drug*, where such provision is needed for the

immediate treatment of that patient before a provision can otherwise be obtained; and

339.2 may provide to a patient any drug, medicine or appliance, not being a *Scheduled drug*, which he personally administers or applies to that patient,

Private fees and charges

Regulations

Terms

24. (1) The contract must contain terms relating to fees and charges which have the same effect as those set out in paragraphs (2) to (4).

(2) The contractor shall not, either itself or through any other person, demand or accept from any patient of its a fee or other remuneration, for its own or another's benefit, for –
  (a) the provision of any treatment whether under the contract or otherwise; or
  (b) any prescription or repeatable prescription for any drug, medicine or appliance,
except in the circumstances set out in Schedule 5.

(3) Where a person applies to a contractor for the provision of essential services and claims to be on that contractor's list of patients, but fails to produce his medical card on request and the contractor has reasonable doubts about that person's claim, the contractor shall give any necessary treatment and shall be entitled to demand and accept a reasonable fee in accordance with paragraph 1(e) of Schedule 5[d] subject to the provision for repayment contained in paragraph (4).

(4) Where a person from whom a contractor received a fee under paragraph 1(e) of Schedule 5[d] applies to the PCT for a refund within 14 days of payment of the fee (or such longer period not exceeding a month as the PCT may allow if it is satisfied that the failure to apply within 14 days was reasonable) and the PCT is satisfied that the person was on the contractor's list of patients when the treatment was given, the PCT may recover the amount of the fee from the contractor, by deduction from its remuneration or otherwise, and shall pay that amount to the person who paid the fee.

Demand or accept a fee or other remuneration

1. The contractor may demand or accept a fee or other remuneration –
   (a) from any statutory body for services rendered for the purposes of that body's statutory functions;
   (b) from any body, employer or school for a routine medical examination of persons for whose welfare the body, employer or school is responsible, or an examination of such persons for the purpose of advising the body, employer or school of any administrative action they might take;
   (c) for treatment which is not primary medical services or otherwise required to be provided under the contract and which is given –
      (i) pursuant to the provisions of section 65 of the Act (accommodation and services for private patients), or
      (ii) in a registered nursing home which is not providing services under that Act,
      if, in either case, the person administering the treatment is serving on the staff of a hospital providing services under the Act as a specialist providing treatment of the kind the patient requires and if, within 7 days of giving the treatment, the contractor or the person providing the treatment supplies the PCT, on a form provided by it for the purpose, with such information about the treatment as it may require;
   (d) under section 158 of the Road Traffic Act 1988 (payment for emergency treatment of traffic casualties);
   (e) when it treats a patient under regulation 24(3), in which case it shall be entitled to demand and accept a reasonable fee (recoverable in certain circumstances under regulation 24(4)) for any treatment given, if it gives the patient a receipt;
   (f) for attending and examining (but not otherwise treating) a patient –
      (i) at his request at a police station in connection with possible criminal proceedings against him,
      (ii) at the request of a commercial, educational or not-for-profit organisation for the purpose of creating a medical report or certificate,
      (iii) for the purpose of creating a medical report required in connection with an actual or potential claim for compensation by the patient;
   (g) for treatment consisting of an immunisation for which no remuneration is payable by the PCT and which is requested in connection with travel abroad;
   (h) for prescribing or providing drugs, medicines or appliances (including a collection of such drugs, medicines or appliances in the form of a travel kit) which a patient requires to have in his possession

solely in anticipation of the onset of an ailment or occurrence of an injury while he is outside the United Kingdom but for which he is not requiring treatment when the medicine is prescribed;

(i) for a medical examination –

    (i) to enable a decision to be made whether or not it is inadvisable on medical grounds for a person to wear a seat belt, or

    (ii) for the purpose of creating a report –

        (aa) relating to a road traffic accident or criminal assault, or

        (bb) that offers an opinion as to whether a patient is fit to travel;

(j) for testing the sight of a person to whom none of paragraphs (a), (b) or (c) of section 38(1) of the Act (arrangements for general ophthalmic services) applies (including by reason of regulations under section 38(6) of that Act);

(k) where it is a contractor which is authorised or required by a PCT under regulation 20 of the Pharmaceutical Regulations or paragraphs 47 or 49 of Schedule 6 to provide drugs, medicines or appliances to a patient and provides for that patient, otherwise than by way of pharmaceutical services or dispensing services, any Scheduled drug;

(l) for prescribing or providing drugs or medicines for malaria chemoprophylaxis.

Standard Contract

482. The Contractor shall not, either itself or through any other person, demand or accept from any patient of its a fee or other remuneration for its own or another's benefit –

    482.1 for the provision of any treatment whether under the Contract or otherwise, or

    482.2 for any prescription or repeat prescription for any drug, medicine or appliance,

except in the circumstances set out in clause 483.

483. The Contractor may demand or accept a fee or other remuneration –

    483.1 from any statutory body for services rendered for the purposes of that body's statutory functions;

    483.2 from any body, employer or school for a routine medical examination of persons for whose welfare the body, employer or school is responsible, or an examination of such persons for the purpose of advising the body, employer or school of any administrative action they might take;

    483.3 for treatment which is not primary medical services or otherwise required to be provided under the Contract and which is given –

        483.3.1 pursuant to the provisions of section 65 of *the Act*, or

483.3.2 in a registered nursing home which is not providing services under that Act,

if, in either case, the person administering the treatment is serving on the staff of a hospital providing services under *the Act* as a specialist providing treatment of the kind the patient requires and if, within 7 days of giving the treatment, the Contractor or the person providing the treatment supplies the PCT, on a form provided by it for the purpose, with such information about the treatment as it may require;

483.4 under section 158 of the Road Traffic Act 1988;

483.5 when it treats a patient under clause 484, in which case it shall be entitled to demand and accept a reasonable fee from the patient (recoverable in certain circumstances under clause 485) for any treatment given, if it gives the patient a receipt;

483.6 for attending and examining (but not otherwise treating) a patient-

483.6.1 at his request at a police station in connection with possible criminal proceedings against him,

483.6.2 at the request of a commercial, educational or not-for-profit organisation for the purpose of creating a medical report or certificate, or

483.6.3 for the purpose of creating a medical report required in connection with an actual or potential claim for compensation by the patient;

483.7 for treatment consisting of an immunisation for which no remuneration is payable by the PCT and which is requested in connection with travel abroad;

483.8 for prescribing or providing drugs, medicines or appliances (including a collection of such drugs, medicines or appliances in the form of a travel kit) which a patient requires to have in his possession solely in anticipation of the onset of an ailment or occurrence of an injury while he is outside the United Kingdom but for which he is not requiring treatment when the medicine is prescribed;

483.9 for a medical examination to enable a decision to be made whether or not it is inadvisable on medical grounds for a person to wear a seat belt, or for the purpose of creating a report relating to a road traffic accident or criminal assault, or that offers an opinion as to whether a patient is fit to travel;

483.10 for testing the sight of a person to whom none of paragraphs (a), (b) or (c) of section 38(1) of *the Act* applies (including by reason of regulations under section 38(6) of that Act);

483.11 where the Contractor is authorised or required by a PCT under regulation 20 of the *Pharmaceutical Regulations* or clauses 305 to

       314 and clauses 321 to 225to provide drugs, medicines or
       appliances to a patient and provides for that patient, otherwise
       than by way of pharmaceutical services or dispensing services,
       any Scheduled drug;

    483.12 for prescribing or providing drugs for malaria chemoprophylaxis.

484.   Where a person applies to the Contractor for the provision of *essential
services* and claims to be on the Contractor's list of patients, but fails to
produce his *medical card* on request and the Contractor has reasonable
doubts about that person's claim, the Contractor shall give any necessary
treatment and shall be entitled to demand and accept a reasonable fee in
accordance with clause 483.5, subject to the provision for repayment
contained in clause 4850.

485.   Where a person from whom the Contractor received a fee under
clause 483.5 applies to the PCT for a refund within 14 days of payment
of the fee (or such longer period not exceeding a month as the PCT
may allow if it is satisfied that the failure to apply within 14 days
was reasonable) and the PCT is satisfied that the person was on the
Contractor's list of patients when the treatment was given, the PCT
may recover the amount of the fee from the Contractor, by deduction
from its remuneration or otherwise, and shall pay that amount to the
person who paid the fee.

486.   Part 18 shall survive the expiry or termination of the Contract to the
extent that it prohibits the Contractor from, either itself or through any
other person, demanding or accepting from any patient of it's a fee or
other remuneration for its own or another's benefit –

    486.1 for the provision of any treatment, whether under the Contract or
          otherwise, that was provided during the existence of the Contract;
          or

    486.2 for any prescription or repeat prescription for any drug, medicine
          or appliance, that was provided during the existence of the
          Contract.[61]

Guidance

(iv) Charging for services

2.24   Primary medical services for NHS patients remain free at the point of
delivery. The existing prohibition on charging NHS patients, except for a

---

61   This clause is not mandatory but it is recommended.

very limited range of circumstances, remains under the new GMS contract. The GMS contract regulations outline and clarify those circumstances. Currently, travel vaccines are provided free for infectious diseases where there is a risk that, on return, the traveller could pass the disease to members of the home population, namely, vaccination against typhoid, poliomyelitis and hepatitis A.

2.25 The prohibitions, with certain stated exceptions, not only apply to those services a contractor has contracted to provide under GMS but also to any other service it could contract to provide under the NHS. For example a GMS contractor opting out of vaccinations and immunisations may not charge any registered patients for that immunisation if they were eligible to receive the immunisation on the NHS. The application of rules on charging to APMS contractors will be covered in the February 2004 guidance.

Provision of information

Regulations

77. Provision of information

(1) Subject to sub-paragraph (2), the contractor shall, at the request of the PCT, produce to the PCT or to a person authorised in writing by the PCT or allow it, or a person authorised in writing by it, to access –
(a) any information which is reasonably required by the PCT for the purposes of or in connection with the contract; and
(b) any other information which is reasonably required in connection with the PCT's functions.

(2) The contractor shall not be required to comply with any request made in accordance with sub-paragraph (1) unless it has been made by the PCT in accordance with directions relating to the provision of information by contractors given to it by the Secretary of State under section 17 of the Act (Secretary of State's directions: exercise of functions).

78. Requests for information from Patients' Forums

(1) Subject to sub-paragraph (2), where the contractor receives a written request from the Patients' Forum established for the PCT to produce any information which appears to the Forum to be necessary for the effective carrying out of its functions it shall comply with that request promptly

and in any event no later than the twentieth working day following the date the request was made.

(2) The contractor shall not be required to produce information under sub-paragraph (1) which –
(a) is confidential and relates to a living individual, unless at least one of the conditions specified in sub-paragraph (3) applies; or
(b) is prohibited from disclosure by or under any enactment or any ruling of a court of competent jurisdiction or is protected by the common law, unless sub-paragraph (4) applies.

(3) The conditions referred to in sub-paragraph (2)(a) are –
(a) the information can be disclosed in a form from which the identity of the individual cannot be ascertained; or
(b) the individual consents to the information being disclosed.

(4) This paragraph applies where –
(a) the prohibition of the disclosure of information arises because the information is capable of identifying an individual; and
(b) the information can be disclosed in a form from which the identity of the individual cannot be ascertained.

(5) In a case where the information falls within –
(a) sub-paragraph (2)(a) and the condition in sub-paragraph (3)(a) applies; or
(b) sub-paragraph (2)(b) and sub-paragraph (4) applies,
a Patients' Forum may require the contractor to disclose the information in a form from which the identity of the individual concerned cannot be ascertained.

79. Inquiries about prescriptions and referrals

(1) The contractor shall, subject to sub-paragraphs (2) and (3), sufficiently answer any inquiries whether oral or in writing from the PCT concerning –
(a) any prescription form or repeatable prescription issued by a prescriber;
(b) the considerations by reference to which prescribers issue such forms;
(c) the referral by or on behalf of the contractor of any patient to any other services provided under the Act; or
(d) the considerations by which the contractor makes such referrals or provides for them to be made on its behalf.

(2) An inquiry referred to in sub-paragraph (1) may only be made for the purpose either of obtaining information to assist the PCT to discharge its

functions or of assisting the contractor in the discharge of its obligations under the contract.

(3) The contractor shall not be obliged to answer any inquiry referred to in sub-paragraph (1) unless it is made –
(a) in the case of sub-paragraph (1)(a) or (b), by an appropriately qualified health care professional; or
(b) in the case of sub-paragraph (1)(c) or (d), by an appropriately qualified medical practitioner,
appointed in either case by the PCT to assist it in the exercise of its functions under this paragraph and that person produces, on request, written evidence that he is authorised by the PCT to make such an inquiry on its behalf.

80. Reports to a medical officer

(1) The contractor shall, if it is satisfied that the patient consents –
(a) supply in writing to a medical officer within such reasonable period as that officer, or an officer of the Department for Work and Pensions on his behalf and at his direction, may specify, such clinical information as the medical officer considers relevant about a patient to whom the contractor or a person acting on the contractor's behalf has issued or has refused to issue a medical certificate; and
(b) answer any inquiries by a medical officer, or by an officer of the Department for Work and Pensions on his behalf and at his direction, about a prescription form or medical certificate issued by the contractor or on its behalf or about any statement which the contractor or a person acting on the contractor's behalf has made in a report.

(2) For the purpose of satisfying himself that the patient has consented as required by paragraph (1), the contractor may (unless it has reason to believe the patient does not consent) rely on an assurance in writing from the medical officer, or any officer of the Department for Work and Pensions, that he holds the patient's written consent.

Annual return and review

81. (1) The contractor shall submit an annual return relating to the contract to the PCT which shall require the same categories of information from all persons who hold contracts with that Trust.
(2) Following receipt of the return referred to in sub-paragraph (1), the PCT shall arrange with the contractor an annual review of its performance in relation to the contract.

(3) Either the contractor or the PCT may, if it wishes to do so, invite the Local Medical Committee for the area of the PCT to participate in the annual review.

(4) The PCT shall prepare a draft record of the review referred to in sub-paragraph (2) for comment by the contractor and, having regard to such comments, shall produce a final written record of the review.

(5) A copy of the final record referred to in sub-paragraph (4) shall be sent to the contractor.

Standard Contract

Provision of information

438. Subject to clause 439, the Contractor shall, at the request of the PCT, produce to the PCT or to a person authorised in writing by the PCT or allow it, or a person authorised in writing by it, to access, on request –
438.1 any information which is reasonably required by the PCT for the purposes of or in connection with the Contract; and
438.2 any other information which is reasonably required in connection with the PCT's functions.

439. The Contractor shall not be required to comply with any request made in accordance with clause 438 unless it has been made by the PCT in accordance with directions relating to the provision of information by contractors given to the PCT under section 17 of *the Act*.

Requests for information from PCT Patients' Forums

440. Subject to clause 440, if the Contractor receives a written request from the PCT Patients' Forum established for the PCT to produce any information which appears to the Forum to be necessary for the effective carrying out of its functions, it shall comply with that request promptly and in any event no later than the twentieth working day following the date the request was made.

441. The Contractor shall not be required to produce information under clause 440 which –
441.1 is confidential and relates to a living individual, unless at least one of the conditions specified in clause 442 applies; or
441.2 is prohibited by disclosure by or under any enactment or any ruling of a court of competent jurisdiction or is protected by the common law, unless clause 443 applies.

442. The conditions referred to in clause 441.1 are –

442.1 the information can be disclosed in a form from which the identity of the individual cannot be ascertained taking account of other information which is in the possession of, or likely to come into the possession of, the person to whom the information is to be disclosed; or

442.2 the individual consents to the information being disclosed.

443. This clause and clause 444 apply where –
    443.1 the prohibition of the disclosure of the information arises because the information is capable of identifying an individual; and
    443.2 the information is or can be disclosed in a form from which the identity of the individual cannot be ascertained.

444. In a case where the information falls within –
    444.1 clause 444.1 and the condition in clause 442.1 applies; or
    444.2 clause 441.2 and clause 443 applies,
    the PCT Patients' Forum may require the Contractor to put the information in a form from which the identity of the individual concerned cannot be ascertained.

Inquiries about prescriptions and referrals

445. The Contractor shall, subject to clauses 446 and 447, sufficiently answer any inquiries whether oral or in writing from the PCT concerning –
    445.1 any *prescription form* or *repeatable prescription* issued by a *prescriber*;
    445.2 the considerations by reference to which *prescribers* issue such forms;
    445.3 the referral by or on behalf of the Contractor of any patient to any other services provided under *the Act*; or
    445.4 the considerations by which the Contractor makes such referrals or provides for them to be made on its behalf.

446. An inquiry referred to in clause 445 may only be made for the purpose either of obtaining information to assist the PCT to discharge its functions or of assisting the Contractor in the discharge of its obligations under the Contract.

447. The Contractor shall not be obliged to answer any inquiry referred to in clause 445 unless it is made –
    447.1 in the case of clause 445.1 or 445.2 by an appropriately qualified *health care professional*; or
    447.2 in the case of clause 445.3 or 445.4, by an appropriately qualified medical practitioner,
    appointed in either case by the PCT to assist it in the exercise of its functions under clause 445 and 446 who produces, on request, written

evidence that that person is authorised by the PCT to make such an inquiry on its behalf.

Reports to a *medical officer*

448. The Contractor shall, if it is satisfied that the patient consents –

448.1 supply in writing to a *medical officer* within such reasonable period as that officer, or an officer of the Department for Work and Pensions on his behalf and at his direction, may specify, such clinical information as the medical officer considers relevant about a patient to whom the Contractor or a person acting on the Contractor's behalf has issued or has refused to issue a medical certificate; and

448.2 answer any inquiries by a *medical officer*, or by an officer of the Department for Work and Pensions on his behalf and at his direction, about a *prescription form* or medical certificate issued by the Contractor or on its behalf or about any statement which the Contractor or a person acting on the Contractor's behalf has made in a report.

449. For the purpose of satisfying itself that the patient has consented as required by clause 448, the Contractor may (unless it has reason to believe the patient does not consent) rely on an assurance in writing from the medical officer, or any officer of the Department for Work and Pensions, that he holds the patient's written consent.

Annual return and review

450. The Contractor shall submit an annual return relating to the Contract to the PCT which shall require the same categories of information from all persons who hold contracts with the PCT.

451. Following receipt of the return referred to in clause 450, the PCT shall arrange with the Contractor an annual review of its performance in relation to the Contract.

452. Either the Contractor or the PCT may, if it wishes to do so, invite the *Local Medical Committee* for the area of the PCT to participate in the annual review.

453. The PCT shall prepare a draft record of the review referred to in clause 450 for comment by the Contractor and, having regard to such comments, shall produce a final written record of the review. A copy of the final record shall be sent to the Contractor.

Quality and outcomes – annual review

Guidance

3.39 *Investing in General Practice* makes clear that Primary Care Trusts (PCTs) should visit their contractors annually to review each contractor's achievement against the quality and outcomes framework (QOF) indicators. The frequency and intensity of visits may decrease in future years if the PCT is confident of the contractor's performance against the QOF indicators, subject to the mandatory requirements for financial audit. Equally, the frequency of visits may increase where there is serious concern about, for example, data accuracy or suspected fraud.

3.40 Experience from existing local quality incentive schemes shows that these visits will involve significant preparation and organisation for PCTs. It is therefore important that PCTs and contractors plan this process thoroughly and well in advance. PCTs will want to:
   (i) nominate a QOF lead who is responsible for planning of visits, and ensuring consistency of the visiting approach and reporting of visits
   (ii) produce a schedule of planned contractor visits by August of each year, for visits to take place between 1 October and 31 January. This timetable is necessary to allow sufficient time before achievement payments are made for remedial plans, if need be, to be drawn up, agreed, implemented and reviewed. A delay by the PCT in visiting the contractor should not delay payment of achievement at the end of the year
   (iii) bear in mind that their visits will require considerable workforce capacity involving trained assessors. National training will be provided for a number of assessors per PCT in summer 2004

3.41 The exact process to be followed during the QOF annual review visit is important, and we have therefore commissioned the School of Health and Related Research (ScHARR) at the University of Sheffield to develop proposals. In the light of these the Department of Health and the NHS Confederation will develop guidance with GPC. This will be published by April 2004.

3.42 The following principles will inform the annual review process:
   (i) the process will build on best practice of existing review and inspection mechanisms
   (ii) PCTs will have the flexibility to timetable review visits as they wish, within the October to January window. Either contractors or PCTs

are able to involve the Local Medical Committee (LMC) if they wish but where a mutually convenient date cannot be found, the visit should not be delayed. The scheduling of visits should bear in mind, wherever possible, any other visits to the contractor, e.g. by Patients' Forums, to minimise burdens on contractors

(iii) contractors will need to submit the written evidence set out in *Supplementary Documents* a month in advance of the visit date. Contractors must report the number of exceptions (initially, the aggregate number, prior to the development of Read Codes for each exception) used for each indicator, and are advised to note the requirement of the statement of financial entitlement (SFE) that all information submitted must be accurate. There will be some form of verification of exception reporting during every QOF visit

(iv) each review visit must cover all of the QOF domains for which the practice plans to submit an achievement claim. Not all indicators will be assessed in equal detail on every visit. The process developed by ScHARR will include a mechanism to ensure balance between covering the breadth of the QOF and inspecting some indicators in detail

(v) practices which have been and remain accredited for Version 7 of the Royal College of General Practitioners' Quality Practice Award will not need to submit evidence for the quality review in relation to the organisational indicators. PCTs should ensure that the review of organisational indicators for accredited providers is very light touch, focusing on a few areas only (e.g. significant event review). Further organisational quality schemes may be accredited for use with the QOF, and details of these will be sent to contractors and PCTs. Each accredited scheme will have listed the QOF organisational domain indicators it can be used against. All schemes will need to involve a visit to the contractor for contractor accreditation to take place

(vi) assessors will have access to patient records in order to check contractor achievement against the QOF. However, this will be subject to a code of practice, which is currently being developed

(vii) assessors will be selected on the basis of meeting certain competencies and will be appropriately trained. One of the assessors will normally be a lay person or patient representative (who is not a patient from that practice) and normally at least one will be a doctor. There may be occasional circumstances where it may not be appropriate for the clinician to be medically qualified, and in these circumstances an assessor could be another appropriately qualified healthcare professional, where both the PCT and contractor agree. Assessors need not be PCT employees; the key requirements are that they have been appropriately trained and meet the necessary competencies. The competencies, roles and responsibilities of the assessors will be defined in the April 2004 guidance. National training will be offered for a certain number of assessors per PCT. It will then be for PCTs or other bodies to commission further training as necessary, within national guidelines

(viii) following the visit, the assessment team will provide the contractor with their assessment of the contractor's likely achievement against the QOF, and a written report of the visit. This report will be sent in draft to the contractor

(ix) the contractor's aspiration for the following year will also be discussed at the annual review visit.

3.43 The PCT should also visit the contractor for the annual contract review, and this is discussed in more detail in chapter 6. This can be combined with the QOF annual review if the contractor so wishes.

Quality and outcomes – review

Guidance

3.79 The Quality and Outcomes Framework should not remain static and will need to be updated, particularly in the light of changes to the evidence base, advances in healthcare, changes in legislation or regulation and the need for further clarity, or so as to include new areas. *Investing in General Practice* makes clear that there will be a formal review process through which changes to the quality and outcomes framework (QOF) will be recommended by a UK-wide independent expert group. This process will be in place before the end of 2004, with the precise arrangements confirmed next summer. However, no changes to the QOF will be made before April 2006, other than in the case of a sudden change in the evidence base or the law that made a particular current indicator inappropriate.

3.80 It is expected that the review group will consider all aspects of the QOF from the twin aims of improving care to patients, whilst recognising changes to practice workload. The group will consider:

(i) whether new indicators should be added, existing indicators revised, dropped or combined

(ii) what the workload implications might be of such changes and how the indicators might be adapted to reflect this

(iii) all aspects of the prevalence adjustment arrangements.

Quality and outcomes framework (QOF) – general

Guidance

3.4 The quality and outcomes framework (QOF) provides substantial financial rewards for GMS providers to provide high quality care. This will bring benefits to patients and the NHS. PCTs should see, for example, fewer avoidable hospital admissions where chronic diseases are better managed. This is just one of the ways that the contract will benefit the whole NHS, and PCTs should keep this in mind when developing commissioning arrangements that will be reflected in Local Development Plans.

3.5 The QOF measures achievement against a scorecard of 146 evidence-based indicators, allowing a possible maximum score of 1050 points. Chapter 3 of *Investing in General Practice* and part 8 of the *New GMS Contract Supplementary Documents* set out the detail. In summary, the QOF comprises:

(i) the clinical domain: 76 indicators in 10 areas (coronary heart disease, stroke or transient ischaemic attack, cancer, hypothyroidism, diabetes, hypertension, mental health, asthma, chronic obstructive pulmonary disease and epilepsy), worth up to 550 points

(ii) the organisational domain: 56 indicators in 5 areas (records & information, patient communication, education & training, practice management, and medicines management), worth up to 184 points

(iii) the patient experience domain: 4 indicators within 2 areas (patient survey and consultation length), worth up to 100 points

(iv) the additional services domain: 10 indicators within 4 areas (cervical screening, child health surveillance, maternity services, contraceptive services), worth up to 36 points.

3.6 The QOF also rewards breadth of care through (i) holistic care payments (which measure overall clinical achievement and are worth up to 100 points) and (ii) quality practice payments (which measure overall achievement in the organisational, patient experience and additional services domains, and are worth up to 30 points). The QOF also rewards achievement against the access standards through 50 bonus points.

3.7 PCTs should note that the core philosophy underpinning the QOF is that incentives are the best method of resourcing work, driving up standards and recognising achievement. The QOF is not about performance management of GMS contractors but resourcing and rewarding good practice. Participation in the QOF is entirely voluntary for GMS contractors.

3.8 Development activities to support the introduction of the QOF are described in chapter 7. PCTs are encouraged to arrange expert seminars for all their contractors to explain how the QOF will work and suggest ways in which practices can maximise achievement. These can be supported by local Modernisation Agency facilitators. PCTs should contact their Strategic Health Authority (SHA) lead for help in arranging such roadshows. If a contractor is not achieving as high a score as it had aspired to, it may welcome an opportunity to see how other contractors in its PCT area (or outside) are managing to achieve, for example 1000 points, so that it can learn from the experience, maximise income and improve services to patients. PCTs should consider what support they might offer to facilitate this if there is local demand, for example, through funding protected time for benchmarking contractors to share learning.

Quality improvement cycle (annual) – quality and outcomes

Guidance

3.10 The QOF reflects a cycle of continuous quality improvement. This involves (i) planning, then (ii) action, then (iii) assessment and then (iv) learning, which in turn leads into the next cycle. This is illustrated in Figure 1.

Key activities and timetable for 2004/05

3.11 A sequence of key activities will make the QOF fully operational in 2004/05. This is illustrated in Figure 2. Key activities, which are described in further detail later in this chapter, are:
(i) agreeing aspiration levels by the end of February 2004
(ii) lump sum payments for Quality Preparation and for Quality Information Preparation DES for 2004/05 being made by the end of April 2004
(iii) the QOF starting in April 2004
(iv) aspiration payments being made in monthly instalments from April 2004

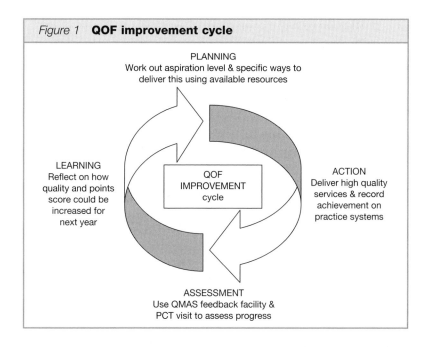

Figure 1 **QOF improvement cycle**

PLANNING
Work out aspiration level & specific ways to
deliver this using available resources

LEARNING
Reflect on how
quality and points
score could be
increased for
next year

QOF
IMPROVEMENT
cycle

ACTION
Deliver high quality
services & record
achievement on
practice systems

ASSESSMENT
Use QMAS feedback facility &
PCT visit to assess progress

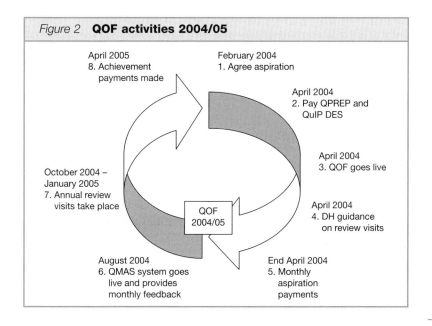

Figure 2 **QOF activities 2004/05**

April 2005
8. Achievement
payments made

February 2004
1. Agree aspiration

April 2004
2. Pay QPREP and
QuIP DES

April 2004
3. QOF goes live

October 2004 –
January 2005
7. Annual review
visits take place

QOF
2004/05

April 2004
4. DH guidance
on review visits

August 2004
6. QMAS system goes
live and provides
monthly feedback

End April 2004
5. Monthly
aspiration
payments

(v)   publication of guidance on annual review visits by the end of April 2004

(vi) the new central Quality and Outcomes Framework Management and Analysis System (QMAS), which calculates achievement and prevalence using links to clinical systems, going live in August 2004

(vii) QOF annual review visits taking place from October 2004 to January 2005

(viii) achievement payments being made by the end of April 2005.

● Quality Information Preparation (QuIP) – Directed Enhanced Services (DES)

Statement of Financial Entitlement

7.1   Direction 3(1)(b) of the directed enhanced services (DES) Directions requires each Primary Care Trust (PCT) to establish (if it has not already done so), operate and, as appropriate, revise a Quality Information Preparation Scheme (QuIPS) for its area, the underlying purpose of which is to summarise and improve the quality of medical records held by PMS or GMS contractors in its area. QuIPSs are to come to an end on 31 March 2005.

7.2   As part of its QuIPS, a PCT must, in respect of the financial year 2004/05 offer to enter into arrangements with each contractor in its area (unless it already has such arrangements with the contractor), thereby affording the contractor a reasonable opportunity to participate in the Scheme. However, before entering into any such arrangements, the PCT must satisfy itself of the matters set out in direction 3(2)(a) and (b) of the DES Directions.

7.3   The plan setting out the arrangements that the PCT enters into with a particular contractor (a "QuIPS plan") must cover the matters set out in direction 5(2)(a) and (b) of the DES Directions.

● Quality Information Preparation Scheme Payments

7.4   If, as part of a GMS contract a contractor and a PCT have agreed a Quality Information Preparation Scheme (QuIPS) plan under which payment is due in respect of the financial year 2004/05, the Primary Care

Trust (PCT) must in respect of the financial year 2004/05 pay to the contractor under the GMS contract a QuIPS Payment. The amount of this payment is to be –

(a) not less than £1000 multiplied by the contractor's CPI; but

(b) not more than £5000 multiplied by the contractor's CPI.

7.5 The precise figure is to depend on the amount of work that needs doing, having regard to the fact that QuIPS payments are not intended to cover the full cost of ensuring that contractors' records are appropriately summarised and edited.

7.6 The payment is to fall due –

(a) if the plan was agreed on or before 1 April 2004, or takes effect on 1 April 2004, on 30 April 2004; and

(b) if the plan is agreed after 1 April 2004, on the first date after the plan is agreed on which one of the contractor's Payable Global Sum Monthly Payments (GSMPs) falls due.

Guidance

3.15 The purpose of the QuIP DES is to provide a contribution to contractors' costs in summarising those medical records that have not already been summarised and in continuing to summarise those that have been. PCTs must offer separate QuIP schemes to all GMS (and PMS) contractors for both 2003/04 and 2004/05.

3.16 Key aspects of the QuIP DES, as laid out in the specification, are:

(i) it is a plan agreed by PCT and contractor

(ii) it must include a protocol for how the summarising is to be done and arrangements for ongoing maintenance. Non-medical personnel must (a) be fully trained, (b) not take medical records away from the practice premises, (c) have appropriate access to GP performers when they have queries, (d) sign a confidentiality agreement and (e) be appropriately supervised

(iii) the payment each year must by law be no less than £1000 and no more than £5000 for a contractor with average national list size. The precise figure depends on both list size and the amount of work that needs doing, bearing in mind the payment is not intended to cover the full cost. As an enhanced service, it is funded through existing unified budget allocations

(iv) for 2003/04 PCTs must, by 1 January 2004, offer the DES to all GMS contractors and agree a plan for implementation. For 2004/05, if the scheme has been agreed on or before 1 April 2004, the payment is due by 30 April 2004. If agreed after 1 April 2004 then it is due in a lump sum on the date the contractors next monthly payment is due. PCTs will want to use the revised Exeter payment system to make the payments.

Quality Preparation (QPREP) Payment

Statement of Financial Entitlement

4.1 Quality preparation (QPREP) payments are to fund the initial collection of data to establish the contractor's current position, and to assist contractors in preparing for the Quality and Outcomes Framework (QOF), which is Annex E to this statement of financial entitlement (SFE).

4.2 Individual practitioners will have received a QPREP payment during the financial year 2003/04 as a Standard Capitation Fee Supplement. For the financial year 2004/05, as capitation fees have been abolished, the way in which QPREP payments are paid is to change.

Calculation of QPREP payments

4.3 The QPREP Payment is an annual amount. In order to calculate it, the PCT must first establish the CRP of the contractor –
(a) if the contract takes effect on 1 April 2004 – or is treated as taking effect for payment purposes on 1 April 2004, which will be the case for GMS contracts replacing default contracts – on that date; or
(b) if the contract takes effect (for payment purposes) after 1 April 2004, on the date the contract takes effect.

4.4 From this number, the contractor's Contractor Population Index (CPI) is to be calculated (which is the number produced by dividing a contractor's most recently established Contractor Registered Population (CRP) by 5891). The contractor's CPI is then multiplied by £3250 which, unless the contract takes effect after 1 April 2004, is the amount of the contractor's QPREP payment.

4.5 If the contract takes effect after 1 April 2004, the amount is to be adjusted by the fraction produced by dividing the number of days during the financial year 2004/05 for which the contract is to have effect by 365.

4.6 Once the amount of a contractor's QPREP payment has been established, the PCT must pay it to the contractor under its GMS contract. The payment is to fall due at the same time as the contractor's first payable global sum monthly payment (GSMP) falls due.

Condition attached to QPREP Payments

4.7 QPREP payments are only payable in respect of GMS contracts that take effect on or before 1 February 2005 if the contractor agrees an Aspiration Points Total with the PCT for the financial year 2004/05. They are only payable in respect of GMS contracts agreed after 1 February 2005 if the contractor has agreed to participate in the QOF.

Guidance

3.13 £9000 per GMS contractor (that is, per practice rather than per GP) with average national list size was available in 2003/04. This should have been paid in November 2003. The final quality preparation payment at an average of £3250 per GMS contractor will be available in 2004/05. This is in line with the joint letter of 30 May 2003 from Mike Farrar and Dr John Chisholm.

3.14 Key aspects of this payment for 2004/05, as set out in the SFE, are:
   (i)   the payment should normally be made by the end of April 2004. This will be done through the revised Exeter payment system
   (ii) however, payment in 2004/05 is conditional on the contractor agreeing to participate in the QOF, usually as shown through having an aspiration points total
   (iii) *pro-rata* payments would be made to new contractors in year except where these arise from practice splits (such practices would have already received their payment)
   (iv) this will be the final payment; QPREP will not be available in 2005/06.

● Recruitment and retention

Guidance

4.14 This will be supported by:
   (i)   the out-of-hours changes. GPs and other primary care professionals can expect a better work/life balance. The transfer of responsibility by the end of December 2004 for out of hours to the Primary Care Trust (PCT) will make general practice a more attractive place to work. Contractors will also benefit from the new ability to manage workload through the ability to opt-out of certain additional services and the new procedures to reduce assignments to contractors with closed lists

(ii)   increased investment in primary care which will support workforce expansion. The devolution of primary care funding to PCTs, combined with the introduction of the PCT provider and alternative provider routes, gives PCTs the ability to develop new services in areas that have historically been under-doctored, and the ability to develop innovative ways of employing GPs, nurses and practice managers to support GMS and PMS providers

(iii) new opportunities for GPs to become salaried to GMS contractors, to PCTs and to out-of-hours providers, where this better suits their particular circumstances. This is supported by the introduction of the model salaried contract which includes a pay range and flexibility for PCTs and contractors to offer salaries commensurate with local labour market conditions. Details are set out in *Supplementary Documents*

(iv)   new opportunities for nurses, allied health professionals, practice managers and others (including consultants) through (a) the introduction of a practice-based contract, (b) the delivery of a wider range of services through the enhanced services route, and (c) delivery of better chronic disease management and organisational standards through the quality and outcomes framework. In a way that is similar to PMS, it will be possible to have nurse-managed, or therapist-managed GMS services. Salaried staff will also be supported through the introduction of Agenda for Change principles in general practice. Whilst Agenda for Change is not mandatory, GMS contractors will be expected to implement its principles and they will want to work closely with their PCTs on this, particularly in relation to the effective use of the Job Evaluation Scheme and the Knowledge and Skills Framework or equivalents

(v)   the continuation of specific supply-side incentives: golden hellos in 2004/05, the GP returners' scheme, the retainer scheme, and the Flexible Careers Scheme. These remain as entitlements in the 2004/05 Statement of Financial Entitlements (SFE). The Flexible Careers Scheme offers opportunities for flexible and part-time working. The returners' scheme offers tailored refresher training and a co-ordinated way back to practice for retired doctors or doctors not currently working in primary care who wish to return to the NHS. The golden hello scheme was introduced in 2001 as a time-limited measure to improve conversion rates of GP registrars and to improve recruitment in historically under-doctored areas. Its efficacy in achieving these objectives will be reviewed during 2004/05 with a view to refocusing it from 2005/06 to provide incentives more targeted towards the most under-doctored areas. The Department of Health or its agents will consult the GPC on these proposals

(vi) ongoing development and support to improve working lives, which is considered further below.

Ongoing support and development

4.15 Ways in which PCTs will be able to help provide ongoing support and development include through:

(i) application of the Department's human resources strategy, including the skills escalator and career pathways. Specialist interest development is a key aspect and will be supported through the commissioning of more specialised services using the enhanced services budget

(ii) promoting best employment practice set out in the Improving Working Lives (IWL) Standard http://www.doh.gov.uk/iwl. PCTs will want to encourage GMS contractors, particularly larger practices, to consider pursuing IWL accreditation. This will help support recruitment and retention, job satisfaction, and also contribute towards achieving points in the organisational standards within the quality and outcomes framework (e.g. education and training and patient communication)

(iv) supporting the appraisal of all staff. Extensive guidance is available on the preparation for, and conduct of, the appraisal process. This can be found at http://www.appraisaluk.info. An on-line appraisal toolkit for GPs can be found at http://www.appraisals.nhs.uk

(v) provision of locum support through PCT locum banks, and partial reimbursement for locum costs where necessary for maternity, paternity, adoptive leave, sickness leave, to cover for suspended doctors, or for the prolonged study leave scheme. Details of minimum requirements are included in the draft Statement of Financial Entitlements. The costs will be funded from the PCT-administered budget described in chapter 5. PCTs will also be under a new legal obligation from 1 April 2004 to develop and seek to agree with the Local Medical Committee (LMC) a policy for locum cover and payment arrangements. This should include what proportion of the maximum funding would be available to those with a less than full working commitment. This is because the existing Red Book rules on that point have been simplified to allow greater local flexibility. PCTs may wish to use the 37.5 hours in the model salaried GP contract as a guide to full-time working. The Department advises that PCTs should develop policies and consult LMCs during March 2004

(vi) initial development of sabbatical schemes. £8.5 million was notionally included within the national PCT-administered funding stream. PCTs will want to consider how best to use this money to develop local support arrangements

(vii) the Directed Enhanced Service for those patients who threaten violence or commit violent acts, which PCTs must commission and which will ensure that all PCTs have secure facilities available to see violent patients

(viii) delivering the NHS childcare strategy in primary care so that those working in primary care have the same access to childcare as staff in other parts of the NHS

(ix) new pension flexibilities to support portfolio careers. These are described later in this section

(x) supporting practice management. Practice managers will have an increasingly important role as they become the experts in the operation of the new contract, including all the new mechanisms outlined in this guidance. PCTs are advised to review their support arrangements for practice management during 2004. The Department will also be introducing a practice management toolkit early in 2004

(xi) supporting practice nurses. The Department is producing further guidance during 2004, in consultation with professional bodies, PCTs and nurses. This will form part of a wider guidance document on human resources issues in primary care.

Refusal to register – list or temporary

Regulations

17. Refusal of applications for inclusion in the list of patients or for acceptance as a temporary resident

(1) The contractor shall only refuse an application made under paragraph 15 or 16 if it has reasonable grounds for doing so which do not relate to the applicant's race, gender, social class, age, religion, sexual orientation, appearance, disability or medical condition.

(2) The reasonable grounds referred to in paragraph (1) shall, in the case of applications made under paragraph 15, include the ground that the applicant does not live in the contractor's practice area.

(3) A contractor which refuses an application made under paragraph 15 or 16 shall, within 14 days of its decision, notify the applicant (or, in the case of a child or incapable adult, the person making the application on their behalf) in writing of the refusal and the reason for it.

(4)   The contractor shall keep a written record of refusals of applications made under paragraph 15 and of the reasons for them and shall make this record available to the PCT on request.

Standard Contract

Refusal of applications for inclusion in the list of patients or for acceptance as a *temporary resident*

180.   The Contractor shall only refuse an application made under clauses 170 to 179 if it has reasonable grounds for doing so which do not relate to the applicant's race, gender, social class, age, religion, sexual orientation, appearance, disability or medical condition.

181.   The reasonable grounds referred to in clause 180 shall, in the case of applications made under clauses 170 to 175 include the ground that the applicant does not live in the Contractor's *practice area*.

182.   If the Contractor refuses an application made under clauses 170 to 179, it shall, within 14 days of its decision, notify the applicant (or, in the case of a child or incapable adult, the person making the application on their behalf) in writing of the refusal and the reason for it.

183.   The Contractor shall keep a written record of refusals of applications made under clauses 170 to 175 and of the reasons for them and shall make this record available to the PCT on request.

● Relationship between contracted parties

Standard Contract

5.   The Contract is a contract for the provision of services. The Contractor is an independent provider of services and is not an employee, partner or agent of the Primary Care Trust (PCT). The Contractor must not represent or conduct its activities so as to give the impression that it is the employee, partner or agent of the PCT.

6.   The PCT does not by entering into this Contract, and shall not as a result of anything done by the Contractor in connection with the performance of this Contract, incur any contractual liability to any other person.

7. This Contract does not create any right enforceable by any person not a party to it.[62]

8. In complying with this Contract, in exercising its rights under the Contract and in performing its obligations under the Contract, the Contractor must act reasonably and in good faith.

9. In complying with this Contract, and in exercising its rights under the Contract, the PCT must act reasonably and in good faith and as a responsible public body required to discharge its functions under *the Act*.

10. Clauses 8 and 9 above do not relieve either party from the requirement to comply with the express provisions of this Contract and the parties are subject to all such express provisions.

11. The Contractor shall not give, sell, assign or otherwise dispose of the benefit of any of its rights under this Contract, [save in accordance with Schedule 1][63] [and subject to specific provision made in clauses 393 to 424].[64] The Contract does not prohibit the Contractor from delegating its obligations arising under the Contract where such delegation is expressly permitted by the Contract.

12. The PCT may give, sell, assign or otherwise dispose of the benefit of its rights under this Contract to another PCT.

Remedial and breach notices

Guidance

6.49 Where it believes that a contractor is in default of its obligations under its contract the Primary Care Trust (PCT) can either issue a breach notice or a remedial notice (see paragraph 114 of Schedule 6):
(i) if a contractor breaches any of the terms of the contract and the breach is capable of remedy, the PCT may give notice to the contractor requiring it to remedy the breach. A breach capable of remedy might be a failure to provide a practice leaflet or to make arrangements for a home visiting service. This remedial notice will

---

62 This clause is required by *the Regulations* (see paragraph 126 of Schedule 6).

63 The words indicated in square brackets only need to be included if the Contractor is a partnership and Schedule 1 (partnerships) has therefore been utilised.

64 The words indicated in square brackets only need to be included if clauses 393 to 424 are to be included in the Contract (see Part 14).

specify the details of the breach, the steps to be taken to remedy the breach, and the period within which those steps must be taken

(ii) where a contractor has breached the terms of the contract and the breach is not capable of remedy, for example a one-off act such as a failure to visit a particular patient, the PCT may serve notice on the contractor requiring the contractor not to repeat the breach.

6.50 If, following a breach notice or a remedial notice, the contractor repeats the breach, or otherwise breaches the contract resulting in another breach or remedial notice, the PCT may give notice terminating the contract from such date as may be specified.

6.51 Before issuing such a termination notice the PCT should give careful consideration to the cumulative effect of any breaches. For example, a run of minor breaches over a short period or occasional breaches over a longer period ought not, in themselves, to lead to a termination. However, a persistent stream of minor breaches could justify termination if it was clear to the PCT that the contractor was unwilling or unable to take steps to stem the flow. It is expected that each decision will be taken in the light of the contractor's individual circumstances. Circumstances that might be considered include the likelihood of temporary support from the PCT being helpful, practice workload and the views of patients. The Local Medical Committee (LMC) should be consulted before the PCT reaches a decision under these provisions. A notice terminating the contract should only be issued if the PCT is satisfied that the cumulative effect is such that it would be prejudicial to the efficiency of patient services to allow the contract to continue.

6.52 If the contractor is in breach of any obligation under the contract, and a breach or remedial notice has been issued, the PCT may consider withholding or deducting monies which would otherwise be payable under the contract, but only those monies payable in respect of the contractual obligation that has been breached.

6.53 The contractor may challenge any notice given by the PCT under these provisions through the dispute resolution procedures. If the contractor does raise a dispute within the specified period given in the notice, the contract termination will not take effect until either (i) there has been an initial determination of the dispute by the relevant adjudication authority or competent court, or (ii) the contractor ceases to pursue the dispute, whichever is the sooner.

6.54 A PCT may terminate the contract before the conclusion of the NHS dispute procedures if it is satisfied that it is necessary to do so to protect the safety of patients or to protect itself from material financial loss. However, in doing so the PCT should exercise due care. On terminating a contract, the PCT decision is still subject to challenge and if the resolution of the subsequent dispute were to find in favour of the contractor, the PCT could be liable for damages as it would have wrongly deprived the contractor of its livelihood under a contract that was not limited as to its duration. The scope for damages could be very substantial. PCTs would normally wish to seek legal advice before terminating a GMS contract to limit any risks that it might be exposed to.

Removal of patients from contractor lists

See also: Administrative removals

Regulations

19. Removals from the list at the request of the patient

(1) The contractor shall notify the Primary Care Trust (PCT) in writing of any request for removal from its list of patients received from a registered patient.

(2) Where the PCT –
(a) receives notification from the contractor under sub-paragraph (1); or
(b) receives a request from the patient to be removed from the contractor's list of patients,
it shall remove that person from the contractor's list of patients.

(3) A removal in accordance with sub-paragraph (2) shall take effect –
(a) on the date on which the PCT receives notification of the registration of the person with another provider of essential services (or their equivalent); or
(b) 14 days after the date on which the notification or request made under sub-paragraph (1) or (2) respectively is received by the PCT,
whichever is the sooner.

(4) The PCT shall, as soon as practicable, notify in writing –
(a) the patient; and
(b) the contractor,
that the patient's name will be or has been removed from the contractor's list of patients on the date referred to in sub-paragraph (3).

(5) In this paragraph and in paragraphs 20(1)(b) and (10), 21(6) and (7), 23 and 26, a reference to a request received from or advice, information or notification required to be given to a patient shall include a request received from or advice, information or notification required to be given to –

(a) in the case of a patient who is a child, a parent or other person referred to in paragraph 15(4)(a); or

(b) in the case of an adult patient who is incapable of making the relevant request or receiving the relevant advice, information or notification, a relative or the primary carer of the patient.

20. Removals from the list at the request of the contractor

(1) Subject to paragraph 21, a contractor which has reasonable grounds for wishing a patient to be removed from its list of patients which do not relate to the applicant's race, gender, social class, age, religion, sexual orientation, appearance, disability or medical condition shall –

(a) notify the PCT in writing that it wishes to have the patient removed; and

(b) subject to sub-paragraph (2), notify the patient of its specific reasons for requesting removal.

(2) Where, in the reasonable opinion of the contractor –

(a) the circumstances of the removal are such that it is not appropriate for a more specific reason to be given; and

(b) there has been an irrevocable breakdown in the relationship between the patient and the contractor,

the reason given under sub-paragraph (1) may consist of a statement that there has been such a breakdown.

(3) Except in the circumstances specified in sub-paragraph (4), a contractor may only request a removal under sub-paragraph (1), if, within the period of 12 months prior to the date of its request to the PCT, it has warned the patient that he is at risk of removal and explained to him the reasons for this.

(4) The circumstances referred to in sub-paragraph (3) are that –

(a) the reason for removal relates to a change of address;

(b) the contractor has reasonable grounds for believing that the issue of such a warning would –

(i) be harmful to the physical or mental health of the patient, or

(ii) put at risk the safety of one or more of the persons specified in sub-paragraph (5); or

(c) it is, in the opinion of the contractor, not otherwise reasonable or practical for a warning to be given.

(5) The persons referred to in sub-paragraph (4) are –

(a) the contractor, where it is an individual medical practitioner;

(b) in the case of a contract with two or more individuals practising in partnership, a partner in that partnership;

(c) in the case of a contract with a company, a legal and beneficial owner of shares in that company;

(d) a member of the contractor's staff;

(e) a person engaged by the contractor to perform or assist in the performance of services under the contract; or

(f) any other person present –

    (i) on the practice premises, or

    (ii) in the place where services are being provided to the patient under the contract.

(6) The contractor shall record in writing –

(a) the date of any warning given in accordance with sub-paragraph (3) and the reasons for giving such a warning as explained to the patient; or

(b) the reason why no such warning was given.

(7) The contractor shall keep a written record of removals under this paragraph which shall include –

(a) the reason for removal given to the patient;

(b) the circumstances of the removal; and

(c) in cases where sub-paragraph (2) applies, the grounds for a more specific reason not being appropriate,

and shall make this record available to the PCT on request.

(8) A removal requested in accordance with sub-paragraph (1) shall, subject to sub-paragraph (9), take effect from –

(a) the date on which the PCT receives notification of the registration of the person with another provider of essential services (or their equivalent); or

(b) the eighth day after the PCT receives the notice referred to in sub-paragraph (1)(a),

whichever is the sooner.

(9) Where, on the date on which the removal would take effect under sub-paragraph (8), the contractor is treating the patient at intervals of less than 7 days, the contractor shall notify the PCT in writing of the fact and the removal shall take effect –

(a) on the eighth day after the Trust receives notification from the contractor that the person no longer needs such treatment; or

(b) on the date on which the PCT receives notification of the registration of the person with another provider of essential services (or their equivalent),

whichever is the sooner.

(10) The PCT shall notify in writing –

(a) the patient; and

(b) the contractor,

that the patient's name has been or will be removed from the contractor's list of patients on the date referred to in sub-paragraph (8) or (9).

21. Removals from the list of patients who are violent

(1) A contractor which wishes a patient to be removed from its list of patients with immediate effect on the grounds that –
(a) the patient has committed an act of violence against any of the persons specified in sub-paragraph (2) or behaved in such a way that any such person has feared for his safety; and
(b) it has reported the incident to the police,
shall notify the PCT in accordance with sub-paragraph (3).

(2) The persons referred to in sub-paragraph (1) are –
(a) the contractor where it is an individual medical practitioner;
(b) in the case of a contract with two or more individuals practising in partnership, a partner in that partnership;
(c) in the case of a contract with a company, a legal and beneficial owner of shares in that company;
(d) a member of the contractor's staff;
(e) a person engaged by the contractor to perform or assist in the performance of services under the contract; or
(f) any other person present –
(i) on the practice premises, or
(ii) in the place where services were provided to the patient under the contract.

(3) Notification under sub-paragraph (1) may be given by any means including telephone or fax but if not given in writing shall subsequently be confirmed in writing within 7 days (and for this purpose a faxed notification is not a written one).

(4) The PCT shall acknowledge in writing receipt of a request from the contractor under sub-paragraph (1).

(5) A removal requested in accordance with sub-paragraph (1) shall take effect at the time that the contractor –
(a) makes the telephone call to the PCT; or
(b) sends or delivers the notification to the PCT.

(6) Where, pursuant to this paragraph, the contractor has notified the PCT that it wishes to have a patient removed from its list of patients, it shall inform the patient concerned unless –
(a) it is not reasonably practicable for it to do so; or
(b) it has reasonable grounds for believing that to do so would –
(i) be harmful to the physical or mental health of the patient, or

        (ii) put at risk the safety of one or more of the persons specified in sub-paragraph (2).

(7)   Where the PCT has removed a patient from the contractor's list of patients in accordance with sub-paragraph (5) it shall give written notice of the removal to that patient.

(8)   Where a patient is removed from the contractor's list of patients in accordance with this paragraph, the contractor shall record in the patient's medical records that the patient has been removed under this paragraph and the circumstances leading to his removal.

22.   Removals from the list of patients registered elsewhere

(1)   The PCT shall remove a patient from the contractor's list of patients if –
     (a) he has subsequently been registered with another provider of essential services (or their equivalent) in the area of the PCT; or
     (b) it has received notice from another PCT, a Local Health Board, a Health Board or a Health and Social Services Board that he has subsequently been registered with a provider of essential services (or their equivalent) outside the area of the PCT.

(2)   A removal in accordance with sub-paragraph (1) shall take effect –
     (a) on the date on which the PCT receives notification of the registration of the person with the new provider; or
     (b) with the consent of the PCT, on such other date as has been agreed between the contractor and the new provider.

(3)   The PCT shall notify the contractor in writing of persons removed from its list of patients under sub-paragraph (1).

23.   Removals from the list of patients who have moved

(1)   Subject to sub-paragraph (2), where the PCT is satisfied that a person on the contractor's list of patients has moved and no longer resides in that contractor's practice area, the PCT shall –
     (a) inform that patient and the contractor that the contractor is no longer obliged to visit and treat the person;
     (b) advise the patient in writing either to obtain the contractor's agreement to the continued inclusion of the person on its list of patients or to apply for registration with another provider of essential services (or their equivalent); and
     (c) inform the patient that if, after the expiration of 30 days from the date of the advice mentioned in paragraph (b), he has not acted in accordance with the advice and informed it accordingly, the PCT will remove him from the contractor's list of patients.

(2) If, at the expiration of the period of 30 days referred to in sub-paragraph (1)(c), the PCT has not been notified of the action taken, it shall remove the patient from the contractor's list of patients and inform him and the contractor accordingly.

24. Where the address of a patient who is on the contractor's list of patients is no longer known to the PCT, the PCT shall –
   (a) give to the contractor notice in writing that it intends, at the end of the period of six months commencing with the date of the notice, to remove the patient from the contractor's list of patients; and
   (b) at the end of that period, remove the patient from the contractor's list of patients unless, within that period, the contractor satisfies the PCT that it is still responsible for providing essential services to that patient.

25. Removals from the list of patients absent from the United Kingdom etc.

(1) The PCT shall remove a patient from the contractor's list of patients where it receives notification that that patient –
   (a) intends to be away from the United Kingdom for a period of at least three months;
   (b) is in Her Majesty's Forces;
   (c) is serving a prison sentence of more than two years or sentences totalling in the aggregate more than that period;
   (d) has been absent from the United Kingdom for a period of more than three months; or
   (e) has died.

(2) A removal in accordance with sub-paragraph (1) shall take effect –
   (a) in the cases referred to in sub-paragraph (1)(a) to (c) from the date of the departure, enlistment or imprisonment or the date on which the PCT first receives notification of the departure, enlistment or imprisonment whichever is the later; or
   (b) in the cases referred to in sub-paragraph (1)(d) and (e) from the date on which the PCT first receives notification of the absence or death.

(3) The PCT shall notify the contractor in writing of patients removed from its list of patients under sub-paragraph (1).

26. Removals from the list of patients accepted elsewhere as temporary residents

(1) The PCT shall remove from the contractor's list of patients a patient who has been accepted as a temporary resident by another contractor or other

provider of essential services (or their equivalent) where it is satisfied, after due inquiry –

(a) that the patient's stay in the place of temporary residence has exceeded three months; and

(b) that he has not returned to his normal place of residence or any other place within the contractor's practice area.

(2) The PCT shall notify in writing of a removal under sub-paragraph (1) –

(a) the contractor; and

(b) where practicable, the patient.

(3) A notification to the patient under sub-paragraph (2)(b) shall inform him of –

(a) his entitlement to make arrangements for the provision to him of essential services (or their equivalent), including by the contractor by which he has been treated as a temporary resident; and

(b) the name and address of the PCT in whose area he is resident.

27. Removals from the list of pupils etc. of a school

(1) Where the contractor provides essential services under the contract to persons on the grounds that they are pupils at or staff or residents of a school, the PCT shall remove from the contractor's list of patients any such persons who do not appear on particulars of persons who are pupils at or staff or residents of that school provided by that school.

(2) Where the PCT has made a request to a school to provide the particulars mentioned in sub-paragraph (1) and has not received them, it shall consult the contractor as to whether it should remove from its list of patients any persons appearing on that list as pupils at, or staff or residents of, that school.

(3) The PCT shall notify the contractor in writing of patients removed from its list of patients under sub-paragraph (1).

Standard Contract

Removals from the list at the request of the patient

186. The Contractor shall notify the PCT in writing of any request for removal from its list of patients received from a *registered patient*.

187. Where the PCT receives notification from the Contractor under clause 186, or receives a request from the patient to be removed from the Contractor's list of patients, it shall remove that person from the Contractor's list of patients.

188. A removal under clause 187 shall take effect –
   188.1 on the date on which the PCT receives notification of the registration of the person with another provider of *essential services* (or their equivalent); or
   188.2 14 days after the date on which the notification or request made under clause 186 or 187 respectively is received by the PCT, whichever is the sooner.

189. The PCT shall, as soon as practicable, notify in writing –
   189.1 the patient; and
   189.2 the Contractor,
   that the patient's name will be or has been removed from the Contractor's list of patients on the date referred to in clause188.

190. In clauses 189, 191, 200.1, 206, 207, 212, 213 and 219 a reference to a request received from, or advice, information or notification required to be given to, a patient shall include a request received from or advice, information or notification required to be given to –
   190.1 in the case of a patient who is a *child*, a *parent* or other person referred to in clause 173.1; or
   190.2 in the case of an adult patient who is incapable of making the relevant request or receiving the relevant advice, information or notification, a relative or the *primary carer* of the patient.

Removals from the list at the request of the Contractor

191. Subject to clauses 201 to 207, where the Contractor has reasonable grounds for wishing a patient to be removed from its list of patients which do not relate to the applicant's race, gender, social class, age, religion, sexual orientation, appearance, disability or medical condition, the Contractor shall –
   191.1 notify the PCT in writing that it wishes to have the patient removed; and
   191.2 subject to clause 192, notify the patient in writing of its specific reasons for requesting removal.

192. Where, in the reasonable opinion of the Contractor, the circumstances of the removal are such that it is not appropriate for a more specific reason to be given, and there has been an irrevocable breakdown in the relationship between the patient and the Contractor, the reason given under clause 191 may consist of a statement that there has been such a breakdown.

193. Except in the circumstances specified in clause194, the Contractor may only request a removal under clause 191, if, within the period of 12 months prior to the date of its request to the PCT, it has warned the

patient that he is at risk of removal and explained to him the reasons for this.

194. The circumstances referred to in clause 193 are that –

194.1 the reason for removal relates to a change of address;

194.2 the Contractor has reasonable grounds for believing that the issue of such a warning would be harmful to the physical or mental health of the patient or would put at risk the safety of one or more of the persons specified in clause 195; or

194.3 it is, in the opinion of the Contractor, not otherwise reasonable or practical for a warning to be given.

195. The persons referred to in clause 194 are –

195.1 if the Contractor is an individual medical practitioner, the Contractor;

195.2 if the Contractor is a partnership, a partner in the partnership;

195.3 if the Contractor is a company, a legal and beneficial owner of shares in that company;

195.4 a member of the Contractor's staff;

195.5 a person engaged by the Contractor to perform or assist in the performance of services under the Contract; or

195.6 any other person present on the *practice premises* or in the place where services are being provided to the patient under the Contract.

196. The Contractor shall record in writing the date of any warning given in accordance with clause 193 and the reasons for giving such a warning as explained to the patient, or the reason why no such warning was given.

197. The Contractor shall keep a written record of removals under clause 191 which shall include the reason for removal given to the patient, the circumstances of the removal and in cases where clause 192 applies, the grounds for a more specific reason not being appropriate, and the Contractor shall make this record available to the PCT on request.

198. A removal requested in accordance with clause 191 shall, subject to clause 199, take effect from the date on which the person is registered with another provider of *essential services*, or the eighth day after the Trust receives the notice, whichever is the sooner.

199. Where, on the date on which the removal would take effect under clause 198, the Contractor is treating the patient at intervals of less than 7 days, the Contractor shall inform the PCT in writing of that fact and the removal shall take effect on the eighth day after the Trust receives notification from the Contractor that the person no longer needs such treatment, or on the date on which the person is registered with another provider of *essential services*, whichever is the sooner.

200. The PCT shall notify in writing –
200.1 the patient; and
200.2 the Contractor
that the patient's name has been or will be removed from the
Contractor's list of patients on the date referred to in clause 198 or 199.

Removals from the list of patients who are violent

201. Where the Contractor wishes a patient to be removed from its list of
patients with immediate effect on the grounds that –
201.1.the patient has committed an act of violence against any of the
persons specified in clause 202 or behaved in such a way that any
such person has feared for his safety; and
201.2 it has reported the incident to the police,
the Contractor shall notify the PCT in accordance with clause 203.

202. The persons referred to in clause 201 are –
202.1 if the Contract is with an individual medical practitioner, that
individual;
202.2 if the Contract is with a partnership, a partner in that partnership;
202.3 if the Contract is with a company, a legal and beneficial owner of
shares in that company;
202.4 a member of the Contractor's staff;
202.5 a person employed or engaged by the Contractor to perform or
assist in the performance of services under the Contract; or
202.6 any other person present on the *practice premises* or in the place
where services were provided to the patient under the Contract.

203. Notification under clause 201 may be given by any means including
telephone or fax but if not given in writing shall subsequently be
confirmed in writing within 7 days (and for this purpose a faxed
notification is not a written one).

204. The PCT shall acknowledge in writing receipt of a request from the
Contractor under clause 201.

205. A removal requested in accordance with clause 201 shall take effect at the
time the Contractor makes the telephone call to the PCT, or sends or
delivers the notification to the PCT.

206. Where, pursuant to clauses 201 to 205, the Contractor has notified the
PCT that it wishes to have a patient removed from its list of patients, it
shall inform the patient concerned unless –
206.1 it is not reasonably practicable for it to do so; or
206.2 it has reasonable grounds for believing that to do so would be
harmful to the physical or mental health of the patient or would

put at risk the safety of one or more of the persons specified in clause 202.

207. Where the PCT has removed a patient from the Contractor's list of patients in accordance with clause 205 it shall give written notice of the removal to that patient.

208. Where a patient is removed from the Contractor's list of patients in accordance with clauses 201 to 207, the Contractor shall record in the patient's medical records that the patient has been removed under this paragraph and the circumstances leading to his removal.

Removals from the list of patients registered elsewhere

209. The PCT shall remove a patient from the Contractor's list of patients if he has subsequently been registered with another provider of essential services (or their equivalent) in the area of the PCT or it has received notice from another PCT, a *Health Board*, a Local Health Board or a *Health and Social Services Board* that the patient has subsequently been registered with a provider of *essential services* (or their equivalent) outside the area of the PCT.

210. A removal in accordance with clause 209 shall take effect on the date on which notification of acceptance by the new provider was received or with the consent of the PCT, on such other date as has been agreed between the Contractor and the new provider.

211. The PCT shall notify the Contractor in writing of persons removed from its list of patients under clause 209.

Removals from the list of patients who have moved

212. Subject to clause 213, where the PCT is satisfied that a person on the Contractor's list of patients no longer resides in that Contractor's *practice area*, the PCT shall –
   212.1 inform that patient and the Contractor that the Contractor is no longer obliged to visit and treat the patient;
   212.2 advise the patient in writing either to obtain the Contractor's agreement to the continued inclusion of the patient on its list of patients or to apply for registration with another provider of *essential services* (or their equivalent); and
   212.3 inform the patient that if, after the expiration of 30 days from the date of the advice referred to in clause 212.2, he has not acted in accordance with the advice and informed it accordingly, the PCT will remove him from the Contractor's list of patients.

213. If, at the expiration of the period of 30 days referred to in clause 212.3, the PCT has not been notified of the action taken, it shall remove the patient from the Contractor's list of patients and inform him and the Contractor accordingly.

214. Where the address of a patient who is on the Contractor's list is no longer known to the PCT, the PCT shall –
    214.1 give to the Contractor notice in writing that it intends, at the end of the period of 6 months commencing with the date of the notice, to remove the patient from the Contractor's list of patients; and
    214.2 at the end of that period, remove the patient from the Contractor's list of patients unless, within that period, the Contractor satisfies the PCT that it is still responsible for providing *essential services* to that patient.

Removals from the list of patients absent from the United Kingdom etc.

215. The PCT shall remove a patient from the Contractor's list of patients where it receives notification that that patient –
    215.1 intends to be away from the United Kingdom for a period of at least 3 months;
    215.2 is in Her Majesty's Forces;
    215.3 is serving a prison sentence of more than 2 years or sentences totalling in the aggregate more than that period;
    215.4 has been absent from the United Kingdom for a period of more than 3 months; or
    215.5 has died.

216. A removal in accordance with clause 215 shall take effect –
    216.1 in the cases referred to in clauses 215.1 to 215.3 from the date of the departure, enlistment or imprisonment or the date on which the PCT first receives notification of the departure, enlistment or imprisonment whichever is the later;
    216.2 in the cases referred to in clauses 215.4 and 215.5 from the date on which the PCT first receives notification of the absence or death.

217. The PCT shall notify the Contractor in writing of patients removed from its list of patients under clause 215.

Removals from the list of patients accepted elsewhere as *temporary residents*

218. The PCT shall remove from the Contractor's list of patients a patient who has been accepted as a *temporary resident* by another contractor or

other provider of *essential services* (or their equivalent) where it is satisfied, after due inquiry –

218.1 that the patient's stay in the place of temporary residence has exceeded 3 months; and

218.2 that the patient has not returned to his normal place of residence or any other place within the Contractor's *practice area*.

219. The PCT shall notify the Contractor and, where practicable, the patient, of a removal under clause 218.

220. A notification to the patient under clause 219 shall inform him of –

220.1 his entitlement to make arrangements for the provision to him of *essential services* (or their equivalent), including by the Contractor by whom he has been treated as a *temporary resident*; and

220.2 the name and address of the PCT in whose area he is resident.

Removals from the list of pupils etc. of a school

221. Where the Contractor provides *essential services* under the Contract to persons on the grounds that they are pupils at or staff or residents of a school, the PCT shall remove from the Contractor's list of patients any such persons who do not appear on particulars of persons who are pupils at or staff or residents of that school provided by that school.

222. Where the PCT has made a request to a school to provide the particulars mentioned in clause 221 and has not received them, it shall consult the Contractor as to whether it should remove from its list of patients any persons appearing on that list as pupils at, or staff or residents of, that school.

223. The PCT shall notify the Contractor in writing of patients removed from its list of patients under clause 221.

Guidance

2.43 When patients register or stop being registered with the contractor, the contractor must supply the necessary information as soon as practicable to the PCT through the registration system. Where either the PCT or contractors remove patients from lists they must notify the patients and inform them of their right to receive primary medical services from another contractor. Patients may be removed from contractors' lists for a variety of reasons. A simple summary is provided in Table 4 (again, the Contract Regulations provide the definitive statement of law).

Table 4 **Reasons for removing patients**

Reason	Point of removal
1. Patient chooses to register elsewhere	14 days after PCT is notified by the contractor or patient or date when PCT receives notification that patient is registered with another provider, whichever is the sooner
2. Teacher or pupil was receiving primary medical services through a school but has left	When PCT receives list from the school which does not include the patient
3. Patient moves outside the practice area	Date PCT is notified by the contractor or patient or 30 days after writing to patient
4. Patient's address is no longer known	PCT notifies the contractor that the patient's name will be removed from the list after 6 months
5. Patient joins the armed forces	Enlistment date, or date PCT is notified by the contractor or patient, whichever is sooner
6. Patient sentenced to a prison sentence for more than 2 years	Start of sentence, or date PCT is notified by the contractor or patient, whichever is sooner
7. Patient leaves the country for more than 3 months	Date patient leaves UK, or date PCT receives notification from the contractor or patient of intention to leave or that patient has left, whichever is sooner
8. Patient death	Date the PCT is notified by the contractor of the patient's death. Contractors must notify the PCT by the end of the first working day following the death where death occurs on the practice's premises – otherwise as soon as is practicable

Continued

Table 4 – continued	
Reason	**Point of removal**
9. Contractor requests that an individual patient is removed	1. Immediate for violent patients 2. When the patient is accepted by/ assigned to another practice, or 8 days after the date of the request by the contractor to the PCT for removal, whichever is sooner 3. If at the date of removal, a patient is receiving treatment at intervals of 7 days or less, the practice will be required to inform the PCT of this and removal will take place on the eighth day after the PCT has received notification from the practice that the person no longer needs such treatment, or on the date that the person is accepted/ assigned to another practice. Doctors are also under an obligation under *GMC Good Medical Practice* guidance to take steps to ensure the continuing care of patients
10. Contractor requests administrative removal of groups of patients	Removal date

Removals proposed by contractors

2.44   Where contractors remove patients from their lists they must always inform the PCT in writing. For individual cases contractors must have reasonable grounds for wishing a patient to be removed. Those reasons cannot be due to the person's disability or medical condition, appearance, age, race, gender, social class, age, religion, or sexual orientation. Legitimate grounds for removal may include for example:

(i)   violence, or threatening behaviour. This could involve, for example in relation to home visits, the patient, a relative, a household member or pets such as unchained dogs

(ii)   crime and deception, for example fraudulently obtaining drugs for non-medical reasons, stealing from the premises or causing criminal damage

(iii) where the relationship between the contractor/practitioner and patient has been broken to the extent that it is necessary to end the professional relationship with the patient. Contractors should note they should not remove patients simply because they are exacting or highly dependent, exhibit high levels of anxiety or demand about perceived serious symptoms, or because they have made a complaint against a practitioner or the contractor.

Warnings and giving reasons for removal

2.45 Contractors should warn the patients before steps are taken for their removal. They may do so by any means they feel appropriate in the circumstances. It may not always be practically possible for a warning to be given to the patient, for example where a warning could result in physical or mental harm to the patient, or put at risk the safety of other people. Warnings should be recorded in writing. This record should note the date that the warning was given. Where a removal does take place and no warning was given, the contractor should also record why. A warning is not required where a patient is removed from a list because that patient moves out of the practice area.

2.46 Contractors will be required to explain in writing to patients their specific reasons for taking action for removing them from their list. In certain cases it may be sufficient to say that there has been a breakdown of the doctor–patient relationship. The Contract Regulations also require the contractor to keep a written record of the reasons and the circumstances for removing a patient, and these records should be shown to the PCT if it so requests.

● Retainer scheme

Statement of Financial Entitlement

17.1 This is an established Scheme designed to keep doctors who are not working in general practice in touch with general practice.

Payments in respect of sessions undertaken by members of the Scheme

17.2 Where –
(a) a contractor who is considered as a suitable employer of members of

the Doctors' Retainer Scheme by the Regional Dean employs or engages a member of the Doctors' Retainer Scheme; and

(b) the service sessions for which the member of the Doctors' Retainer Scheme is employed or engaged by that contractor have been arranged by the local Director of Postgraduate GP Education,

the Primary Care Trust (PCT) must pay to that contractor under its GMS contract £57.33 in respect of each full session that the member of the Doctors' Retainer Scheme undertakes for the contractor in any week, up to a maximum of four sessions per week.

Payment conditions

17.3 Payments under this section are to fall due at the end of the month in which the session to which the payment relates takes place. However, the payments, or any part thereof, are only payable if the contractor satisfies the following conditions –

(a) the contractor must inform the PCT of any change to the member of the Doctors' Retainer Scheme's working arrangements that may affect the contractor's entitlement to a payment under this section; and

(b) the contractor must inform the PCT if the doctor in respect of whom the payment is made ceases to be a member of the Doctors' Retainer Scheme, or if it ceases to be considered a suitable employer of members of the Doctors' Retainer Scheme by the Regional Dean.

17.4 If a contractor breaches any of these conditions, the PCT may, in appropriate circumstances, withhold payment of any payment otherwise payable under this Section.

● Returner scheme

Statement of Financial Entitlement

15.1 This is an established Scheme designed to facilitate the return of qualified GPs to the NHS. It is managed locally by Postgraduate Deaneries, each of which has a local Return Co-ordinator responsible for admitting doctors to the Scheme.

Returners' scheme doctor payments

15.2 If a GP performer has been employed or engaged by a contractor, and that GP performer is a doctor who is a member of the Returners' Scheme

(RS), the PCT must, in respect of that doctor, pay to the contractor an annual RS Doctor Payment of £1050.

15.3 If –
(a) a RS doctor's membership of the RS ceases during a year of membership; or
(b) a RS doctor moves to new employer during a year of membership of the RS, or becomes a partner or shareholder in a different contractor, but remains a member,
the amount of the RS Doctor Payment payable to the contractor is to be adjusted as follows. Multiply the amount of the payment otherwise payable by the following fraction: the number of days for which the RS doctor is contracted to work for the contractor during the membership year, divided by 365.

15.4 Payments under this Section to the contractor are to fall due –
(a) if the doctor joins the RS on or after 1 April 2004 on the last day of the month during which the date on which he joins the scheme falls; and
(b) if the doctor joined the RS before 1 April 2004, on the last day of the month during which the anniversary of the date on which he joined the scheme falls.

Conditions attached to Returners' Scheme Doctor Payments and overpayments

15.5 RS Doctor Payments, or any part thereof, are only payable if the following conditions are satisfied –
(a) a contractor who receives a RS Doctor Payment in respect of a GP performer must give that payment to that GP performer –
(i) within one calendar month of it receiving that payment, and
(ii) as an element of the personal income of that doctor, subject to any lawful deduction of income tax, national insurance and superannuation contributions,
once it has secured from the doctor an enforceable undertaking that he will repay to the contractor any amount repayable by the contractor to the PCT under this Section in respect of him;
(b) the contractor must inform the PCT if the GP performer in respect of whom the payment is made ceases to be a member of the RS.

15.6 If a contractor breaches these conditions, the PCT may require repayment of the payment paid, or may withhold payment of any other payment payable to the contractor under this Statement of Financial Entitlement (SFE), to the value of the payment paid.

15.7   If as a result of a doctor leaving the RS, the PCT has paid a larger amount
        to the contractor in respect of that doctor's RS Doctor Payment than the
        amount to which the contractor is entitled under this Section, the PCT
        may require repayment of the excess paid, or may withhold payment of
        any other payment payable to the contractor under this SFE, to the value
        of the excess paid.

15.8   Where, pursuant to paragraph 15.6 or 15.7, a contractor is required to
        repay any or any part of a RS Doctor Payment, the arrangements by
        which the contractor may seek to enforce the undertaking referred to in
        paragraph 15.5(a) as a consequence of that repayment are a matter for
        the contractor.

● Seniority

Statement of Financial Entitlement

13.   Seniority payments

13.1   Seniority payments are payments to a contractor in respect of individual
        GP providers in eligible posts. They reward experience, based on years of
        Reckonable Service.

Eligible posts

13.2   Contractors will only be entitled to a Seniority Payment in respect of a
        GP provider if the GP provider has served for at least 2 years in an
        eligible post, or for an aggregate of 2 years in more than one eligible
        post – part-time and full-time posts counting the same. The first date
        after the end of this 2-year period is the GP provider's qualifying date.
        For the purposes of this Section, a post is an eligible post –
        (a) in case of posts held prior to 1 April 2004, if the post-holder
            provided unrestricted general medical services and was eligible for a
            basic practice allowance under the Red Book; or
        (b) in the case of posts held on or after 1 April 2004, if the post-holder
            performs primary medical services and is –
            (i)   himself a GMS contractor (i.e. a sole practitioner),
            (ii) a partner in a partnership that is a GMS contractor, or
            (iii) a shareholder in a company limited by shares that is a GMS
                  contractor.

Service that is Reckonable Service

13.3   Work shall be counted as Reckonable Service if –

(a) it is clinical service as a doctor within the NHS or service as a doctor in the health care system of another EEA Member State;

(b) it is clinical service as a doctor or service as a medical officer within the prison service or the civil administration (which includes the Home Civil Service) of the United Kingdom, or within the prison service or the civil administration of another EEA Member State;

(c) it is service as a medical officer –

(i) in the armed forces of an EEA Member State (including the United Kingdom) or providing clinical services to those forces in a civilian capacity, or

(ii) in the armed forces under the Crown other than the United Kingdom armed forces or providing clinical services to those forces in a civilian capacity,

if accepted by the PCT or endorsed by the Secretary of State for Health as Reckonable Service;

(d) it is service with the Foreign and Commonwealth Office as a medical officer in a diplomatic mission abroad, if accepted by the PCT or endorsed by the Secretary of State for Health as Reckonable Service; or

(e) it is clinical service outside the United Kingdom that, prior to 1 April 2004, was counted as Reckonable Service for the purposes of a seniority payment under the Red Book.

Calculation of years of Reckonable Service

13.4   Claims in respect of years of service are to be made to the PCT, and should be accompanied by appropriate details, including dates, of relevant clinical service. Where possible, claims should be authenticated from appropriate records, which may in appropriate circumstances include superannuation records. If the PCT is unable to obtain authentication of the service itself, the onus is on the GP provider to provide documentary evidence to support his claim (although payments may be made while verification issues are being resolved). PCTs should only count periods of service in a calculation of a GP provider's Reckonable Service if they are satisfied that there is sufficient evidence to include that period of service in the calculation.

13.5   In determining a GP provider's length of Reckonable Service –

(a) only clinical service is to count towards Reckonable Service;

(b) only clinical service since the date on which the GP provider first became registered (be it temporarily, provisionally, fully or with limited registration) with the General Medical Council, or an equivalent authority in another EEA Member State, is to count towards Reckonable Service, with the exception of Reckonable Service prior to registration that is taken into account by virtue of paragraph 13.3(e);

(c) periods of part-time and full-time working count the same; and

(d) generally, breaks in service are not to count towards Reckonable Service, but periods when doctors were taking leave of absence (i.e. they were absent from a post but had a right of return) due to compulsory national service, maternity leave, paternity leave, adoption leave, parental leave, holiday leave, sick leave or study leave, or because of a secondment elective or similar temporary attachment to a post requiring the provision of clinical services, are to count towards Reckonable Service.

13.6 Claims in respect of service in or on behalf of armed forces pursuant to paragraph 13.3(c) are to be considered in the first instance by the PCT, and should be accompanied by appropriate details, including dates and relevant postings. If the PCT is not satisfied that the service should count towards the GP provider's Reckonable Service as a doctor, it is to put the matter to the Secretary of State for Health, together with any comments it wishes to make.

13.7 Before taking his decision on whether or not to endorse the claim, the Secretary of State will then consult the Ministry of Defence. Generally, the only service that will be endorsed is service where the GP provider undertook clinical or medical duties (whether on military service or in a civilian capacity), and the Secretary of State has received acceptable confirmation of the nature and scope of the duties performed by the GP provider from the relevant authorities.

13.8 Claims in respect of clinical service for or on behalf of diplomatic missions abroad pursuant to paragraph 13.3(d) are to be considered in the first instance by the PCT, and should be accompanied by appropriate details, including dates and relevant postings. If the PCT is not satisfied that the service should count towards the GP provider's Reckonable Service as a doctor, it is to put the matter to the Secretary of State for Health, together with any comments it wishes to make.

13.9 Before taking his decision on whether or not to endorse the claim, the Secretary of State will consult the Foreign and Commonwealth Office. Generally, the only service that will be endorsed is service where the GP provider undertook clinical duties for –

(a) members of the Foreign and Commonwealth Office and their families;

(b) members of the Overseas Development Administration and their families;

(c) members of the British Council and their families;

(d) British residents, official visitors and aid workers;

(e) Commonwealth and EEA Member State official visitors; or

(f) staff and their families of other Commonwealth, EEA Member State or friendly State diplomatic missions,

and the Secretary of State has received acceptable confirmation of the nature and scope of the clinical duties performed by the GP provider from the relevant authorities.

Determination of the relevant dates

13.10 Once a GP provider's years of Reckonable Service have been determined, a determination has to be made of two dates –

(a) the date a GP provider's Reckonable service began, which is the date on which his first period of Reckonable Service started (his "Seniority Date"); and

(b) the GP provider's qualifying date (see paragraph 13.2).

Calculation of the full annual rate of Seniority Payments

13.11 Once a GP provider has reached his qualifying date, he is entitled to a Seniority Payment in respect of his service as a GP provider thereafter. The amount of his Seniority Payment will depend on two factors: his Superannuable Income Fraction, and his number of years of Reckonable Service.

13.12 At the end of each quarter, the PCT is to make an assessment of the Seniority Payments to be made in respect of individual GP providers working for or on behalf of its GMS contractors. If –

(a) a GP provider's Seniority Date is on the first date of that quarter, or falls outside that quarter, his Years of Reckonable Service are the number of complete years since his first Seniority Date, and the full annual rate of the Seniority Payment payable in respect of him is the full annual rate opposite his Years of Reckonable Service in the Table below; and

(b) if the GP provider's Seniority Date falls in that quarter on any date other than the first date of that quarter, the full annual rate of the Seniority Payment payable in respect of him changes on his Seniority Date – and so in respect of that quarter, the full annual rate of the Seniority Payment payable in respect of him is to be calculated as follows–

(i) calculate the daily rate of the full annual rate of payment for the first total of Years of Reckonable Service relevant to him (i.e. divide the annual rate by 365), and multiply that daily rate by the number of days in that quarter before his Seniority Date, and

(ii) calculate the daily rate of the full annual rate of payment for the second total of Years of Reckonable Service relevant to him (i.e. divide the annual rate by 365), and multiply that daily rate by the number of days in that quarter after and including his Seniority Date,

then add the totals produced by the calculations in heads (i) and (ii) together, and multiply by four.

Years of Reckonable Service	Full annual rate of payment per practitioner in 2004/05
0	0
1	0
2	0
3	0
4	0
5	0
6	0
7	600
8	630
9	662
10	695
11	729
12	766
13	804
14	844
15	886
16	3185
17	3344
18	3511
19	3687
20	3871
21	4065
22	6785
23	6989
24	7198
25	7414
26	7637
27	7866
28	8225

Years of Reckonable Service	Full annual rate of payment per practitioner in 2004/05
29	8447
30	8675
31	8909
32	9150
33	9397
34	9651
35	9911
36	10,179
37	10,454
38	10,736
39	11,026
40	11,324
41	11,629
42	11,943
43	12,266
44	12,597
45	12,937
46	13,286
47	13,645

13.13 If, for any GP provider, the full annual rate payable in respect of him, as calculated above, is less than the total amount due to him –

(a) on 31 March 2003 as the full annual rate of his Seniority Payment under the Red Book; plus

(b) on 31 March 2004 as the full annual rate of his Delayed Retirement Scheme payment under the Red Book,

that GP provider is entitled to at least that total amount as the full annual rate of his Seniority Payments in the financial year 2004/05.

Superannuable Income Fractions

13.14 In all cases, the full annual rate of a Seniority Payment for a GP provider is only payable under this SFE in respect of a GP provider who has a Superannuable Income Fraction of at least two-thirds.

13.15 For these purposes, a GP provider's Superannuable Income Fraction is the fraction produced by dividing–

(a) his NHS profits from all sources for the financial year 2004/05, excluding –
  (i) superannuable income which does not appear on his certificate submitted to the PCT in accordance with paragraph 22.10 (i.e. NHS income already superannuated elsewhere), and
  (ii) any amount in respect of Seniority Payments; by
(b) the Average Adjusted Superannuable Income.

13.16 The Average Adjusted Superannuable Income is to be calculated as follows –
  (a) all the NHS profits of the type mentioned in paragraph 13.15(a) of all the GP providers in England who have submitted certificates to a PCT in accordance with paragraph 22.10 by [a date still to be fixed] are to be aggregated; then
  (b) this aggregate is then to be divided by the number of GP providers in respect of which the aggregate was calculated; then
  (c) the total produced by sub-paragraph (b) is to be adjusted to take account of the shift towards less than full-time working. The index by which the amount is to be adjusted is to be the same as the index for the financial year 2004/05 by which the uprating factor for pensions is to be adjusted to take account of the shift towards less than full-time working,
  and the total produced by sub-paragraph (c) is the Average Adjusted Superannuable Income amount for the calculation in paragraph 13.15.

13.17 If the GP provider has a Superannuable Income Fraction of one-third or between one-third and two-thirds, only 60% of the full annual amount payable in respect of a GP provider with his Reckonable Service is payable under this SFE in respect of him. If he has a Superannuable Income Fraction of less than one-third, no Seniority Payment is payable under this SFE in respect of him.

Amounts payable

13.18 Once a GP provider's full annual rate in respect of a quarter has been determined, and any reduction to be made in respect of his Superannuable Income Fraction has been made, the resulting amount is to be divided by four, and that quarterly amount is the Quarterly Superannuation Payment that the PCT must pay to the contractor under his GMS contract in respect of the GP provider.

13.19 If, however, the GP provider's –
  (a) qualifying date falls in that quarter, the quarterly amount is instead to be calculated as follows: the annual amount (taking account of any reduction in accordance with the GP provider's Superannuable

Income Fraction) is to be divided by 365, and then multiplied by the number of days in the quarter after and including his qualifying date; and

(b) retirement date falls in that quarter, the quarterly amount is instead to be calculated as follows: the annual amount (taking account of any reduction in accordance with the GP provider's Superannuable Income Fraction) is to be divided by 365, and then multiplied by the number of days in the quarter prior to the GP provider's retirement date.

13.20 Payment of the Quarterly Seniority Payment is to fall due on the last day of the quarter to which it relates (but see paragraph 21.8).

Conditions attached to payment of Quarterly Seniority Payments

13.21 A Quarterly Seniority Payment, or any part thereof, is only payable to a contractor if the following conditions are satisfied –

(a) if a GP provider receives a Quarterly Seniority Payment from more than one contractor, those payments taken together must not amount to more than one-quarter of the full annual rate of Seniority Payment in respect of him;

(b) the contractor must make available to the PCT any information which the PCT does not have but needs, and the contractor either has or could reasonably be expected to obtain, in order to calculate the payment;

(c) all information provided pursuant to or in accordance with sub-paragraph (a) must be accurate; and

(d) a contractor who receives a Seniority Payment in respect of a GP provider must give that payment to that doctor –

(i) within one calendar month of it receiving that payment, and

(ii) as an element of the personal income of that GP provider subject (in the case of a GP provider who is a shareholder in a contractor that is a company limited by shares) to any lawful deduction of income tax and national insurance.

13.22 If the conditions set out in paragraph 13.21(a) to (c) are breached, the PCT may in appropriate circumstances withhold payment of any or any part of a payment to which the conditions relate that is otherwise payable.

13.23 If a contractor breaches the condition in paragraph 13.21(c), the PCT may require repayment of any payment to which the condition relates, or may withhold payment of any other payment payable to the contractor under this SFE, to the value of the payment to which the condition relates.

Service of notice

See also: Notice/notification

Standard Contract

614. Save as otherwise specified in this Contract or where the context otherwise requires, any notice or other information required or authorised by this Contract to be given by either party to the other party must be in writing and may be served:
    614.1 personally;
    614.2 by post, or in the case of any notice served pursuant to Part 25, registered or recorded delivery post;
    614.3 by telex, or facsimile transmission (the latter confirmed by telex or post);
    614.4 unless the context otherwise requires and except in clause 528, electronic mail; or
    614.5 by any other means which the Primary Care Trust (PCT) specifies by notice to the Contractor.

615. Any notice or other information shall be sent to the address specified in the Contract or such other address as the PCT or the Contractor has notified to the other.

616. Any notice or other information shall be deemed to have been served or given:
    616.1 if it was served personally, at the time of service;
    616.2 if it was served by post, two *working days* after it was posted; and
    616.3 if it was served by telex, electronic mail or facsimile transmission, if sent during *normal hours* then at the time of transmission and if sent outside *normal hours* then on the following *working day*.

617. Where notice or other information is not given or sent in accordance with clauses 614 to 616, such notice or other information is invalid unless the person receiving it elects, in writing, to treat it as valid.

Severence

Standard Contract

611. Subject to clauses 612 and 613, if any term of this Contract, other than a *mandatory term*, is held to be invalid, illegal or unenforceable by any

court, tribunal or other competent authority, such term shall, to the extent required, be deemed to be deleted from this Contract and shall not affect the validity, lawfulness or enforceability of any other terms of the Contract.

612.   If, in the reasonable opinion of either party, the effect of such a deletion is to undermine the purpose of the Contract or materially prejudice the position of either party, the parties shall negotiate in good faith in order to agree a suitable alternative term to replace the deleted term or a suitable amendment to the Contract.

613.   If the parties are unable to reach agreement as to the suitable alternative term or amendment within a reasonable period of commencement of the negotiations, then the parties may refer the dispute for determination in accordance with the *NHS dispute resolution procedure* set out in clauses 520 to 527.

Sickness locum costs

Statement of Financial Entitlement

10.   Payments for locums covering sickness leave

10.1   Employees of contractors will, if they qualify for it, be entitled to statutory sick pay for 28 weeks of absence on account of sickness in any 3 years. The rights of partners in partnership agreements to paid sickness leave is a matter for their partnership agreement.

10.2   If an employee or partner who takes any sickness leave is a performer under a GMS contract, the contractor may need to employ a locum to maintain the level of services that it normally provides. Even if the Primary Care Trust (PCT) is not directed in this Statement of Financial Entitlement (SFE) to pay for such cover, it may do so as a matter of discretion – and indeed, it may also provide locum support for performers who are returning from sickness leave or for those who are at risk of needing to go on sickness leave. It should in particular consider exercising its discretion –
(a)   where there is an unusually high rate of sickness in the area where the performer performs services; or
(b)   to support contractors in rural areas where the distances involved in making home visits make it impracticable for a GP performer returning from sickness leave to assume responsibility for the same number of patients for which he previously had responsibility.

Entitlement to payments for covering sickness leave

10.3   In any case where a contractor actually and necessarily engages a locum (or more than one such person) to cover for the absence of a GP performer on sickness leave, and –
(a) the leave of absence is for more than 1 week;
(b) if the performer on leave is employed by the contractor, the contractor must –
   (i) be required to pay statutory sick pay to that performer, or
   (ii) be required to pay the performer on leave his full salary during absences on sick leave under his contract of employment;
(c) if the GP performer's absence is as a result of an accident, the contractor must be unable to claim any compensation from whoever caused the accident towards meeting the cost of engaging a locum to cover for the GP performer during the performer's absence. But if such compensation is payable, the PCT may loan the contractor the cost of the locum, on the condition that the loan is repaid when the compensation is paid unless –
   (i) no part of the compensation paid is referable to the cost of the locum, in which case the loan is to be considered a reimbursement by the PCT of the costs of the locum which is subject to the following provisions of this Section, or
   (ii) only part of the compensation paid is referable to the cost of the locum, in which case the liability to repay shall be proportionate to the extent to which the claim for full reimbursement of the costs of the locum was successful;
(d) the locum is not a partner or shareholder in the contractor, or already an employee of the contractor, unless the performer on leave is a job-sharer; and
(e) the contractor is not already claiming another payment for locum cover in respect of the performer on leave pursuant to this Part,
then subject to the following provisions of this Section, the PCT must provide financial assistance to the contractor under its GMS contract in respect of the cost of engaging that locum (which may or may not be the maximum amount payable, as set out in paragraph 10.5).

10.4   It is for the PCT to determine whether or not it was in fact necessary to engage the locum, or to continue to engage the locum, but it is to have regard to the following principles –
(a) it should not normally be considered necessary if the PCT has offered to provide the locum cover itself and the contractor has refused that offer without good reason;
(b) it should not normally be considered necessary to employ a locum if the performer on leave had a right to return but that right has been extinguished; and

(c) it should not normally be considered necessary to employ a locum if the contractor has engaged a new employee or partner to perform the duties of the performer on leave and it is not carrying a vacancy in respect of another position which the performer on leave will fill on his return;

(d) it should not normally be considered necessary for a contractor with two or more GP performers to engage a locum to replace a GP performer, unless the absence of the performer on leave leaves each of the other GP performers *(not including members of the Doctor's Retainer Scheme)* with average numbers of patients as follows –

Absences lasting or expected to last	Full-time GP	Three-quarter time GP	Half-time GP
Not more than 2 weeks	3600+ patients	2700+ patients	1800+ patients
Not more than 6 weeks	3100+ patients	2325+ patients	1550+ patients
Longer than 6 weeks	2700+ patients	2025+ patients	1350+ patients

(e) it should normally be considered necessary that a single-handed GP performer or a job-sharer fulfilling the role of a single-handed GP performer will need to be replaced, if they are on sickness leave, by a locum.

Ceilings on the amounts payable

10.5 The maximum amount payable under this Section by the PCT in respect of locum cover for a GP performer is £948.33 per week.

10.6 However, in any 12-month period, the maximum periods in respect of which payments under this Section are payable in relation to a particular GP performer are –
(a) 6 months for the full amount of the sum that the PCT has determined is payable; and
(b) a further 6 months for half the full amount of the sum the PCT initially determined was payable.

Payment arrangements

10.7 The contractor is to submit to the PCT claims for costs actually incurred during a month at the end of that month, and any amount payable is to fall due on the same day of the following month that the contractor's Payable global sum monthly payment (GSMP) falls due.

Statutory requirements – minimum
Guidance

Conditions attached to the amounts payable

10.8 Payments under this Section, or any part thereof, are only payable if the following conditions are satisfied –

(a) the contractor must obtain the prior agreement of the PCT to the engagement of the locum (but its request to do so must be determined as quickly as possible by the PCT), including agreement as to the amount that is to be paid for the locum cover;

(b) the contractor must, without delay, supply the PCT with medical certificates in respect of each period of absence for which a request for assistance with payment for locum cover is being made;

(c) the contractor must, on request, provide the PCT with written records demonstrating the actual cost to it of the locum cover;

(d) once the locum arrangements are in place, the contractor must inform the PCT –

   (i) if there is to be any change to the locum arrangements, or

   (ii) if, for any other reason, there is to be a change to the contractor's arrangements for performing the duties of the performer on leave, at which point the PCT is to determine whether it still considers the locum cover necessary;

(e) if the locum arrangements are in respect of a performer on leave who is or was entitled to statutory sick pay, the contractor must inform the PCT immediately if it stops paying statutory sick pay to that employee;

(f) the performer on leave must not engage in conduct that is prejudicial to his recovery; and

(g) the performer on leave must not be performing clinical services for any other person, unless under medical direction and with the approval of the PCT.

10.9 If any of these conditions are breached, the PCT may, in appropriate circumstances, withhold payment of any sum otherwise payable under this Section.

Statutory requirements – minimum

Guidance

3.2 The contract regulations set out the full list of statutory requirements for contractors. Table 10 summarises those that most directly relate to minimum quality standards.

Table 10	**Statutory requirements relating to quality**
Subject area	**Contractor requirement**
1. Clinical governance	Must have: • effective system of clinical governance in place • named clinical governance lead who is performing or managing services
2. General skill and care	Must carry out its obligations under the contract with "reasonable skill and care"
3. Complaints	Must: • operate a complaints procedure in accordance with the NHS complaints procedure • provide the PCT with information on the number, subject matter and handling of complaints
4. Professional indemnity insurance	Must hold adequate insurance against liability arising from negligent performance of clinical services
5. Qualification and skills of performers	Must ensure: • performers (i) are suitably qualified, (ii) are competent, (iii) have the necessary clinical experience and training, (iv) are registered on the Primary Care Performers List (where appropriate) • performers have arrangements in place to maintain and update skills and knowledge • GP performers participate in appraisal • compliance with National Clinical Assessment Authority (NCAA) assessment when requested by PCT
6. Premises	Must be (i) suitable for the delivery of services, (ii) sufficient to meet the reasonable needs of patients and (iii) comply with the requirements of the Disability Discrimination Act
7. Record keeping	Must keep adequate patient records and ensure patient lists are kept up to date. Where records are computerised: • systems used must be RFA99 compliant • security measures must be enabled

Continued

Table 10 – continued	
Subject area	Contractor requirement
	• contractor must have regard to guidelines for GP electronic patient records
	Must have named Caldicott Guardian, who leads on the practices and procedures for handling the confidentiality of patient records.
8. Practice leaflet	Must: • compile a practice leaflet in line with regulations • review it at least every 12 months and ensure it is accurate • make a copy available to its patients and prospective patients
9. Infection control	Must have effective arrangements in place for appropriate infection control and decontamination

3.3 This list is not exhaustive. GMS providers must also comply with all other relevant legislation, e.g. that covering employment, discrimination, data protection, child protection, medicines and health and safety matters. Arrangements for dealing with contract breaches are set out in chapter 6 on contracting process.

● Study leave payments

Statement of Financial Entitlement

12.1 GP performers may be entitled to take Prolonged Study Leave, and in these circumstances, the contractor for whom they have been providing services under its GMS contract may be entitled to two payments –
(a) an educational allowance, to be forwarded to the GP performer taking Prolonged Study Leave; and
(b) the cost of, or a contribution towards the cost of, locum cover.

Types of study in respect of which prolonged study leave may be taken

12.2   Payments may only be made under this Section in respect of Prolonged Study Leave taken by a GP performer where –
   (a) the study leave is for at least 10 weeks but not more than 12 months;
   (b) the educational aspects of the study leave have been approved by the local Director of Postgraduate GP Education, having regard to any guidance on Prolonged Study Leave that Directors of Postgraduate GP Education have agreed nationally; and
   (c) the PCT has determined that the payments to the contractor under this Section in respect of the Prolonged Study Leave are affordable, having regard to the budgetary targets it has set for itself for the financial year 2004/05.

The educational allowance payment

12.3   Where the criteria set out in paragraph 12.2 are met, in respect of each week for which the GP performer is on Prolonged Study Leave, the Primary Care Trust (PCT) must pay the contractor an Educational Allowance Payment of £129.50 per week, subject to the condition that where the contractor is aware of any change in circumstances that may affect its entitlement to the Educational Allowance Payment, it notifies the PCT of that change in circumstances.

12.4   If the contractor breaches the condition set out in paragraph 12.3, the PCT may, in appropriate circumstances, withhold payment of any or any part of an Educational Allowance Payment that is otherwise payable.

Locum cover in respect of doctors on Prolonged Study Leave

12.5   In any case where a contractor actually and necessarily engages a locum (or more than one such person) to cover for the absence of a GP performer on Prolonged Study Leave, then subject to the following provisions of this Section, the PCT must provide financial assistance to the contractor under its GMS contract in respect of the cost of engaging that locum (which may or may not be the maximum amount payable, as set out in paragraph 12.7).

12.6   It is for the PCT to determine whether or not it was in fact necessary to engage the locum, or to continue to engage the locum, but it is to have regard to the following principles –
   (a) it should not normally be considered necessary to employ a locum if the PCT has offered to provide the locum cover itself and the contractor has refused that offer without good reason;

(b) it should not normally be considered necessary to employ a locum if the performer on leave had a right to return but that right has been extinguished; and

(c) it should not normally be considered necessary to employ a locum if the contractor has engaged a new employee or partner to perform the duties of the performer on leave and it is not carrying a vacancy in respect of another position which the performer on leave will fill on his return.

12.7   The maximum amount payable under this Section by the PCT in respect of locum cover for a GP performer is £948.33 per week.

Payment arrangements

12.8   The contractor is to submit to the PCT claims for costs actually incurred during a month at the end of that month, and any amount payable is to fall due on the same day of the following month that the contractor's Payable GSMP falls due.

Conditions attached to the amounts payable

12.9   Payments in respect of locum cover under this Section, or any part thereof, are only payable if the following conditions are satisfied –

(a) the contractor must obtain the prior agreement of the PCT to the engagement of the locum (but its request to do so must be determined as quickly as possible by the PCT), including agreement as to the amount that is to be paid for the locum cover;

(b) the locum must not be a partner or shareholder in the contractor, or already an employee of the contractor, unless the performer on leave is a job-sharer;

(c) the contractor must, on request, provide the PCT with written records demonstrating the actual cost to it of the locum cover; and

(d) once the locum arrangements are in place, the contractor must inform the PCT –

(i) if there is to be any change to the locum arrangements, or

(ii) if, for any other reason, there is to be a change to the contractor's arrangements for performing the duties of the performer on leave,

at which point the PCT is to determine whether it still considers the locum cover necessary.

12.10 If any of these conditions are breached, the PCT may, in appropriate circumstances, withhold payment of any sum in respect of locum cover otherwise payable under this Section.

Sub-contracting

Regulations

69. Sub-contracting of clinical matters

(1) Subject to sub-paragraph (2), the contractor shall not sub-contract any of its rights or duties under the contract in relation to clinical matters unless –
   (a) in all cases, including those which fall within paragraph 70, it has taken reasonable steps to satisfy itself that –
      (i) it is reasonable in all the circumstances; and
      (ii) that person is qualified and competent to provide the service; and
   (b) except in cases which fall within paragraph 70, it has notified the PCT in writing of its intention to sub-contract as soon as reasonably practicable before the date on which the proposed sub-contract is intended to come into force.

(2) Sub-paragraph (1)(b) shall not apply to a contract for services with a health care professional for the provision by that professional personally of clinical services.

(3) The notification referred to in sub-paragraph (1)(b) shall include –
   (a) the name and address of the proposed sub-contractor;
   (b) the duration of the proposed sub-contract;
   (c) the services to be covered; and
   (d) the address of any premises to be used for the provision of services.

(4) Following receipt of a notice in accordance with sub-paragraph (1)(b), the PCT may request such further information relating to the proposed sub-contract as appears to it to be reasonable and the contractor shall supply such information promptly.

(5) The contractor shall not proceed with the sub-contract or, if it has already taken effect, shall take appropriate steps to terminate it, where, within 28 days of receipt of the notice referred to in sub-paragraph (1)(b), the PCT has served notice of objection to the sub-contract on the grounds that –
   (a) the sub-contract would –
      (i) put at serious risk the safety of the contractor's patients, or
      (ii) put the Trust at risk of material financial loss; or
   (b) the sub-contractor would be unable to meet the contractor's obligations under the contract.

(6)   Where the PCT objects to a proposed sub-contract in accordance with sub-paragraph (5), it shall include with the notice of objection a statement in writing of the reasons for its objection.

(7)   Sub-paragraphs (1) and (3) to (6) shall also apply in relation to any renewal or material variation of a sub-contract in relation to clinical matters.

(8)   Where a PCT does not object to a proposed sub-contract under paragraph (5), the parties to the contract shall be deemed to have agreed a variation of the contract which has the effect of adding to the list of practice premises any premises whose address was notified to it under sub-paragraph (3)(d) and paragraph 104(1) shall not apply.

(9)   A contract with a sub-contractor must prohibit the sub-contractor from sub-contracting the clinical services it has agreed with the contractor to provide.

70.   Sub-contracting of out-of-hours services

(1)   A contractor shall not, otherwise than in accordance with the written approval of the PCT, sub-contract all or part of its duty to provide out-of-hours services to any person other than those listed in sub-paragraph (2) other than on a short-term occasional basis.

(2)   The persons referred to in sub-paragraph (1) are –
(a) a person who holds a general medical services contract with a PCT which includes out-of-hours services;
(b) a section 28C provider who is required to provide the equivalent of essential services to his patients during all or part of the out-of-hours period;
(c) a health care professional, not falling within paragraph (a) or (b), who is to provide the out-of-hours services personally under a contract for services; or
(d) a group of medical practitioners, whether in partnership or not, who provide out-of-hours services for each other under informal rota arrangements.

(3)   An application for approval under sub-paragraph (1) shall be made by the contractor in writing to the PCT and shall state –
(a) the name and address of the proposed sub-contractor;
(b) the address of any premises to be used for the provision of services;
(c) the duration of the proposed sub-contract;
(d) the services to be covered by the arrangement; and
(e) how it is proposed that the sub-contractor will meet the contractor's obligations under the contract in respect of the services covered by the arrangement.

(4) Within 7 days of receipt of an application under sub-paragraph (3), a PCT may request such further information relating to the proposed arrangements as seem to it to be reasonable.

(5) Within 28 days of receipt of an application which meets the requirements specified in sub-paragraph (3) or the further information requested under sub-paragraph (4) (whichever is the later), the PCT shall –
(a) approve the application;
(b) approve the application with conditions; or (c) refuse the application.

(6) The PCT shall not refuse the application if it is satisfied that the proposed arrangement will, in respect of the services to be covered, enable the contractor to meet satisfactorily its obligations under the contract and will not –
(a) put at serious risk the safety of the contractor's patients; or
(b) put the Trust at risk of material financial loss.

(7) The PCT shall inform the contractor by notice in writing of its decision on the application and, where it refuses an application, it shall include in the notice a statement of the reasons for its refusal.

(8) Where a PCT approves an application under this paragraph the parties to the contract shall be deemed to have agreed a variation of the contract which has the effect of adding to the list of practice premises, for the purposes of the provision of services in accordance with that application, any premises whose address was notified to it under sub-paragraph (3)(b) and paragraph 104(1) shall not apply.

(9) Sub-paragraphs (1) to (8) shall also apply in relation to any renewal or material variation of a sub-contract in relation to out-of-hours services.

(10) A contract with a sub-contractor must prohibit the sub-contractor from sub-contracting the out-of-hours services it has agreed with the contractor to provide.

71. Withdrawal and variation of approval under paragraph 70

(1) Without prejudice to any other remedies which it may have under the contract, where a PCT has approved an application made under paragraph 70(3) it shall, subject to paragraph 72, be entitled to serve notice on the contractor withdrawing or varying that approval, from a date specified in the notice, if it is no longer satisfied that the proposed arrangement will enable the contractor to meet satisfactorily its obligations under the contract.

(2) The date specified in the notice shall be such as appears reasonable in all the circumstances to the PCT.

(3)   The notice referred to in sub-paragraph (1) shall take effect on whichever
is the later of –
(a) the date specified in the notice; or
(b) (if applicable) the date of the final determination of the NHS dispute
resolution procedure (or any court proceedings) relating to the
notice in favour of the PCT.

72.

(1)   Without prejudice to any other remedies which it may have under the
contract, where a PCT has approved an application made under
paragraph 70(3) it shall be entitled to serve notice on the contractor
withdrawing or varying that approval with immediate effect if –
(a) it is no longer satisfied that the proposed arrangement will enable
the contractor to meet satisfactorily its obligations under the
contract; and
(b) it is satisfied that immediate withdrawal or variation is necessary to
protect the safety of the contractor's patients.

(2)   An immediate withdrawal of approval under sub-paragraph (1) shall take
effect on the date on which the notice referred to in that sub-paragraph is
received by the contractor.

Standard Contract

Sub-contracting of clinical matters

369.   Subject to clause 370, the Contractor shall not sub-contract any of its
rights or duties under the Contract unless-
369.1 in all cases, including those which fall within clauses 378 to 392 it
has taken reasonable steps to satisfy itself that it is reasonable in all
the circumstances and that person is qualified and competent to
provide the service; and
369.2 except in cases which fall within clauses 378 to 392, it has notified
the PCT in writing of its intention to sub-contract as soon as
reasonably practicable before the date on which the proposed sub-
contract is intended to come into force.

370.   Clause 369.2 shall not apply to a contract for services with a *health care
professional* for the provision by that professional personally of clinical
services.

371.   The notification referred to in clause 369.2 shall include –
371.1 the name and address of the proposed sub-contractor;
371.2 the duration of the proposed sub-contract;

371.3 the services to be covered; and
371.4 the address of any premises to be used for the provision of services.

372. Following receipt of a notice in accordance with clause 369.2, the PCT may request such further information relating to the proposed sub-contract as appears to it to be reasonable and the Contractor shall supply such information promptly.

373. The Contractor shall not proceed with the sub-contract or, if it has already taken effect, shall take steps to terminate it, where, within 28 days of the notice referred to in clause 369.2, the PCT has served a notice of objection to the sub-contract on the grounds that –
373.1 the sub-contract would –
    (a) put at serious risk the safety of the Contractor's *patients*, or
    (b) put the PCT at risk of material financial loss; or
373.2 the sub-contractor would be unable to meet the Contractor's obligations under the contract.

374. Where the PCT objects to a proposed sub-contract in accordance with clause 373, it shall include with the notice of objection a statement in writing of the reasons for its objection.

375. Clauses 369, 371 to 374 shall also apply in relation to any renewal or material variation of a sub-contract in relation to clinical matters.

376. Where the PCT does not object to a proposed sub-contract under clause 373, the parties to the Contract shall be deemed to have agreed to a variation of the contract which has the effect of adding to the list of *practice premises* any premises whose address was notified to it under clause 371.4 and clause 528 shall not apply.

377. A contract with a sub-contractor must prohibit the sub-contractor from sub-contracting the clinical services it has agreed with the Contractor to provide.

Sub-contracting of out-of-hours services[65]

378. The Contractor shall not, otherwise than in accordance with the written approval of the PCT, sub-contract all or part of its duty to provide *out-of-hours services* to any person other than those listed in clause 379 other than on a short-term occasional basis.

---

65 Clauses 378 to 392 only need to be included in the Contract if the Contractor is providing *out-of-hours services* under the Contract. Articles 21 and 22 of *the Transitional Order* are also relevant to these clauses.

379. The persons referred to in clause 378 are –
   379.1 a person who holds a *general medical services contract* or *a default contract* with a PCT which includes *out-of-hours services*;
   379.2 a person who is a party to contractual arrangements made under article 15 of *the Transitional Order*;
   379.3 a *section 28C provider* who is required to provide the equivalent of *essential services* to his patients during all or part of the *out-of-hours period*;
   379.4 a *health care professional*, not falling within clause 379.1 to 379.3, who is to provide the *out-of-hours* services personally under a contract for services; or
   379.5 a group of medical practitioners, whether in partnership or not, who provide *out-of-hours services* for each other under informal rota arrangements.

380. An application for approval under clause 378 shall be made by the Contractor in writing to the PCT and shall state –
   380.1 the name and address of the proposed sub-contractor;
   380.2 the address of any premises to be used for the provision of services;
   380.3 the duration of the proposed sub-contract;
   380.4 the services to be covered by the arrangement; and
   380.5 how it is proposed that the sub-contractor will meet the Contractor's obligations under the Contract in respect of the services covered by the arrangement.

381. Within 7 days of receipt of an application under clause 380, the PCT may request such further information relating to the proposed arrangements as seem to it to be reasonable.

382. Within 28 days of receipt of an application which meets the requirements of clause 380 or the further information requested under clause 381 (whichever is the later), the PCT shall –
   382.1 approve the application;
   382.2 approve the application with conditions; or
   382.3 refuse the application.

383. The PCT shall not refuse the application if it is satisfied that the proposed arrangement will, in respect of the services to be covered, enable the Contractor to meet satisfactorily its obligations under the Contract and will not –
   383.1 put at serious risk the safety of the Contractor's patients; or
   383.2 put the PCT at risk of material financial loss.

384. The PCT shall inform the Contractor by notice in writing of its decision on the application and, where it refuses an application, it shall include in the notice a statement of the reasons for its refusal.

385. Where the PCT approves an application pursuant to clause 382 the parties to the Contract shall be deemed to have agreed a variation of the contract which has the effect of adding to the list of *practice premises*, for the purposes of the provision of services in accordance with that application, any premises whose address was notified to it under clause 380.20 and clause 528 shall not apply.

386. Clauses 378 to 385 shall also apply in relation to any renewal or material variation of a sub-contract in relation to *out-of-hours services*.

387. A contract with a sub-contractor must prohibit the sub-contractor from sub-contracting the *out-of-hours services* it has agreed with the Contractor to provide.

388. Without prejudice to any other remedies which it may have under the Contract, where the PCT has approved an application made under clause 380 it shall, subject to clauses 391 and 392, be entitled to serve notice on the Contractor withdrawing or varying that approval from a date specified in the notice if it is no longer satisfied that the proposed arrangement will enable the Contractor to meet satisfactorily its obligations under the Contract.

389. The date specified pursuant to clause 388 shall be such as appears reasonable in all the circumstances to the PCT.

390. The notice referred to in clause 388 shall take effect on whichever is the later of –
    390.1 the date specified in the notice; or
    390.2 the date on which any dispute relating to the notice is finally determined.

391. Without prejudice to any other remedies which it may have under the Contract, where the PCT has approved an application made under clause 378 it shall be entitled to serve notice on the Contractor withdrawing or varying that approval with immediate effect if –
    391.1 it is no longer satisfied that the proposed arrangement will enable the Contractor to meet satisfactorily its obligations under the Contract; and
    391.2 it is satisfied that immediate withdrawal or variation is necessary to protect the safety of the Contractor's patients.

392. An immediate withdrawal of approval under clause 391 shall take effect on the date on which the notice referred to in that clause is received by the Contractor.

Temporary arrangements for transfer of obligations and liabilities in relation to certain *out-of-hours services*[66]

393.   Where the Contractor is required to provide *out-of-hours services* under the Contract pursuant to regulation 30 or 31 of *the Regulations*, it may, with the approval of the PCT, make an arrangement with one of the persons specified in clause 369, as if regulations 1 to 11 of the *Out-of-hours* Regulations (subject to the modifications in clause 397) were still in force.

394.   Any arrangement made pursuant to clause 393 shall cease to have effect on 1 January 2005.

395.   An arrangement made in accordance with clause 393 shall, for so long as it continues, or is not suspended under clause 423, relieve the Contractor of –
395.1 its obligations to provide *out-of-hours services* pursuant to the Contract; and
395.2 all liabilities under the Contract in respect of those services.

396.   The persons referred to in clause 393 are –
396.1 an *accredited service provider*; or
396.2 a person who holds a *general medical services contract* or a *default contract* with a PCT which includes the provision of *out-of-hours services*, or a person who is a party to contractual arrangements made under article 15 of *the Transitional Order*.

397.   The modifications referred to in clause 393 are –
397.1 as if *out-of-hours period* had the meaning given in regulation 2 of the regulations;
397.2 as if the requirements relating to an assessing authority in regulation 4(5) to (8) did not apply in cases where, in the opinion of the accrediting authority, it was appropriate and safe to dispense with them;
397.3 as if the reference to a medical practitioner in regulation 11(2)(c) was a reference to the Contractor;
397.4 as if the reference to section 44 in regulation 11(2)(d) was to section 45A of *the Act*; and
397.5 as if the reference to a medical list or supplementary list in paragraph 7 of the Schedule was to a *medical performers list* and the words "or he is named in an agreement under section 2 of the 1997 Act as a performer of personal medical services" were omitted.

---

66   Clauses 393 to 424 only need to be included in the Contract if the Contractor is providing *out-of-hours services* under the Contract pursuant to Regulations 30 or 31 of *the Regulations*: see Schedule 7 to *the Regulations*. Articles 21 and 22 of the Transitional Order are also relevant to these clauses.

398. The Contractor may make more than one *out-of-hours arrangement* and may do so (for example) with different *transferee doctors* or *accredited service providers* and in respect of different patients, different times and different parts of its *practice area*.

399. The Contractor may retain responsibility for, or make separate *out-of-hours arrangements* in respect of, the provision to any patients of *maternity medical services* during the *out-of-hours period* which the Contractor is required to provide pursuant to regulation 30 or 31 and any separate *out-of-hours arrangements* it makes may encompass all or any part of the *maternity medical services* it provides.

400. Nothing in clauses 393 to 399 shall prevent the Contractor from retaining or resuming its obligations in relation to named patients.

Application for approval of an *out-of-hours arrangement*

401. An application to the PCT for approval of an *out-of-hours arrangement* shall be made in writing and shall state –
   401.1 the name and address of the *accredited service provider* or the proposed *transferee doctor*;
   401.2 the periods during which the Contractor's obligations under the Contract are to be transferred;
   401.3 how the *accredited service provider* or proposed *transferee doctor* intends to meet the Contractor's obligations during the periods specified in clause 401.2;
   401.4 the arrangements for the transfer of the Contractor's obligations under the Contract to and from the *accredited service provider* or *transferee doctor* at the beginning and end of the period specified under clause 401.2;
   401.5 whether the proposed arrangement includes the Contractor's obligations in respect of *maternity medical services*; and
   401.6 how long the proposed arrangements are intended to last and the circumstances in which the Contractor's obligations under the Contract during the periods specified in clause 401.2 would revert to it.

402. The PCT shall determine the application before the end of the period of 28 days beginning with the day on which the PCT received it.

403. The PCT shall grant approval to a proposed *out-of-hours arrangement* if it is satisfied –
   403.1 having regard to the overall provision of primary medical services provided in the *out-of-hours period* in its area, that the arrangement is reasonable and will contribute to the efficient provision of such services in the area;

403.2 having regard, in particular, to the interests of the Contractor's patients, that the arrangement is reasonable;

403.3 having regard, in particular, to all reasonably foreseeable circumstances that the arrangement is practicable and will work satisfactorily;

403.4 that any arrangement with a person referred to in clause 396.2 will be of an equivalent standard to an arrangement with a person referred to in clause 396.1;

403.5 that in the case of an arrangement with a person referred to in clause 396.1, the practice premises are within the geographical area in respect of which approval is given under regulation 5 of the *Out-of-hours Regulations*;

403.6 that it will be clear to the Contractor's patients how to seek primary medical services during the *out-of-hours period*;

403.7 where *maternity medical services* are to be provided under the *out-of-hours arrangement*, that they will be performed by a medical practitioner who has such medical experience and training as are necessary to enable him properly to perform such services; and

403.8 that if the arrangement comes to an end, the Contractor has in place proper arrangements for the immediate resumption of its responsibilities,

and shall not refuse to grant approval without first consulting the *Local Medical Committee* (if any) for its area.

404. The PCT shall give notice to the Contractor of its determination and, where it refuses an application, it shall send to the Contractor a statement in writing of the reasons for its determination.

405. If the Contractor wishes to refer the matter in accordance with the *NHS dispute resolution procedure*, it must do so before the end of the period of 30 days beginning with the day on which the PCT's notification under clause 404 was sent.

Effect of approval of an arrangement where the Contractor is the *transferee doctor*

406. If the Contractor acts as a *transferee doctor*, in accordance with an *out-of-hours arrangement* approved by the PCT in relation to another contractor (including a contractor who is a party to a *default contract*), the PCT and the Contractor shall be deemed to have agreed a variation of the Contract which has the effect of including in it, from the date on which the *out-of-hours arrangement* commences, and for so long as that arrangement is not suspended or terminated, the services covered by that arrangement, and clause 528 shall not apply.

Review of approval

407. Where it appears to the PCT that it may no longer be satisfied of any of the matters referred to in clauses 403.1 to 403.8, it may give notice to the Contractor that it proposes to review its approval of the *out-of-hours arrangement*.

408. On any review under clause 407, the PCT shall allow the Contractor a period of 30 days, beginning with the day on which the PCT sent the notice, within which to make representations in writing to the PCT.

409. After considering representations made in accordance with clause 408, the PCT may determine to –
409.1 continue its approval,
409.2 withdraw its approval following a period of notice; or
409.3 if it appears to the PCT that it is necessary in the interests of the Contractor's patients, withdraw its approval immediately.

410. Except in the case of an immediate withdrawal of approval, the PCT shall not withdraw its approval without first consulting the *Local Medical Committee* (if any) for its area.

411. The PCT shall give notice to the Contractor of its determination under clause 409.

412. Where the PCT withdraws its approval, whether immediately or on notice, its shall include with the notice a statement in writing of the reasons for its determination.

413. If the Contractor wishes to refer the matter in accordance with the *NHS dispute resolution procedure*, it must do so before the end of 30 days beginning with the day on which the PCT's notification under clause 411 was sent.

414. Where the PCT determines to withdraw its approval following a period of notice, the withdrawal shall take effect at the end of the period of 2 months beginning with –
414.1 the date on which the notice referred to in clause 412 was sent, or
414.2 where there has been a dispute which has been referred under the *NHS dispute resolution procedure* and the dispute is determined in favour of withdrawal, the date on which the Contractor receives notice of the determination.

415. Where the PCT determines to withdraw its approval immediately, the withdrawal shall take effect on the day on which the notice referred to in clause 411 is received by the Contractor.

Suspension of approval

416. Where the PCT suspends its approval of an *accredited service provider* under regulation 9 of the *Out-of-Hours Regulations*, or receives notice suspension of such approval under regulation 11 of those Regulations, it shall forthwith suspend its approval of any *out-of-hours arrangement* made by the Contractor with that *accredited service provider*.

417. A suspension of approval under clause 416 shall take effect on the day on which the Contractor receives notice of suspension of approval of the *accredited service provider* under regulation 11 of the *Out-of-Hours Regulations*.

Immediate withdrawal of approval other than following review

418. The PCT shall withdraw its approval of an *out-of-hours arrangement* immediately –
    418.1 in the case of an arrangement with a person referred to in clause 396.1, if it withdraws its approval of the *accredited service provider* under regulation 8 of the *Out-of-Hours Regulations* or receives notice of withdrawal of such approval under regulation 11 of those Regulations;
    418.2 in the case of an arrangement with a person referred to in clause 396.2, if the person with whom it is made ceases to hold a *general medical services contract* or a *default contract* with the PCT which includes the provision of *out-of-hours services*, or ceases to be a party to contractual arrangements made under article 15 of *the Transitional Order*; or
    418.3 where, without any review having taken place under clauses 407 to 415, it appears to the PCT that it is necessary in the interests of the Contractor's patients to withdraw its approval immediately.

419. The PCT shall give notice to the Contractor of a withdrawal of approval under clause 418.2 or 418.3 and shall include with the notice a statement in writing of the reasons for its determination.

420. An immediate withdrawal of approval under clause 418 shall take effect –
    420.1 in the case of a withdrawal under clause 418.1, on the day on which the Contractor receives notice of withdrawal of approval of the *accredited service provider* under regulation 11 of the *Out-of-Hours Regulations*; or
    420.2 in the case of a withdrawal under clauses 418.2 or 418.3, on the day on which the notice referred to in clause 419 is received by the Contractor.

421. The PCT shall notify the *Local Medical Committee* (if any) for its area of a withdrawal of approval under clause 418.3.

422. If the Contractor wishes to refer a withdrawal of approval under clause 418.3 in accordance with the *NHS dispute resolution procedure*, it must do so before the end of the period of 30 days beginning with the day on which the PCT's notification under clause 419 was sent.

Suspension or termination of an *out-of-hours arrangement*

423. The Contractor shall suspend an arrangement with an *accredited service provider* under clause 393 on receipt of the notice of suspension of approval of that provider under regulation 11 of the *Out-of-Hours Regulations*.

424. The Contractor shall terminate an *out-of-hours arrangement* made under clause 393 with effect from the date of the taking effect of the withdrawal of the PCT's approval of that arrangement under clauses 407 to 415 or clauses 418 to 422.

● Superannuation

Statement of Financial Entitlement

PCTs' responsibilities in respect of contractors', employer's and employee's superannuation contributions

22.1 Under the NHS Pension Scheme Regulations, contractors are responsible for paying the employer's superannuation contributions of practice staff who are members of the NHS Pension Scheme, and collecting and forwarding to the NHS Pensions Agency both employer's and employee's superannuation contributions in respect of their practice staff.

22.2 Employer's superannuation contributions in respect of GP Registrars – who are subject to separate funding arrangements from those in respect of other GP performers – are the responsibility of Primary Care Trusts (PCTs), which act as their employer for superannuation purposes.

22.3 PCTs are also responsible for paying the employer's superannuation contributions of a contractor's members of the NHS Pension Scheme who are –
(a) GP performers who are not GP Registrars;

(b) non-practising GP partners and non-GP partners, if the contractor is a partnership; or

(c) non-practising GP shareholders and non-GP shareholders, if the contractor is a company limited by shares,

in respect of their NHS superannuable profits from all sources – unless superannuated for the purposes of the NHS Pension Scheme elsewhere – whether or not these earnings are derived from payments under this statement of financial entitlement (SFE). In this Section, the three categories of people set out in sub-paragraphs (a) to (c) are referred as "partner/GPs".

22.4 The cost of paying partner/GPs' employer's and employee's superannuation contributions relating to the income of partner/GPs which is derived from the revenue of a GMS contract has been or will be included in the national calculations of the levels of the payments in respect of services set out in this SFE. It is also to be assumed that –

(a) any other arrangements that the contractor has entered into to provide medical services to the NHS, whether or not under its GMS contract, will have included provision for all the payable superannuation contributions in respect of its partner/GPs in the contract price; and

(b) the payments from the PCT to the contractor in respect of services under the GMS contract, together with the contract price of any other contract to provide medical services to the NHS that the contractor has entered into, also cover the cost of any additional voluntary contributions that the PCT is obliged, as its partner/GPs' employer for superannuation purposes, to make to the NHS Pensions Agency or an Additional Voluntary Contributions Provider on the partner/GPs' behalf.

22.5 Accordingly, the costs of paying the employer's and employee's superannuation contributions of a contractor's partner/GPs under the NHS Pensions Scheme in respect of their NHS superannuable profits from all sources – unless superannuated for the purposes of the NHS Pension Scheme elsewhere – are all to be deducted by the PCT from the money the PCT pays to the contractor pursuant to this SFE.

Monthly deductions in respect of superannuation contributions

22.6 The deductions are to be made in two stages. First, PCTs must, as part of the calculation of the net amount (as opposed to the gross amount) of a contractor's Payable global sum monthly payments (GSMPs), deduct an amount that represents a reasonable approximation of a monthly proportion of –

(a) the PCT's liability for the financial year 2004/05 in respect of the employer's superannuation costs under the NHS Pension Scheme relating to any of the contractor's partner/GPs who are members of the Scheme;

(b) those partner/GPs' related employee's superannuation contributions; and

(c) any payable additional voluntary contributions in respect of those partner/GPs.

Before determining the monthly amount to be deducted, the PCT must take all reasonable steps to agree with the contractor what that amount should be, and it must duly justify the amount that it does determine as the monthly deduction.

22.7 An amount equal to the monthly amount that the PCT deducts must be remitted to NHS Pensions Agency and any relevant Money Purchase Additional Voluntary Contributions Providers no later than –

(a) the 19th day of the month after the month in respect of which the amount was deducted; or

(b) in the case of Money Purchase Additional Voluntary Contributions, 7 days after an amount in respect of them is deducted pursuant to paragraph 22.6.

End-year adjustments

22.8 Then, after the end of the financial year, the final amount of each partner/ GP's superannuable income in respect of the financial year will need to be determined.

22.9 For these purposes, the superannuable income of –

(a) a salaried GP who is an employee of the contractor, or of a partner/GP who is a shareholder in a contractor that is a company limited by shares, will be –

(i) his earnings – less expenses, bonuses or overtime – from his contract of employment with the contractor, and

(ii) his income from any Golden Hello Payment, Returners' Scheme Doctor Payment, Flexible Career Scheme Doctor Payment or Seniority Payment paid in respect of him to the contractor pursuant to Part 4; or

(b) any other partner/GP will be –

(i) in the case of a sole practitioner, his NHS profits from all sources, and

(ii) in the case of a partner in a partnership, his share of the partnership's NHS profits, together with his income from any Golden Hello Payment, Returners' Scheme Payment or Seniority Payment paid in respect of him to the contractor pursuant to Part 4.

22.10 As regards contractors that are partnerships, sole practitioners or companies limited by shares, it is a condition of all the payments payable pursuant to Parts 1 to 3 of this SFE – if any of the contractor's partner/GPs are members of the NHS Pension Scheme – that the contractor ensures that its partner/GPs (other than those who are neither members of the NHS Pension Scheme nor due Seniority Payments) prepare, sign and forward to the PCT within what, in all the circumstances, is a reasonable time an accurate certificate, in the standard format provided nationally, which provides the following information –

(a) the contractor's NHS superannuable profits in respect of the financial year 2004/05 (i.e. for the tax year, which may be different from the contractor's own accounting year);

(b) in the case of –
(i) a partner in a partnership, his own share of those profits, or
(ii) a shareholder in a company limited by shares, his earnings – less expenses, bonuses or overtime – from his contract of employment with the contractor; and

(c) his NHS profits from all other sources, if these are not superannuated (for the purposes of the NHS Pension Scheme) elsewhere.

22.11 Seniority Payments have to be separately identifiable in the certificate for the purposes of the calculation of Average Adjusted Superannuable Income, which is necessary for the determination of the amount of GP providers' Seniority Payments. Seniority Payment figures in the certificates forwarded to PCTs will necessarily be provisional (unless they are submitted too late for the information they contain to be included in the Average Adjusted Superannuable Income calculation), but the forwarding of certificates must not be delayed simply because of this. Partner/GPs who are not members of the NHS Pension Scheme but in respect of whom a claim for a Quarterly Seniority Payment is to be made must prepare, sign and forward the certificate to the PCT so that the correct amount of their Seniority Payments for the financial year 2004/05 may be determined.

22.12 Once a contractor's partner/GPs' superannuable earnings in respect of the financial year 2004/05 have been agreed, the PCT must –

(a) pay any outstanding NHS Pension Scheme employer's and employee's superannuation contributions due in respect of those earnings to the NHS Pensions Agency or any relevant Additional Voluntary Contributions Provider (having regard to the payments it has already made on account in respect of those partner/GPs for the financial year 2004/05); and

(b) if its deductions from the contractor's Payable GSMPs during the financial year 2004/05 relating to the superannuation contributions in respect of those earnings –

(i) did not cover the cost of all the employer's and employee's superannuation contributions that are payable by the PCT or the partner/GPs in respect of those earnings –

    (aa) deduct the amount outstanding from any payment payable to the contractor under its GMS contract pursuant to this SFE (and for all purposes the amount that is payable in respect of that payment is to be reduced accordingly), or

    (bb) obtain payment (where no such deduction can be made) from the contractor of the amount outstanding, and it is a condition of the payments made pursuant to this SFE that the contractor must pay to the PCT the amount outstanding, or

(ii) were in excess of the amount payable by the PCT and the partner/GP to the NHS Pensions Agency or a relevant Money Purchase Additional Voluntary Contributions Provider in respect of those earnings, repay the excess amount to the contractor promptly (unless, in the case of an excess amount in respect of Money Purchase Additional Voluntary Contributions, the contributor elects for that amount to be a further contribution and he is entitled to so elect).

Locums

22.13 There are different arrangements for superannuation contributions of locums, and these are not covered by this SFE.

● Suspended doctor payments

Statement of Financial Entitlement

11.1 Primary Care Trusts (PCTs) have powers to suspend GP performers from their medical performers list. They may also, on 1 April 2004, still be considering cases of GP performers who are on but suspended from their medical performers lists because prior to 1 April 2004 they were suspended from a medical list, a services list or a supplementary list.

11.2 A GP performer who is suspended from a medical performers list either –

(a) on or after 1 April 2004; or

(b) by virtue of being suspended from a medical list, a services list or a supplementary list, may be entitled to payments directly from the PCT that suspended him. This is covered by a separate determination under regulation 13(17) of the Performers List Regulations.

Eligible cases

11.3 In any case where a contractor –
(a) either –
   (i) is a sole practitioner who is suspended from his PCT's medical performers list and is not in receipt of any financial assistance from his PCT under section 28Y of the 1977 Act as a contribution towards the cost of the arrangements to provide primary medical services under his GMS contract during his suspension,
   (ii) is paying a suspended GP performer –
      (aa) who is a partner in the contractor, at least 90% of his normal monthly drawings (or a *pro rata* amount in the case of part months) from the partnership account, or
      (bb) who is an employee of the contractor, at least 90% of his normal salary (or a *pro rata* amount in the case of part months), or
   (iii) paid a suspended GP performer the amount mentioned in paragraph (ii)(aa) or (bb) for at least 6 months of his suspension, and the suspended GP performer is still a partner in or employee of the contractor;
(b) actually and necessarily engages a locum (or more than one such person) to cover for the absence of the suspended GP performer;
(c) the locum is not a partner or shareholder in the contractor, or already an employee of the contractor, unless the absent performer is a job-sharer; and
(d) the contractor is not also claiming a payment for locum cover in respect of the absent performer under another Section in this Part,
then subject to the following provisions of this Section, the PCT must provide financial assistance to the contractor under its GMS contract in respect of the cost of engaging that locum (which may or may not be the maximum amount payable, as set out in paragraph 11.5).

11.4 It is for the PCT to determine whether or not it is or was in fact necessary to engage the locum, or to continue to engage the locum, but it is to have regard to the following principles –
(a) it should not normally be considered necessary to employ a locum if the PCT has offered to provide the locum cover itself and the contractor has refused that offer without good reason;

(b) it should not normally be considered necessary to employ a locum if the absent performer had a right to return but that right has been extinguished; and

(c) it should not normally be considered necessary to employ a locum if the contractor has engaged a new employee or partner to perform the duties of the absent performer and it is not carrying a vacancy in respect of another position which the absent performer will fill on his return.

Ceilings on the amounts payable

11.5   The maximum amount payable under this Section by the PCT in respect of locum cover for a GP performer is £948.33 per week.

Payment arrangements

11.6   The contractor is to submit claims for costs actually incurred after they have been incurred, at a frequency to be agreed between the PCT and the contractor, or if agreement cannot be reached, within 14 days of the end of month during which the costs were incurred. Any amount payable falls due 14 days after the claim is submitted.

Conditions attached to the amounts payable

11.7   Payments under this Section, or any part thereof, are only payable if the contractor satisfies the following conditions –

(a) the contractor must, on request, provide the PCT with written records demonstrating–

   (i) the actual cost to it of the locum cover, and

   (ii) that it is continuing to pay the suspended GP performer the full amount of the income to which he was entitled before the suspension (i.e. his normal drawings from the partnership account or his normal salary); and

(b) once the locum arrangements are in place, the contractor must inform the PCT –

   (i) if there is to be any change to the locum arrangements, or

   (ii) if, for any other reason, there is to be a change to the contractor's arrangements for performing the duties of the absent performer,

at which point the PCT is to determine whether it still considers the locum cover necessary.

11.8   If the contractor breaches any of these conditions, the PCT may, in appropriate circumstances, withhold payment of any sum otherwise payable under this Section.

● Temporary patients

Regulations

16. Temporary residents

(1) The contractor may, if its list of patients is open, accept a person as a temporary resident provided it is satisfied that the person is –
(a) temporarily resident away from his normal place of residence and is not being provided with essential services (or their equivalent) under any other arrangement in the locality where he is temporarily residing; or
(b) moving from place to place and not for the time being resident in any place.

(2) For the purposes of sub-paragraph (1), a person shall be regarded as temporarily resident in a place if, when he arrives in that place, he intends to stay there for more than 24 hours but not more than 3 months.

(3) A contractor which wishes to terminate its responsibility for a person accepted as a temporary resident before the end of –
(a) 3 months; or
(b) such shorter period for which it agreed to accept him as a patient, shall notify him either orally or in writing and its responsibility for that patient shall cease 7 days after the date on which the notification was given.

(4) At the end of 3 months, or on such earlier date as its responsibility for the temporary resident has come to an end, the contractor shall notify the Primary Care Trust (PCT) in writing of any person whom it accepted as a temporary resident.

Standard Contract

176. The Contractor may if its list of patients is *open* accept a person as a *temporary resident* provided it is satisfied that the person is –
176.1 temporarily resident away from his normal place of residence and is not being provided with *essential services* under any other arrangement in the locality where he is temporarily residing; or
176.2 moving from place to place and not for the time being resident in any place.

177. For the purposes of clause 176, a person shall be regarded as temporarily resident in a place if, when he arrives in that place, he intends to stay there for more than 24 hours but not more than 3 months.

178. Where the Contractor wishes to terminate its responsibility for a person accepted as a *temporary resident* before the end of 3 months or such shorter period for which it had agreed to accept him as a patient, the Contractor shall notify the patient either orally or in writing and its responsibility for that person shall cease 7 days after the date on which the notification was given.

Guidance

2.21 The obligation on contractors to provide treatment to patients who are not registered with them remains in the new contract. Fees for providing Emergency Treatment, Immediately Necessary Treatment and the care of Temporary Residents have been simplified into a single off-formula adjustment in the global sum, described in annex B. This is calculated on the basis of the average number of claims in the practice over the previous 5 years. If PCTs and contractors agree that the incidence of non-registered patients at the practice is insufficiently accounted for within the global sum, funding could be supplemented through an enhanced services contract.

2.22 There are three different types of circumstances when a contractor must accept temporary patients for treatment:
   (i) ordinarily, services will be provided where: (a) a contractor's list is open, and (b) services are requested by a person who is temporarily away from his or her normal place of residence and, (c) that person is not being provided with essential services (or their equivalent) under any other arrangement in the locality where he or she is residing, or who is moving from place to place, and is not for the time being resident in any place. For this purpose persons are temporarily resident if when they arrive they intend to stay for more than 24 hours but for not more than 3 months
   (ii) in core hours a contractor must also provide for the necessary treatment for a period of up to 14 days of a person whose application to be accepted as a temporary patient has been refused
   (iii) finally a contractor must provide in core hours immediately necessary treatment for a person to whom the contractor has been requested to provide treatment owing to an accident or emergency at any place in its practice area.

● Termination of responsibility for patients not on list

Regulations

28. Termination of responsibility for patients not registered with the contractor

(1)   Where a contractor –
    (a) has received an application for the provision of medical services other than essential services –
        (i) from a person who is not included in its list of patients,
        (ii) from a person whom it has not accepted as a temporary resident, or
        (iii) on behalf of a person mentioned in sub-paragraph (i) or (ii), from one of the persons specified in paragraph 15(4); and
    (b) has accepted that person as a patient for the provision of the service in question,
its responsibility for that patient shall be terminated in the circumstances referred to in sub-paragraph (2).

(2)   The circumstances referred to in sub-paragraph (1) are –
    (a) the patient informs the contractor that he no longer wishes it to be responsible for provision of the service in question;
    (b) in cases where the contractor has reasonable grounds for terminating its responsibility which do not relate to the person's race, gender, social class, age, religion, sexual orientation, appearance, disability or medical condition, the contractor informs the patient that it no longer wishes to be responsible for providing him with the service in question; or
    (c) it comes to the notice of the contractor that the patient –
        (i) no longer resides in the area for which the contractor has agreed to provide the service in question, or
        (ii) is no longer included in the list of patients of another contractor to whose registered patients the contractor has agreed to provide that service.

(3)   A contractor which wishes to terminate its responsibility for a patient under sub-paragraph (2)(b) shall notify the patient of the termination and the reason for it.

(4)   The contractor shall keep a written record of terminations under this paragraph and of the reasons for them and shall make this record available to the PCT on request.

(5)   A termination under sub-paragraph (2)(b) shall take effect –
   (a) from the date on which the notice is given where the grounds for
       termination are those specified in paragraph 21(1); or
   (b) in all other cases, 14 days from the date on which the notice is given.

Standard Contract

Termination of responsibility for patients not registered with the Contractor

224.   Where the Contractor –
   224.1 has received an application for the provision of medical services
        other than *essential services* –
        224.1.1 from a person who is not included in its list of patients,
        224.1.2 from a person whom it has not accepted as a *temporary
                resident*, or
        224.1.3 on behalf of a person mentioned in clause 224.1.1 or
                224.1.2, from one of the persons specified in clause 173;
                and
   224.2 has accepted that person as a patient for the provision of the
        service in question
   its responsibility for that patient shall be terminated in the circumstances
   referred to in clause 225.

225.   The circumstances referred to in clause 224 are –
   225.1 the patient informs the Contractor that he no longer wishes it to be
        responsible for provision of the service in question;
   225.2 in cases where the Contractor has reasonable grounds for
        terminating its responsibility which do not relate to the person's
        race, gender, social class, age, religion, sexual orientation,
        appearance, disability or medical condition, the Contractor
        informs the patient that it no longer wishes to be responsible for
        providing him with the service in question; or
   225.3 it comes to the notice of the Contractor that the patient –
        225.3.1 no longer resides in the area for which the Contractor has
                agreed to provide the service in question; or
        225.3.2 is no longer included in the list of patients of another
                contractor to whose *registered patients* the Contractor has
                agreed to provide that service.

226.   If the Contractor wishes to terminate its responsibility for a patient
      under clause 225.2, it shall notify the patient of the termination and the
      reason for it.

227. The Contractor shall keep a written record of terminations under clauses 224 to 226 and of the reasons for them and shall make this record available to the PCT on request.

228. A termination under clause 225.2 shall take effect –
228.1 from the date on which the notice is given where the grounds for termination are those specified in clause 201; or
228.2 in all other cases, 14 days from the date on which the notice is given.

Third-party rights

Regulations

126. The contract shall not create any right enforceable by any person not a party to it.

Vaccines – storage of

Regulations

8. The contractor shall ensure that –
(a) all vaccines are stored in accordance with the manufacturer's instructions; and
(b) all refrigerators in which vaccines are stored have a maximum/minimum thermometer and that readings are taken on all working days.

Standard Contract

39.1 The Contractor shall ensure that –
39.1 all vaccines are stored in accordance with the manufacturer's instructions; and
39.2 all refrigerators in which vaccines are stored have a maximum/minimum thermometer and that readings are taken on all working days.

Variation of contracts

See also: Contract sanctions · Contract variations

Regulations

104. Variation of a contract: general

(1)   Subject to Schedule 3, paragraphs 69(8), 70(8), 105, 106 and 117 and paragraph 3 of Schedule 7, no amendment or variation shall have effect unless it is in writing and signed by or on behalf of the PCT and the contractor.

(2)   In addition to the specific provision made in paragraphs 105(6), 106(6) and 117, the PCT may vary the contract without the contractor's consent where it –

(a) is reasonably satisfied that it is necessary to vary the contract so as to comply with the Act, any regulations made pursuant to that Act, or any direction given by the Secretary of State pursuant to that Act; and

(b) notifies the contractor in writing of the wording of the proposed variation and the date upon which that variation is to take effect,

and, where it is reasonably practicable to do so, the date that the proposed variation is to take effect shall be not less than 14 days after the date on which the notice under paragraph (b) is served on the contractor.

105. Variation provisions specific to a contract with an individual medical practitioner

(1)   If a contractor which is an individual medical practitioner proposes to practise in partnership with one or more persons during the existence of the contract, the contractor shall notify the PCT in writing of –

(a) the name of the person or persons with whom it proposes to practise in partnership; and

(b) the date on which the contractor wishes to change its status as a contractor from that of an individual medical practitioner to that of a partnership, which shall be not less than 28 days after the date upon which it has served the notice on the PCT pursuant to this sub-paragraph.

(2)   A notice under sub-paragraph (1) shall in respect of the person or each of the persons with whom the contractor is proposing to practise in partnership, and also in respect of itself as regards the matters specified in paragraph (c) –

(a) confirm that he is either –
    (i) a medical practitioner, or
    (ii) a person who satisfies the conditions specified in section 28S(2)(b)(i) to (iv) of the Act;
(b) confirm that he is a person who satisfies the conditions imposed by regulations 4 and 5; and
(c) state whether or not it is to be a limited partnership, and if so, who is to be a limited and who a general partner,

and the notice shall be signed by the individual medical practitioner and by the person, or each of the persons (as the case may be), with whom he is proposing to practise in partnership.

(3) The contractor shall ensure that any person who will practise in partnership with it is bound by the contract, whether by virtue of a partnership deed or otherwise.

(4) If the PCT is satisfied as to the accuracy of the matters specified in sub-paragraph (2) that are included in the notice, the PCT shall give notice in writing to the contractor confirming that the contract shall continue with the partnership entered into by the contractor and its partners, from a date that the PCT specifies in that notice.

(5) Where it is reasonably practicable, the date specified by the PCT pursuant to sub-paragraph (4) shall be the date requested in the notice served by the contractor pursuant to sub-paragraph (1), or, where that date is not reasonably practicable, the date specified shall be a date after the requested date that is as close to the requested date as is reasonably practicable.

(6) Where a contractor has given notice to the PCT pursuant to sub-paragraph (1), the PCT –
(a) may vary the contract but only to the extent that it is satisfied is necessary to reflect the change in status of the contractor from an individual medical practitioner to a partnership; and
(b) if it does propose to so vary the contract, it shall include in the notice served on the contractor pursuant to sub-paragraph (4) the wording of the proposed variation and the date upon which that variation is to take effect.

106. Variation provisions specific to a contract with two or more individuals practising in partnership

(1) Subject to sub-paragraph (4), where a contractor consists of two or more individuals practising in partnership in the event that the partnership is terminated or dissolved, the contract shall only continue with one of the former partners if that partner is –

(a) nominated in accordance with sub-paragraph (3); and

(b) a medical practitioner who meets the condition in regulation 4(2)(a), and provided that the requirements in sub-paragraphs (2) and (3) are met.

(2) A contractor shall notify the PCT in writing at least 28 days in advance of the date on which the contractor proposes to change its status from that of a partnership to that of an individual medical practitioner pursuant to sub-paragraph (1).

(3) A notice under sub-paragraph (2) shall –
(a) specify the date on which the contractor proposes to change its status from that of a partnership to that of an individual medical practitioner;
(b) specify the name of the medical practitioner with whom the contract will continue, which must be one of the partners; and (c) be signed by all of the persons who are practising in partnership.

(4) If a partnership is terminated or dissolved because, in a partnership consisting of two individuals practising in partnership, one of the partners has died, sub-paragraphs (1), (2) and (3) shall not apply and –
(a) the contract shall continue with the individual who has not died only if that individual is a medical practitioner who meets the condition in regulation 4(2)(a); and
(b) that individual shall in any event notify the PCT in writing as soon as is reasonably practicable of the death of his partner.

(5) When the PCT receives a notice pursuant to sub-paragraph (2) or (4)(b), it shall acknowledge in writing receipt of the notice, and in relation to a notice served pursuant to sub-paragraph (2), the Trust shall do so before the date specified pursuant to sub-paragraph (3)(a).

(6) Where a contractor gives notice to the PCT pursuant to sub-paragraph (2) or (4)(b), the PCT may vary the contract but only to the extent that it is satisfied is necessary to reflect the change in status of the contractor from a partnership to an individual medical practitioner.

(7) If the PCT varies the contract pursuant to sub-paragraph (6), it shall notify the contractor in writing of the wording of the proposed variation and the date upon which that variation is to take effect.

Standard Contract

Variation of the Contract: general

528. Subject to Part 10 of the Contract (opt-outs of *additional* and *out-of-hours services*), clauses 85, 86, 376, 385 and 406, and this Part (variation

and termination of the Contract), no amendment or variation shall have effect unless it is in writing and signed by or on behalf of the PCT and the Contractor.

529.   In addition to the specific provision made in clauses 536, 541 and 576, the PCT may vary the Contract without the Contractor's consent so as to comply with *the Act*, any regulations made pursuant to that Act, or any direction given by *the Secretary of State* pursuant to that Act where it –
    529.1 is reasonably satisfied that it is necessary to vary the Contract in order so to comply; and
    529.2 notifies the Contractor in writing of the wording of the proposed variation and the date upon which that variation is to take effect.

530.   Where it is reasonably practicable to do so, the date that the proposed variation is to take effect shall be not less than 14 days after the date on which the notice under clause 529.2 is served on the Contractor.

Variation provisions specific to a contract with an individual medical practitioner[67]

531.   Where the Contractor is an individual medical practitioner and proposes to practise in partnership with one or more persons during the existence of the Contract, the Contractor shall notify the PCT in writing of –
    531.1 the name of the person or persons with whom it proposes to practise in partnership;
    531.2 the date on which the Contractor wishes to change its status from that of an individual medical practitioner to that of a partnership, which shall be not less than 28 days after the date upon which it has served the notice on the PCT pursuant to this clause.

532.   A notice under clause 531 shall, in respect of the person or each of the persons with whom the Contractor is proposing to practise in partnership, and also in respect of the Contractor as regards the matters specified in clause 532.2 –
    532.1 confirm that he is either a medical practitioner or a person who satisfies the conditions specified in section 28S(2)(b)(i) to (iv) of *the Act*,
    532.2 confirm that he is a person who satisfies the conditions imposed by regulations 4 and 5 of *the Regulations*; and
    532.3 state whether or not it is to be a *limited partnership*, and if so, who is to be a limited partner and who a general partner,

---

67   If the Contractor is not an individual medical practitioner, then this clause does not need to be included.

and the notice shall be signed by the Contractor, and by the person or each of the persons with whom it is proposing to practice in partnership.

533. The Contractor shall ensure that any person who will practise in partnership with it is bound by the Contract, whether by virtue of a partnership deed or otherwise.

534. If the PCT is satisfied as to the accuracy of the matters specified in the notice referred to in clause 531, the PCT shall give notice in writing to the Contractor confirming that the Contract shall continue with the partnership entered into by the Contractor and its partners, from a date that the PCT specifies in that notice.

535. The date specified by the PCT pursuant to clause 534 shall be the date requested in the notice served by the Contractor pursuant to clause 531, or, where that date is not reasonably practicable, the date closest to the requested date as is reasonably practicable.

536. Where the Contractor has given notice to the PCT pursuant to clause 531, the PCT may vary the Contract but only to the extent that it is satisfied is necessary to reflect the change in status of the Contractor from an individual medical practitioner to a partnership. If the PCT does propose so to vary the Contract, it shall include in the notice served on the Contractor pursuant to clause 534 the wording of the proposed variation and the date upon which that variation is to take effect.

Variation provisions specific to a contract with a Partnership[68]

537. Subject to clause 539 where the Contractor consists of two or more individuals practising in partnership, in the event that the partnership is terminated or dissolved, the Contract shall only continue with one of the former partners if that partner is –
537.1 nominated in accordance with clause 538; and
537.2 a medical practitioner who meets the condition in regulation 4(2)(a) of the Regulations,
and provided that the other requirements in clause 538 are met.

538. The Contractor shall notify the PCT in writing at least 28 days in advance of the date on which the Contractor proposes to change its status from that of a partnership to that of an individual medical practitioner. The notice shall:
538.1 specify the date on which the Contractor proposes to change its status from that of a partnership to that of an individual medical practitioner;

---

68 If the Contractor is not a partnership, then this clause does not need to be included.

538.2 specify the name of the medical practitioner with whom the Contract will continue, which must be one of the partners; and

538.3 be signed by all the persons who are practising in partnership.

539. If the partnership is terminated or dissolved because, in a partnership consisting of two individuals practising in partnership, one of the partners has died –

539.1 clauses 537 and 538 shall not apply; and

539.2 the Contract shall continue with the individual who has not died only if that individual is a medical practitioner who meets the condition in regulation 4(2)(a) of *the Regulations*, and that individual shall in any event notify the PCT in writing as soon as is reasonably practicable of the death of his partner.

540. When the PCT receives a notice pursuant to clause 538 or 539, it shall acknowledge in writing receipt of the notice, and in relation to a notice served pursuant to clause 538, the PCT shall do so as soon as reasonably practicable, and in any event before the date specified pursuant to clause 538.1.

541. Where the Contractor gives notice to the PCT pursuant to clause 538 or 539, the PCT may vary the Contract but only to the extent that it is satisfied is necessary to reflect the change in status of the Contractor from a partnership to an individual medical practitioner. If the PCT varies the Contract, it shall notify the Contractor in writing of the wording of the proposed variation and the date upon which that variation is to take effect.

● Waiver, delay or failure to exercise rights

Standard Contract

606. The failure or delay by either party to enforce any one or more of the terms or conditions of this Contract shall not operate as a waiver of them, or of the right at any time subsequently to enforce all terms and conditions of this Contract.

Warranties

Standard Contract

20. Each of the parties warrants that it has power to enter into this Contract and has obtained any necessary approvals to do so.

21. The Contractor warrants that:
    21.1 all information in writing provided to the PCT in seeking to become a party to this Contract was, when given, true and accurate in all material respects, and in particular, that the Contractor satisfied the conditions set out in regulations 4 and 5 of *the Regulations*;
    21.2 no information has been omitted which would make the information that was provided to the PCT materially misleading or inaccurate;
    21.3 no circumstances have arisen which materially affect the truth and accuracy of such information;
    21.4 it is not aware as at the date of this Contract of anything within its reasonable control which may or will materially adversely affect its ability to fulfil its obligations under this Contract.

22. The PCT warrants that:
    22.1 all information in writing which it provided to the Contractor specifically to assist the Contractor to become a party to this Contract was, when given, true and accurate in all material respects;
    22.2 no information has been omitted which would make the information that was provided to the Contractor materially misleading or inaccurate;
    22.3 no circumstances have arisen which materially affect the truth and accuracy of such information.

23. The PCT and the Contractor have relied on, and are entitled to rely on, information provided by one party to the other in the course of negotiating the Contract.

Workforce planning

Guidance

4.12 Contractors will have freedom to spend their overall budget as they see fit. They will be rewarded for the outcomes they deliver under the quality and outcomes framework, rather than be constrained in relation to specific input conditions such as those that existed under old GMS, through for example the GP basic practice allowance. This autonomy and flexibility, combined with the increased investment described in chapter 5, and the change in out-of-hours arrangements described in chapter 2, are likely to lead to increases in primary care workforce capacity and changes in skill-mix.

4.13 PCTs are advised to consider the workforce planning implications of the new contract, the changes to PMS described in December 2003 guidance, and the new PCT and alternative provider delivery routes described in chapter 2. They will want, during contract discussions in January and February 2004, to ascertain the intentions of their contractors about, for example, plans to recruit additional staff to support the implementation of the quality and outcomes framework. PCTs will then want to ensure that this information is fed into their local SHA workforce directorate, which brings together local NHS and non-NHS employers to plan the whole health care workforce.